Bioactive Molecules from
Marine Microorganisms

Bioactive Molecules from Marine Microorganisms

Editors

Hanna Mazur-Marzec
Anna Toruńska-Sitarz

MDPI • Basel • Beijing • Wuhan • Barcelona • Belgrade • Manchester • Tokyo • Cluj • Tianjin

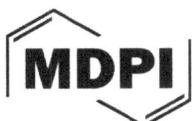

Editors
Hanna Mazur-Marzec
University of Gdańsk
Poland

Anna Toruńska-Sitarz
University of Gdańsk
Poland

Editorial Office
MDPI
St. Alban-Anlage 66
4052 Basel, Switzerland

This is a reprint of articles from the Special Issue published online in the open access journal *Marine Drugs* (ISSN 1660-3397) (available at: https://www.mdpi.com/journal/marinedrugs/special_issues/Bioactive_Molecules_Marine_Microorganisms).

For citation purposes, cite each article independently as indicated on the article page online and as indicated below:

LastName, A.A.; LastName, B.B.; LastName, C.C. Article Title. *Journal Name* **Year**, *Volume Number*, Page Range.

ISBN 978-3-0365-0620-3 (Hbk)
ISBN 978-3-0365-0621-0 (PDF)

© 2021 by the authors. Articles in this book are Open Access and distributed under the Creative Commons Attribution (CC BY) license, which allows users to download, copy and build upon published articles, as long as the author and publisher are properly credited, which ensures maximum dissemination and a wider impact of our publications.

The book as a whole is distributed by MDPI under the terms and conditions of the Creative Commons license CC BY-NC-ND.

Contents

About the Editors vii

Preface to "Bioactive Molecules from Marine Microorganisms" ix

Samuel Cavalcante do Amaral, Patrick Romano Monteiro, Joaquim da Silva Pinto Neto, Gustavo Marques Serra, Evonnildo Costa Gonçalves, Luciana Pereira Xavier and Agenor Valadares Santos
Current Knowledge on Microviridin from Cyanobacteria
Reprinted from: *Mar. Drugs* **2021**, *19*, 17, doi:10.3390/md19010017 1

Anna Fidor, Michał Grabski, Jan Gawor, Robert Gromadka, Grzegorz Wegrzyn and Hanna Mazur-Marzec
Nostoc edaphicum CCNP1411 from the Baltic Sea—A New Producer of Nostocyclopeptides
Reprinted from: *Mar. Drugs* **2020**, *18*, 442, doi:10.3390/md18090442 31

Marta Cegłowska, Karolia Szubert, Ewa Wieczerzak, Alicja Kosakowska and Hanna Mazur-Marzec
Eighteen New Aeruginosamide Variants Produced by the Baltic Cyanobacterium *Limnoraphis* CCNP1324
Reprinted from: *Mar. Drugs* **2020**, *18*, 446, doi:10.3390/md18090446 49

Jing-Shuai Wu, Xiao-Hui Shi, Guang-Shan Yao, Chang-Lun Shao, Xiu-Mei Fu, Xiu-Li Zhang, Hua-Shi Guan and Chang-Yun Wang
New Thiodiketopiperazine and 3,4-Dihydroisocoumarin Derivatives from the Marine-Derived Fungus *Aspergillus terreus*
Reprinted from: *Mar. Drugs* **2020**, *18*, 132, doi:10.3390/md18030132 63

Lu-Ping Chi, Xiao-Ming Li, Li Li, Xin Li and Bin-Gui Wang
Cytotoxic Thiodiketopiperazine Derivatives from the Deep Sea-Derived Fungus *Epicoccum nigrum* SD-388
Reprinted from: *Mar. Drugs* **2020**, *18*, 160, doi:10.3390/md18030160 73

Chiara Lauritano, Kirsti Helland, Gennaro Riccio, Jeanette H. Andersen, Adrianna Ianora and Espen H. Hansen
Lysophosphatidylcholines and Chlorophyll-Derived Molecules from the Diatom *Cylindrotheca closterium* with Anti-Inflammatory Activity
Reprinted from: *Mar. Drugs* **2020**, *18*, 166, doi:10.3390/md18030166 85

Dongbo Xu, Erli Tian, Fandong Kong and Kui Hong
Bioactive Molecules from Mangrove *Streptomyces qinglanensis* 172205
Reprinted from: *Mar. Drugs* **2020**, *18*, 255, doi:10.3390/md18050255 97

Yi Ding, Xiaojing Zhu, Liling Hao, Mengyao Zhao, Qiang Hua and Faliang An
Bioactive Indolyl Diketopiperazines from the Marine Derived Endophytic *Aspergillus versicolor* DY180635
Reprinted from: *Mar. Drugs* **2020**, *18*, 338, doi:10.3390/md18070338 109

Ji-Yeon Hwang, Sung Chul Park, Woong Sub Byun, Dong-Chan Oh, Sang Kook Lee, Ki-Bong Oh and Jongheon Shin
Bioactive Bianthraquinones and Meroterpenoids from a Marine-Derived *Stemphylium* sp. Fungus
Reprinted from: *Mar. Drugs* **2020**, *18*, 436, doi:10.3390/md18090436 121

Yi-Cheng Chu, Chun-Hao Chang, Hsiang-Ruei Liao, Ming-Jen Cheng, Ming-Der Wu, Shu-Ling Fu and Jih-Jung Chen
Rare Chromone Derivatives from the Marine-Derived *Penicillium citrinum* with Anti-Cancer and Anti-Inflammatory Activities
Reprinted from: *Mar. Drugs* **2021**, *19*, 25, doi:10.3390/md19010025 . . . . **141**

About the Editors

Hanna Mazur-Marzec (Prof. Dr.) is a researcher and lecturer at the Institute of Oceanography, University of Gdańsk where she leads the Division of Marine Biotechnology. She studied organic chemistry and did her Ph.D. in marine chemistry at the University of Gdańsk. In 2017–2019, she was also employed as a professor at the Institute of Oceanology, Polish Academy of Science. Throughout her whole research career, she has been involved in studies on bioactive metabolites produced by microorganisms. Initially, she worked on plant growth regulators in microalgae. Then, she became interested in cyanobacteria and cyanotoxins. Her current research interests extend to other bioactive cyanometabolites, especially peptides of pharmaceutical potential. Hanna Mazur-Marzec has published over 80 research articles, reviews and book chapters and has delivered several invited and plenary lectures. In 2019, she won the Polish Award of Smart Growth in the category of scientist of the future. In 2020, she was nominated for the prize of Ambassador of Innovation, awarded by the European Centre of Economy Development in Poland.

Anna Toruńska-Sitarz is currently a researcher, academic teacher and tutor in the Division of Marine Biotechnology at the Institute of Oceanography, University of Gdańsk (Poland). From 2020, she has also been employed at the Marine Research Institute (Klaipeda University, Lithuania). She received her M.Sc. in oceanography, and her Ph.D. in environmental sciences. Her research interests lie in the area of microbial diversity and marine antibacterial compounds. Anna Toruńska-Sitarz has co-authored more than 20 research articles and book chapters. She is also actively involved in various other activities of the academic community, as a conference organizer, reviewer and member of scientific societies

Preface to "Bioactive Molecules from Marine Microorganisms"

Microorganisms live in all types of habitats and under variety of environmental conditions, including extreme ones. They are the most abundant organisms on Earth, highly diverse and classified into different domains. The diversity of marine microorganisms and their products represents high, but still unexplored, pharmaceutical potential. The most frequently observed effects of microbial products include anticancer, anticoagulant, antibacterial, antiviral, neurotoxic and immune-modulating activities. Metabolites of marine microorganisms have also been used as templates for the development of new pharmaceuticals with unique mechanisms of action. Despite the enormous potential offered by marine microorganisms, so far only a few of their metabolites have been successfully developed into FDA-approved drugs or have entered clinical trials. The fact that only a small fraction of marine microorganisms and their bioactive molecules has been discovered gives a great chance to further explore them and develop them into high added value products.

For this Special Issue book, ten papers focusing on novel bioactive molecules from different marine microorganisms, including fungi, cyanobacteria, actinobacteria and diatoms, were selected. The isolated biomolecules represent different structures and showed anticancer, antiviral, antifungal, antibacterial, anti-inflammatory and enzyme-inhibiting activities. One of the papers is a review article on microviridins, a class of bioactive cyanobacterial peptides.

Hanna Mazur-Marzec, Anna Toruńska-Sitarz
Editors

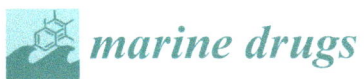

Review

Current Knowledge on Microviridin from Cyanobacteria

Samuel Cavalcante do Amaral [1], Patrick Romano Monteiro [1,2], Joaquim da Silva Pinto Neto [1], Gustavo Marques Serra [1], Evonnildo Costa Gonçalves [2], Luciana Pereira Xavier [1] and Agenor Valadares Santos [1,*]

[1] Laboratory of Biotechnology of Enzymes and Biotransformation, Biological Sciences Institute, Federal University of Pará, Belém 66075-110, Brazil; samuel.amaral@icb.ufpa.br (S.C.d.A.); patrick.monteiro@icb.ufpa.br (P.R.M.); joaquim.neto@icb.ufpa.br (J.d.S.P.N.); gustavo.serra@icb.ufpa.br (G.M.S.); lpxavier@ufpa.br (L.P.X.)

[2] Laboratory of Biomolecular Technology, Biological Sciences Institute, Federal University of Pará, Belém 66075-110, Brazil; ecostag@ufpa.br

* Correspondence: avsantos@ufpa.br; Tel.: +55-91-99177-3164

Abstract: Cyanobacteria are a rich source of secondary metabolites with a vast biotechnological potential. These compounds have intrigued the scientific community due their uniqueness and diversity, which is guaranteed by a rich enzymatic apparatus. The ribosomally synthesized and post-translationally modified peptides (RiPPs) are among the most promising metabolite groups derived from cyanobacteria. They are interested in numerous biological and ecological processes, many of which are entirely unknown. Microviridins are among the most recognized class of ribosomal peptides formed by cyanobacteria. These oligopeptides are potent inhibitors of protease; thus, they can be used for drug development and the control of mosquitoes. They also play a key ecological role in the defense of cyanobacteria against microcrustaceans. The purpose of this review is to systematically identify the key characteristics of microviridins, including its chemical structure and biosynthesis, as well as its biotechnological and ecological significance.

Keywords: cyanobacteria; oligopeptide; microviridin; biotechnology; ecology

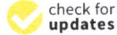

Citation: do Amaral, S.C.; Monteiro, P.R.; Neto, J.d.S.P.; Serra, G.M.; Gonçalves, E.C.; Xavier, L.P.; Santos, A.V. Current Knowledge on Microviridin from Cyanobacteria. *Mar. Drugs* **2021**, *19*, 17. https://doi.org/md19010017

Received: 17 November 2020
Accepted: 17 December 2020
Published: 4 January 2021

Publisher's Note: MDPI stays neutral with regard to jurisdictional claims in published maps and institutional affiliations.

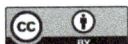

Copyright: © 2021 by the authors. Licensee MDPI, Basel, Switzerland. This article is an open access article distributed under the terms and conditions of the Creative Commons Attribution (CC BY) license (https://creativecommons.org/licenses/by/4.0/).

1. Introduction

Cyanobacteria are among the first living beings to exist on Earth. The oldest fossil cyanobacteria registries date back 3.8 billion years ago. Their presence was crucial to the creation of an aerobic atmosphere, resulting in the emergence of an enormous species variety [1]. They are defined as prokaryotic oxygen photosynthetic microorganisms and are mainly known for their ability to synthesize structurally diverse and biologically active natural products [2]. In addition, similar to other bacteria, these microorganisms are nucleus-free and have an immense morphological diversity. The various structural shapes encountered in these species are the result of their ability to alter their morphology according to the environment allowing for higher energy accumulation and growth [3,4].

These microorganisms are at mercy of various stress situations found in diverse types of environments, including water-based and land-based. The ability to thrive in these heterogeneous environments can be attributed to an enormous secondary metabolite repertory, which has intrigued numerous scientists for its rarity and richness [5,6]. Peptides generated by ribosomal synthesis and produced by large multi-domain enzymes called nonribosomal peptide synthetases (NRPS) are among these metabolites [7,8]. The macrolides present in these photosynthetic species derive from an enzyme complex called polyketide synthase, which is also modular in nature, similar to animal fatty acid synthase. Some molecules are synthesized from the combination of these two metabolic pathways, such as toxin nodularin and microcystin. Products from these two pathways constitute the majority of the secondary metabolites described in cyanobacteria [9].

The ribosomal peptide pathway forms a group very diverse and complex of products, and it is present in all three domains of life. The building blocks used by this pathway are usually limited to 20 proteinogenic amino acids. The enormous structural diversity of these proteinaceous substances can be enriched by post-translational modifications, which are also responsible for the functional diversity contained in this category. Such modifications occur in the side chains and can lead to different forms of macrocyclization [10,11]. The precursor peptide is mainly formed by a leader peptide (LP) and core peptides (CP), which act as recognition and modification sites, respectively. This identification assists post-translational enzymes to focus a biosynthetic effort on a particular precursor peptide. The different types of post-translational modifications (PTMs) are used to differentiate the subfamilies of this group and can enhance the stability of the peptide and its activities [12,13].

Microviridins are among the most promising peptides found in cyanobacteria. These molecules are potent inhibitors of protease found in an enormous variety of cyanobacteria, mainly those of the genus *Microcystis, Planktothrix, Anabaena, Nostoc* and *Nodularia* [14]. An in silico analysis revealed that the occurrence of microviridins in bacteria belonged to other phyla [15,16]. Here, we present a review of the microviridins produced by cyanobacteria and their biotechnological and ecological relevance.

2. Microviridin

Microviridins are one of the most known and largest oligopeptides formed by cyanobacteria. They are ribosomally produced, classified as depsipeptides. Their size can vary from 12 to 20 amino acids, where the N-terminal residue is typically acetylated [17–19]. By post-translational modifications, the side chains of some of these amino acids lead to ω-ester and an ω-amide linkage, which result in distinct ring formations. When completely cyclic, microviridins typically exhibit two ester bonds between the Thr-Asp/Glu and Ser-Asp/Glu side chains and an amide bond formed between the Lys side chain at position 9 and Glu or Asp at position 2. The formation of amide and ester bonds are catalyzed by ATP-grasp enzymes. Mono- and bicyclical structures may also be formed, possibly due to the lack of one of the PTM enzymes or further modification of the tricyclic microviridin [14,15,20]. These oligopeptides are capable of inhibiting the hydrolytic activity of several serine protease, including elastase, trypsin, thrombin and chymotrypsin, as well as tyrosinase. Hence, they have cogitated as promising agent in the treatment of several metabolic disorders [21,22]. Their selectivity can be related to their amino acid sequence, especially that occupying the fifth position from the C-terminal. All known microviridins normally share the TxKxPSD motif and possess Asp, Thr, Ser and Lys residues (Figure 1) [20].

Microviridins have been identified in different cyanobacterial genera, mostly isolated from freshwater. The screening of environmental samples and isolated strains showed a wide distribution and diversity of this oligopeptide [14]. The majority of reports focused mainly on the strains of *Microcystis* and *Planktothrix*, as these genera are bloom-forming and are usually found in the eutrophic ambient. Over the last few years, more microviridin variants have been discovered in phyla other than cyanobacteria [15,16].

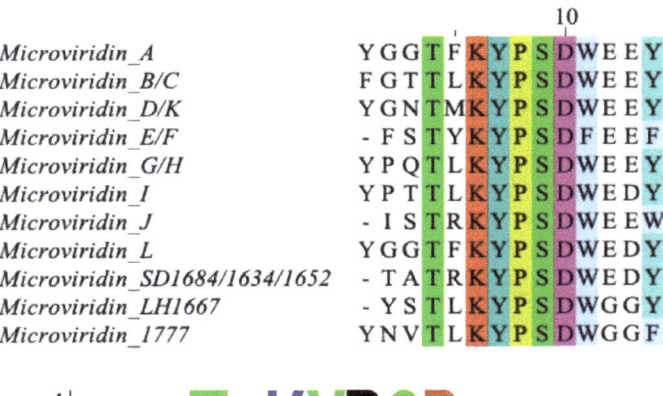
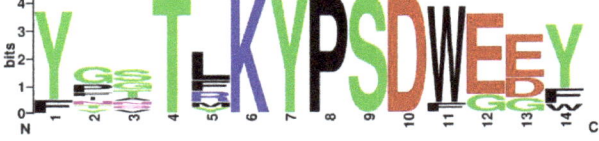

Figure 1. Diversity of microviridin sequences and the conserved KYPSD motif. Multiple alignment was obtained by Clustal Omega (https://www.ebi.ac.uk) and visualized using JalView software (https://www.jalview.org), and the consensus sequence was generated by WebLogo (https://weblogo.berkeley.edu).

3. Microviridin Structure

Microviridin was firstly described in the toxic *Microcystis viridis* (NIES-102), which was isolated from a bloom on Kasumigaura Lake, by Ishitsuka et al. (1990) [21]. Its amino acid sequence was defined as Ac-Tyr (I)-Gly (I)-Gly (I)-Thr-Phe-Lys-Tyr (II)-Pro-Ser-Asp-Trp-Glu (I)-Glu (II)-Tyr-OH, where Lys is bound to Glu (II) through its ε-NH with γ-CO of Glu (II). Thr and Ser amino acids are esterified and form ester bonds with the γ and δ carboxylic moieties of Asp and Glu (I), respectively (Figure 2). After the discovery of microviridin A, Okino et al. (1995) [23] identified a further two novel microviridins in the freshwater cyanobacterium *M. aeruginosa* (NIES-298). They were named microviridin B and C, the former exhibiting high similarity to microviridin A. They differ solely by three amino acid residues: Phe, Thr and Leu, which occupy the same position of Tyr (I), Gly (I) and Phe in microviridin A. The microviridin B amino acid composition was defined as Ac-Phe-Gly-Thr-(I)-Thr (II)-Leu-Lys-Tyr-Pro-Ser-Asp-Trp-Glu-(I)-Glu (II)-Tyr-OH. Microviridin C is closely related to microviridin B, exhibiting the same amino acid composition but containing a methoxy group in the γ carboxylic acid of Glu (I) and one additional hydroxyl group correlated to Ser. In this oligopeptide, neither Ser nor Glu are esterified. The slight difference between anti-elastase activity exhibited by both inhibitors was important to demonstrate that the ester bond between Ser and Glu(I) is not included in the reactive site.

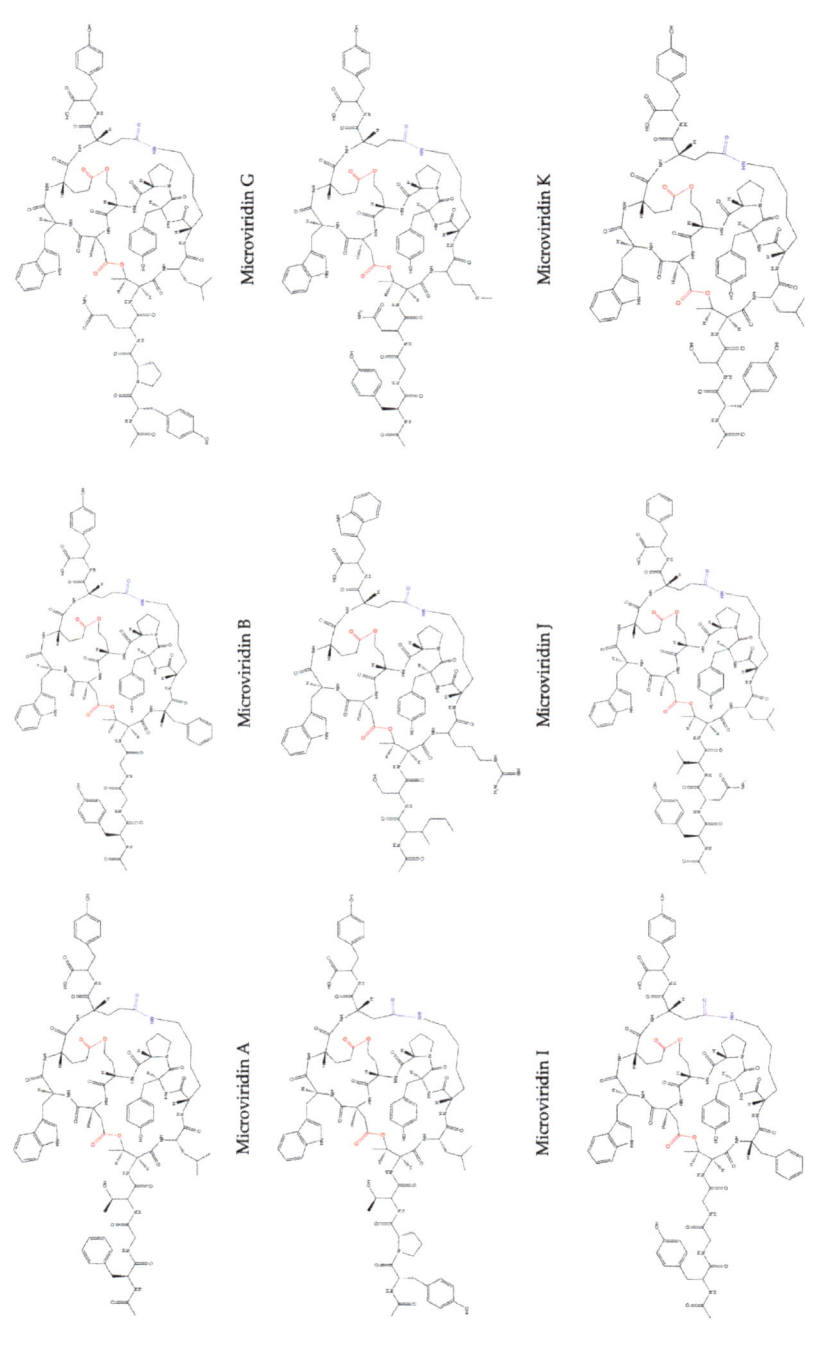

Figure 2. Microviridin structures belonging to group I.

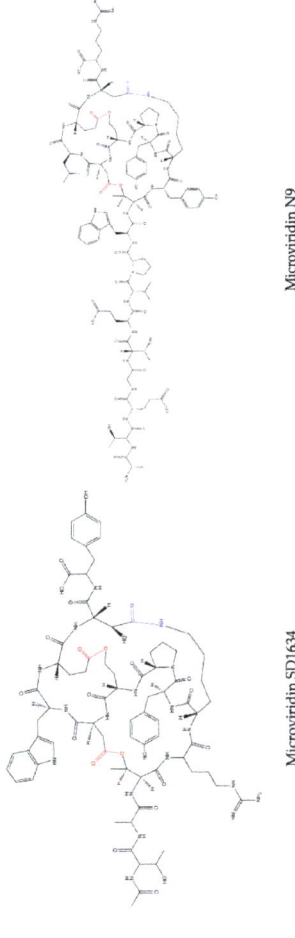

Figure 2. *Cont.*

One year later, Shin et al. (1996) [24] revealed the presence of three novel microviridins in *Planktothrix agardhii* (NIES-2014), known as microviridins D, E and F. Microviridin D is a bicyclic peptide, the N-terminal of which is occupied by an acetylated Tyr. Similar to microviridin A, this metabolite also possesses a ester bond formed between the side chains of the Thr and Asp residues. Differing from the former, microviridin D has Asn and Met residues instead of Gly and Phe, respectively. Furthermore, the ester bond between the γ-carboxyl of the Glu and the Ser hydroxyl group is missing in microviridin D, since γ-carboxyl of the Glu existed as a methyl ester. Microviridin E was the first microviridin composed of 13 amino acids described. In microviridin E, three Phe residues replaced two Tyr and one Trp residues of microviridin D. Unlike the other microviridins mentioned above, which have Glu occupying the second position from the C-terminal, this oligopeptide presents the residue of Asp in this position. Microviridin F seems to be a hydrolyzed microviridin E product with the same amino acid sequence. The absence of an ester bond between Thr and Asp is the main difference compared to other microviridins mentioned above. *Nostoc minutum* (NIES-26) was uncovered in 1997 as a source of two novels microviridins (G and H). Microviridin G is structurally related to microviridins A and B, while microviridin H has its structure closely related to microviridin C. These newly identified peptides have the same amino acid compositions. However, microviridin H does not have an ester bond between the Ser and Glu amino acid residues [25].

Microviridin I was firstly identified in the nontoxic *P. agardhii* strains 2 and 18. This oligopeptide exhibits high similarity to microviridins A, B and G. They share the Lys-Tyr (2)-Pro (2)-Ser-Asp (1)-Trp-Glu amino acid sequence, as can be seen in Figure 1 [26]. Microviridin J was firstly described in *M. aeruginosa* strain UWOCC MRC, being composed of 13 amino acids organized in three rings and two linear side chains. Unlike the previous microviridins, this peptide has arginine residues between Thr and Lys, which confer a special arrangement with the hydrophobic regions formed between the side chain of this residue and other amino acid residues. This novel structure conferred by the Arg residue occupying the fifth position provides ring stabilization and may be associated with a strong inhibition of trypsin, which has been identified solely in this microviridin [27]. The N-acetyl group of microviridin J also contributes to a marginal increase in the inhibition of trypsin by hydrogen bond formation [28]. The greatest amount of this toxin was obtained by utilizing MeOH at a concentration between 40–80%. The lowest yield was achieved by utilizing absolute methanol [27].

Reshef and Carmeli (2006) [29] isolated, for the first time, three microviridins with the nonproteinogenic amino acid β-hydroxyaspartic acid (Has) bound to lysine through an amide bond. These oligopeptides received the names of microviridin SD1684, SD1634 and SD1652 and were isolated from the extract of *M. aeruginosa* (IL-215). All these microviridins exhibit the same amino acid compositions. However, they differ regarding the number of ester bonds. SD1684 has no ester bonds (solely the amide bond), while SD1634 possesses the two-ester bonds and SD1552 contains only one ester bond, Ser-Glu.

Vegman and Carmeli (2014) [30] isolated from the extract of a yellow-brown bloom material composed of *Microcystis* spp. (TAU IL-376) the microviridin LH1667, whose amino acid sequence was defined as Ac-Tyr (I)-Ser(I)-Thr-Leu-Lys-Tyr (II)-Pro-Ser (II)-Asp-Trp-Glu(I)-Glu (II)-Tyr (III), with a Lys side chain amine and Glu (II) side chain carboxylic acid connected via a lactam, Ser (II) side chain hydroxyl and Glu (I) side chain carboxylic acid connected via a lactone and a side chain of Thr forming a lactone ring with a side chain carboxylic acid of Asp [30].

The increased number of genome sequences belonging to cyanobacteria opened the doors to a deeper knowledge about microviridins, allowing the discovery and engineering of new variants. The structure of microviridin K was determined by Philmus et al (2008) [15] in *P. agardhii* CYA126/8. Its amino acid composition is similar to microviridin D. However, the residue of Glu12 is not methylated. This oligopeptide thus contains two rings of lactone. Microviridin L, detected in cyanobacterium *M. Aeruginosa* (NIES843), was one of the first cyanobacterial oligopeptides to be characterized with the assistance of genomic data. The gene cluster of this metabolite was inserted into a fosmid and subsequently expressed in *Escherichia coli* [31].

Microviridins N3−N9 were identified in the model strain *N. punctiforme* PCC73102 via a genomic approach. These unusual microviridins contain between 15 and 20 amino acid residues and are not acetylated. The name was given to highlight the difference between the number of N-terminal amino acids, which can range from three to nine [19].

Two new microviridins have recently been discovered in strain *M. aeruginosa* EAWAG 127A: microviridin 1777 and microviridin O [32]. The former is the most potent chymotrypsin inhibitor of the microviridin class, while the latter was not detected in the extract, although the precursor peptide gene was contained in the genome (EZJ55 03525). An antiSMASH analysis allowed the identification of its gene cluster. This oligopeptide exhibits high similarly with microviridins A, B, G and J. They share the Lys-Tyr (2)-Pro (2)-Ser-Asp (1)-Trp-Glu amino acid sequence. Its peptide sequence is AC-Tyr-Asn-Val-Thr-Leu-Lys-Tyr-Pro-Ser-Asp-Trp-Glu-Glu-Phe.

Based on the number and structure of the ester bonds, microviridins can be classified into four classes. The amide bond is conserved in all of them. Group I consists of microviridins with two ester bonds. The second and third groups have only one ester bond between Thr1-Asp7 and Ser6-Glu9, respectively. In the fourth, microviridins are present with only the amide bond conserved (Figures 2–5).

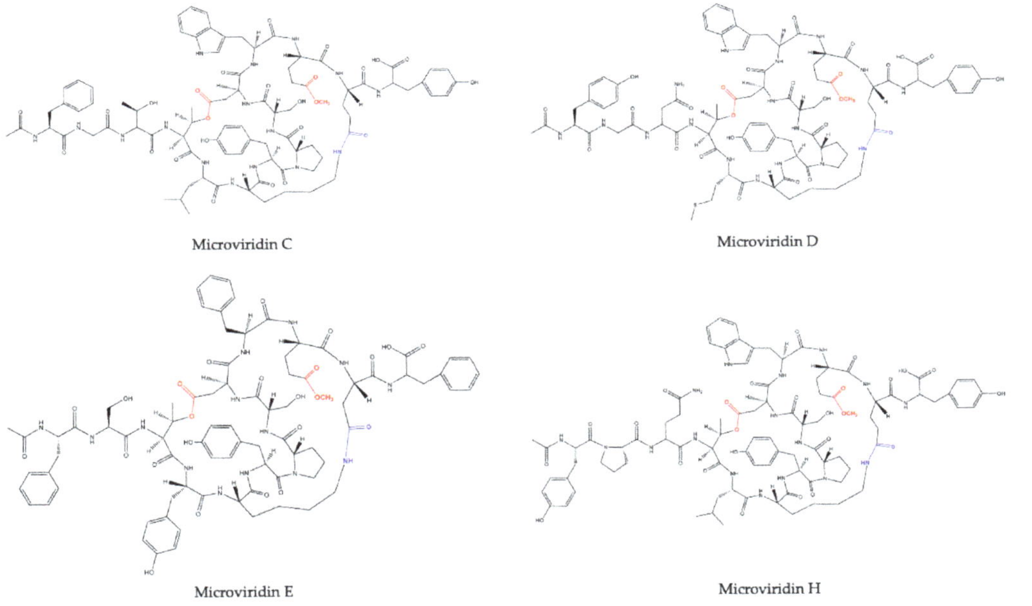

Figure 3. Microviridin structures belonging to group II.

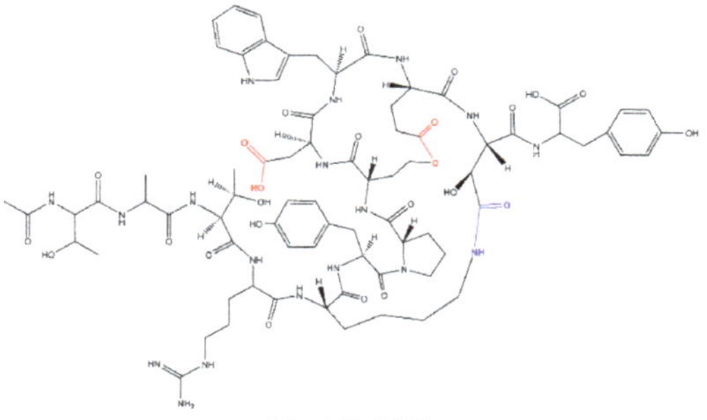

Microviridin SD1652

Figure 4. Microviridin structure belonging to group III.

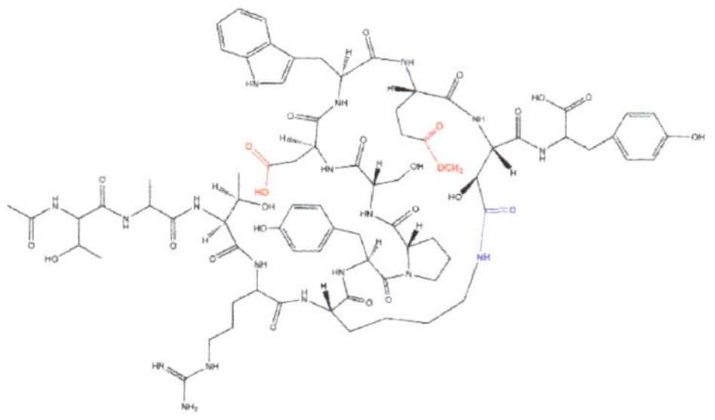

Microviridin F

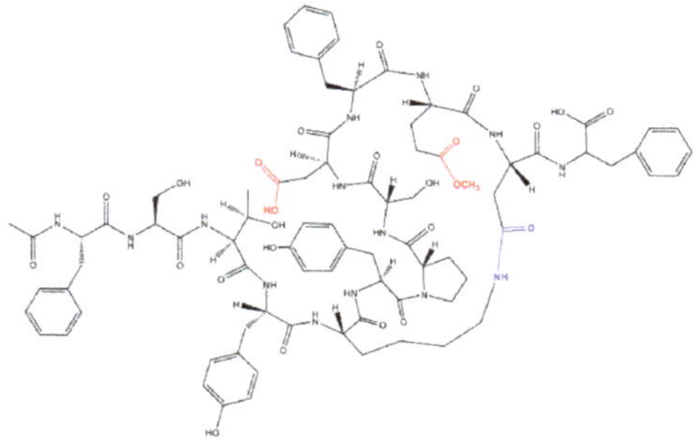

Microviridin SD1684

Figure 5. Microviridin structure belonging to group IV.

4. Microviridin Biosynthesis

Owing to their atypical conformation, microviridins have been mistakenly labeled as nonribosomal peptides. This concept has been discarded, because numerous studies have failed in the quest for biosynthetic gene clusters with mechanisms linked to NRPS genes and being similar to ribosomally biosynthesized peptides, such as cyanobactins (patellamides, tencyclamides and patellins) and trichamide [15,33]. In addition, NRPS products usually have nonproteinogenic amino acids in their structure and can be paired with hydroxy acids. Furthermore, their amino acids can also be in a D-configuration. These characteristics are not usually present in the family of microviridins [15,33]. Microviridins have recently been identified as ω-ester-containing peptides, along with plesiocins and thuringinins of the ribosomally synthesized and post-translationally modified peptide (RiPP) family [34].

Apart from the fact that microviridins have been isolated and characterized since the 1990s, their biosynthesis started to be elucidated by two groups independently using separate approaches in 2008 [14,15]. Firstly, Ziemert et al. [14] pursued a NRPS gene cluster related to microviridin production in *Anabaena*; however, they detected a gene with similar sequence to microviridin, known as *mdnA*. In the immediate proximity of *mdnA*, two additional genes were discovered, named *mdnB* and *mdnC* [14]. In comparison, Philmus et al. 2008 [15] detected similar genes from *Planktothrix agardhii*. This filamentous cyanobacterium possesses a homologous *mdnA* sequence, named *mvdE*, and homologous genes of *mdnB* and *C* encoding two ATP-grasp ligases (*mvdB* and *mvdC*). In addition, an acetyl transferase (*mvdB*) and an ATP-binding cassette transporter (*mvdA*) were detected, which their homologous genes were identified in *Microcystis* named *mdnD* and *mdnE*, respectively (Table 1) [15].

Table 1. Genes involved in microviridins biosynthesis.

Genes	Product	Role
mdnA/mvdE	Microviridin prepeptide	Contains the leader peptide at N-terminal and the core peptide at C-terminal
mdnB/mvdC	Family of carboxylate-amine/thiol ligases belonging to the ATP-grasp fold superfamily	Lactam rings formation through amide bonds.
mdnC/mvdD	Family of carboxylate-amine/thiol ligases belonging to the ATP-grasp fold superfamily	Lactone rings formation through ester bonds
mdnD/mvdB	N-acetyltransferase of the GNAT family	Acetylation of microviridin at N-terminal
mdnE/mvdA	ATP-binding cassette (ABC) transporter	Stabilization of the biosynthetic enzymes

These genes have been analyzed by various methods, confirming their roles during the synthesis of microviridins. The heterologous expression of microviridin B *mdnA-C* genes from *Microcystis* in *E. coli* produced a tricyclic microviridin-lacking leader peptide [14]. Concurrently, the in vitro reconstitution of the MvdB-E enzymes from *P. agardhii* also confirmed that these genes were linked to the production of microviridins [15]. These studies were important to demonstrate that the microviridin biosynthetic clusters have different organizations, with or without different genes (Figure 6) [14,15,35].

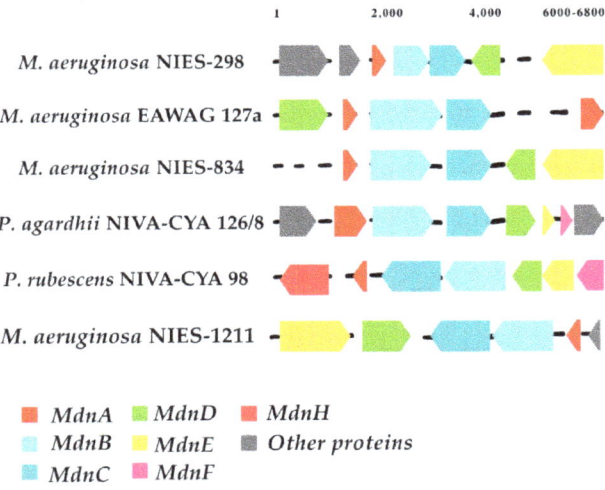

Figure 6. Graphical representation of microviridin biosynthetic clusters. The gene cluster compilation was accomplished through the Gene Graphics application (https://katlabs.cc/genegraphics/app).

Through an extensive bioinformatics study of microviridin biosynthetic gene clusters, a number of variations between them have been identified. The majority of these clusters consisted of *mdnA-C* genes, where *mdnB* and *-C* are normally in strict order. However, *mdnD* is only present in a subset of the clusters found. In comparison, *mdnE* is also absent in microviridin gene clusters or replaced by the C39 peptidase, which is followed by the HlyD3 homolog protein, normally linked to the transport of proteases across membranes.

Several other gene clusters carry additional proteins, likely linked to the noncommon post-translational modification of the core sequence, such as *mdnF* and *G* [21,33].

One of the first steps needed to produce a completely tricyclic N-acetylated microviridin is the production of prepeptide. The microviridin precursor gene (*mdnA*) produces an immature peptide that its leader peptide (LP) has preserved among different variants and possessing a highly conserved PFFARFL motif among the microviridin gene clusters, which has a α-helix structure in a solution (Figure 7) [36]. The core sequence frequently contains Asp, Thr, Ser and Lys residues, as well as the TxKxPSD motif, in which both features are related, to form lactone and lactam rings [20]. When evaluating different cyclized peptides with ω-ester and ω-amide bonds, their core sequences have a high frequency of conserved Thr and Glu residues, which are highly related to lactone ring formations. In addition, when contrasting plesiocin, thuringinins and microviridins, the residues involved in both ester and amide bonds are arranged in a similar order: the nucleophilic residues (Lys, Ser and Thr) always precede the acidic residues (Glu or Asp), indicating their relationship to the directionality of the modification enzymes, as described below [34].

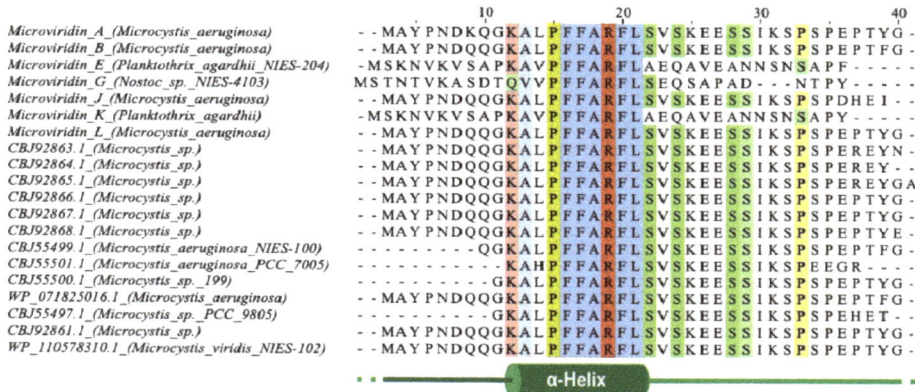

Figure 7. Leader peptide sequences from different microviridins. The PFFARFL motif is highly conversed among them. This sequence and some of its flanking amino acids are structured as an α-helix, responsible for recognition by ATP-grasp ligases. Multiple alignment was obtained by Clustal Omega (https://www.ebi.ac.uk) and visualized using JalView software (https://www.jalview.org).

The PFFARFL motif and its α-helix structure is crucial as a recognition motif for the ATP grasp-type ligases (MdnB and -C), as can be visualized in Figure 8A, considering that both enzymes do not modify the core microviridin peptide when the leader peptide is absent, and lactonization and lactamization occur with the PFFARFL motif presence [36–38]. The PFFARFL motif is also present in the leader peptide of marinostatin, a double-cyclic peptide with serine protease inhibitor activity, which, by a phylogenetic analysis, suggests that this bicyclic peptide is derived from microviridins [20,37]. Nevertheless, the N-terminal ten-residues sequence of MdnA is not relevant for MdnB and C activity, as this modified prepeptide still containing a PFFARFL motif can also be cyclized and processed. However, a N-His$_6$-tagged MdnA with an integral LP fused to three consecutives core peptides was not able to be processed by MdnC from *Anabaena* sp. PCC7120 [36,39].

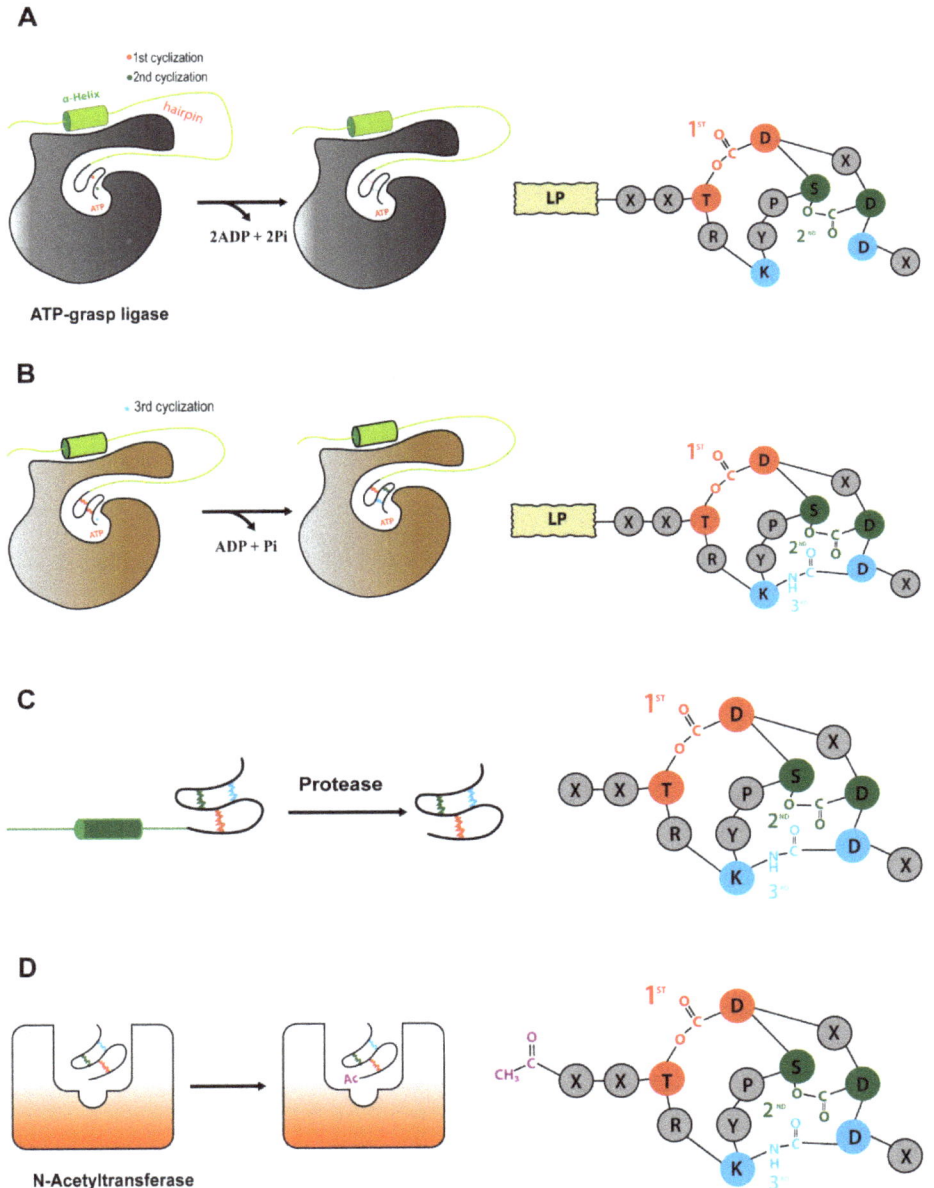

Figure 8. Microviridin biosynthesis. (**A**) Ester bond formations by MvdD/MdnC. (**B**) Amide bond formations by MvdC/MdnB. (**C**) Removal of a peptide leader by a proteolytic enzyme. (**D**) N-acetylation by MvdB/MdnD.

In addition to this motif, a proline-rich segment is present in the C-terminal region of the leader peptide in a variety of microviridins from *Microcystis* organisms, close to those eukaryotic signal peptides normally associated with cleavage sites. In contrast, microviridin K obtained from *Planktothrix aghardii* CYA128/8 possesses only one proline at the same region [15,35,40]. However, the substitution of these prolines in *Microcystis* did not affect the removal of the peptide leader but resulted in the cessation of microviridin production [37], suggesting the necessity of the β-turn of peptide leaders MdnB and C.

Ahmed et al [20] analyzed several *mdnA* sequences among their biosynthetic clusters and divided this gene into three different classes. Class I precursor peptides contain the LP fused to only one core sequence and are often associated with the presence of *mdnE*, which occurs in a majority of the strains. Class II precursor peptides present a single leader peptide for up to five core peptides in tandem, separated or not by double-glycine cleavage sites, and these clusters normally encode a C39 peptidase membrane protein. Finally, class III is identical in length to class II, but the former has its core sequence only at the C-terminal of the prepeptide [20]. This indicates a number of pathways for the genetic organization of *mdnA*.

After *mdnA* has been expressed, prepeptides should be submitted for cycling by the sequential catalysis of the enzymes. Thus, in order to understand the mechanisms related to this stage, Philmus et al. [15,37] were the first to define, through biochemical methods, the steps taken by MvdC and D of *P. agardhii* CYA126/8. Both enzymes are carboxylate-amine/thiol ligases that belong to the ATP-grasp superfamily and act by requiring ATP and Mg^{2+} [38,40] to form a carboxylate–phosphate intermediate, which is then susceptible to nucleophilic attacks to form ester, amide or thioester bonds [17,36]. MvdD/MdnC are responsible for the first step in the formation of both ester bonds (Figure 8A) and, subsequently, lactone rings in the linear prepeptide, while MvdC/MdnB are responsible for the formation of lactam rings by amide bonds [15,35].

Both enzymes are homodimers with related assemblies, similar to most proteins of this family, having three subdomains: N-domain, central domain and C-domain. Besides their overall similarities, there are differences comparing their central and C-domains. MdnC/MvdD possess a two-stranded antiparallel β-sheet forming a hairpin structure, followed by a reasonably ordered α-helix that anchors the leader peptide. Meanwhile, this hairpin region is located at the C-domain of MdnB/MvcC, followed by a flexible loop in the α-helix region. The MdnB has a closed conformation, compared to MdnC, because the antiparallel β-sheet hairpin blocks the pocket site where MdnA interacts. Those differences can be related to their specificity and mode of action, as can be seen below. Regarding the ATP-binding pocket, it is structurally conserved, as confirmed by mutagenesis, where substitution of the key amino acids completely abolished the MdnC reaction [36].

Phylogenetic studies and the study of preserved sequences of different classes of prepeptides forming cyclic structures by the action of ATP-grasp ligases (plesiocins, microviridins and thuringinins) suggest that the enzymes coevolved with their respective precursor peptides due to the specificity of the preserved residues present in the core sequence [36]. Consequently, the association between microviridin production and ATP-grasp enzymes indicates that cyanobacteria recycled primary metabolic enzymes for the production of natural products, such as ribosomal peptides, as most ATP-grasp ligases are engaged to primary metabolism [15,17,35,36]. In addition, MdnC is well-conserved among *Microcystis* species, suggesting its derivation from a common ancestor, as well as its dependence on the core motif KYPSD and threonine and aspartate conservation sites of microviridins, as seen by the mutagenesis and phylogenetic analysis [14,15].

As described by Li et al. (2016) [36], the reaction of the bond formation by MdnC (Protein Data Bank (PDB) code 5IG9) is driven by the interaction with the leader peptide. Thus, the PFFARFL motif structured as a α-helix and its flanking amino acids interact with the MdnC hairpin, inducing its movement towards the linear prepeptide bound to the enzyme, then acting as an allosteric region. Considering the ATP-grasp ligase from *Microcystis aeruginosa*, these interactions occur between the amino acids Arg17 (MdnA) and Glu191, Asp192 and Asn195 (MdnC) and Ser20 (MdnA) and Val182 (MdnC). However, Glu191 is mostly replaced by an aspartate residue among all microviridin macroclases but still bears the negative charge required to recognize the LP [36].

After binding to the peptide leader through the PFFARFL motif, the ester bond formations are strictly required to occur in a specific order in microviridins: MvdD catalyze the lactone ring between Asp44 and Thr38, then Glu46 and Ser43 into the prepeptide, by phosphorylating the carboxyl side chain of Asp and Glu with ATP, thus forming the large then small lactone rings, respectively [37]. These residues participating in the amide bond and ring formation are highly conserved among the cyclic peptides, suggesting their requirement for the correct cyclization and similar catalysis between ATP-grasp ligases from different groups [34].

When a site-directed mutagenesis was applied to produce different variants of MvdE/MdnA, S43A and T38A, it has been noticed that MvdD catalyzes a reaction following a N-terminal-to-C-terminal direction, as the S43A variant is still lactonized, producing a monocyclic microviridin. In addition, the amino acid bearing the hydroxyl group is crucial for the reaction, as it seems that MvdD cannot react when it is moved one position in either the N- or C-terminal direction [15,37,41]. It seems that both ATP-grasp ligases are highly tolerant for nonconserved residues, then being able to catalyze different microviridins. However, they are not flexible to conserved residues that are involved in cyclization [34,35].

For a better understanding of the different MdnC/MvdD enzymes, Zhang et al. [39] characterized a homolog of these enzymes from *Anabaena* sp. PCC7120, AMdnC, which belonged to a biosynthetic cluster with a prepeptide of class II, with a LP followed by three consecutives core sequences (AMdnA). The mode of action of AMdnC indicates a distributive catalysis, where the ATP-grasp ligase dissociates from the processed peptide after each monocyclization, until achieving all lactone ring formations. This feature has been also described in other modification proteins from RiPP pathways, such as the NisB, LctM, LabKC and HalM2 enzymes from lanthipeptides processing; microcin B17 synthetases; ATP-grasp enzyme PsnB and N-methylation enzyme OphA of omphalotin. Additionally, AMdnC also demonstrates a preferential N-to-C directionality when catalyzing the reaction but not unstrict. Thus, this homolog of MdnC can process each core peptide independently from AMdnA. Moreover, the calculated K_m from AMdnC when catalyzing AMdnA or MdnA is comparable to MdnC values when processing MdnA; however, the k_{cat} of the ATP hydrolysis of AMdnC were up to 60 times faster, suggesting a different mechanism for processing a prepeptide with multiple core sequences.

MdnB has a similar structure and mechanism of activation as MdnC, where the PFFARFL motif interacts with the hairpin, resulting in the activation of the enzyme [36]. Then, the bicyclic prepeptide produced by MvdD/MdnC is catalyzed by MndB/MvdC, and the lactam ring is formed through the amide bond formation between the ε-amino group of Lys40 and δ-carboxyl group of Glu47 (Figure 8B). The omega-amide bond is similar to those present in microcin J25 and capistruin; however, the enzymatic mechanism is different, because microviridin K synthesis occurs via an acyl-adenylated intermediate [17].

Both preformed lactone rings are required by MvdC/MdnB, as the linear and monocyclic peptides are not modified. A single mutation in the PFFARFL pattern in the leader peptide prevents the formation of amide bonds, as well as the proper conformation of the β-turn by the proline-rich region at the C-terminal of microviridin from *Microcystis*, suggesting a lower flexibility compared to MndC [39]. In addition, the amino acid sequence of the core peptide can also influence the correct cyclization, even those not well-conserved, requiring the TxKxPSD motif and Lys and Glu residues [41].

MdnC/MvdD is less rigid than MdnB/MvdC, as it can still catalyze both lactone rings besides single and double mutations in the PFFARFL motif and proline-rich region of the leader peptide (in *Microcystis*) but could result in producing different microviridin variants differing at the N-terminal [37]. This versatility is possibly due to the more open conformation of the hairpin structure and to the binding interaction between MdnC and the prepeptide relative to MdnB. As seen in vitro, the binding interaction between LP and MdnC is approximately tenfold higher compared to the LP and MdnB, resulting in a rapid processing of the linear prepeptide compared to the bicyclic modification. It is also believed that this is due to the fact that linear MdnA is less stable, requiring prompt modification [36]. However, this post-translational modification does not seem to be strictly sufficient for further steps, as bicyclic microviridins can still be cleaved and N-acetylated and possessing inhibitory activity against proteases [41]. As seen by bioinformatic analyses, the absence of MdnB is normal and is likely to lead to the formation of marinostatin, a peptide that lacks an amide bond and is closely related to microviridins [20]. Firstly, it was suggested that MdnE, an ABC transporter, could be related to the removal of the leader peptide through peptide cleavage due to the presence of a N-terminal C39 peptidase domain from *Anabaena* PCC7120 [14,37]. However, not all MdnE carry that domain, and the heterologous expression of the microviridin cluster lacking this protein still produces this tricyclic peptide, indicating other roles [14,37]. Comparing the microviridin expression with the presence and absence of MdnE, it was noted that these peptides were not correctly processed at the N-terminal and were incompletely cyclized due to a lack of lactam rings, as was the amount of MdnB observed in the cytoplasmic fraction when the ABC transporter was absent. This pattern then suggests the hypothesis that MdnE is a scaffolding protein, anchoring and stabilizing the microviridin biosynthesis complex on the cytosolic side of the membrane [37]. In addition to its similarity to transporter proteins, its function in exporting microviridin from the cell has not been demonstrated.

Knowledge on the removal of a peptide leader has so far been scarce in the literature. However, the heterologous expression of microviridin suggests that this step can be mediated by a nonspecific proteolytic enzyme (Figure 8C), as *E. coli* expressing only MdnA-C was capable of producing microviridin lacking a LP [14]. Moreover, GluC endoprotease is capable of cleaving peptide bond C-terminals to glutamic acid residues, and during the in vitro production of class II microviridin with three core sequences, this enzyme released all three mono-, bi- and tricyclized microviridins [40]. Finally, another hypothesis related to MdnE was raised. As described above, this enzyme may have a peptidase domain, typically present in class II clusters. This function may be linked to the presence of interspaced regions between the core sequences of MdnA and the release of each individual microviridin [14,20,37,39].

Acetylation is one of the last steps for the development of a fully matured tricyclic microviridin. Microviridin synthesis in vitro has shown that MvdB from *P. aghardii* CYA126/8 does not require the presence of the peptide leader to acetylate the microviridin N-terminal. In addition, MdnD/MvdB can react with mono-, bi- and tricyclic, being more flexible than MdnB and C. Thus, it can be assumed that this step occurs after the peptide leader removal, or this enzyme does not interact with this region (Figure 8D) [38]. In addition, a 12 amino acid-long tricyclic peptide is not N-acetylated by MdnD from *P. aghardii* CYA126/8, but those microviridin with 13/14 amino acids are acetylated, indicating that there a specific size requirement by this enzyme, and it is flexible regarding the core sequence [20], thus suggesting that N-acetylation occurs only after leader peptide removal [15,20,35,38].

5. Occurrence

Genome mining has shown that cyanobacteria have the potential to generate much more microviridin than is typically found under normal growth conditions. A study of this type has contributed to the expansion of knowledge on the chemical and genetic diversity of microviridins. They have been detected in various cyanobacterial genera and species, and these microorganisms are notorious producers of different groups of peptides and can be found in many environments, whether in fresh or salt water (Table 2). Due to this great variety, these bacteria have been evaluated for their significant biotechnological potential. The genus *Microcystis* and the species *M. aeruginosa* are the largest producers of microviridins—currently, of the 25 isolated microviridins, 11 belong to the genus *Microcystis*, and eight of these belong to the species *M. aeruginosa* [21,23,27,29–31]. Microviridin gene clusters have also been found in genomes of a number of bacteria, such as bacteroidetes and proteobacteria phyla [20].

Table 2. Occurrence of microviridins.

Species/Genera	Isolation Source	Trophic State	Sequenced Genome	Microviridins	Mass (Da)	Ref.
Microcystis. viridis NIES-102	Aquatic	Eutrophic	+	Microviridin A	1729.7	[21]
Microcystis. aeruginosa NIES-298	Aquatic	Eutrophic	+	Microviridin B	1723.8	[23]
Microcystis. aeruginosa NIES-298	Aquatic	Eutrophic	+	Microviridin C	1755.8	[23]
Planktothrix agardhii NIES-204	Aquatic	Eutrophic	+	Microviridin D Microviridin E Microviridin F	1802.7 1665.7 1683.7	[24]
Nostoc minutum NIES-26	Terrestrial	Mesotrophic	+	Microviridin G Microviridin H	1806 1838	[24]
Planktothrix agardhii CYA126/8	Aquatic	N.I.	-	Microviridin K	1769	[15]
Planktothrix. agardhii strain 2 & 18	Aquatic	Eutrophic		Microviridin I	1764.7	[26]
Microcystis aeruginosa UWOCC CBS	Aquatic	N.I.	-	Microviridin J	1684.4	[27]
Microcystis aeruginosa NIES-843	Aquatic	Eutrophic	+	Microviridin L	1715	[31]
Planktothrix sp.	Aquatic	Eutrophic	-	Microviridin I Microviridin 1642 Microviridin 1663	1765.8 1642.8 1663.7	[43]
Microcystis aeruginosa	Aquatic	Mesotrophic	-	N.I.	N.I.	[44]
Microcystis sp.	Aquatic	N.I.	-	Microviridin LH1667	1666.7	[30]
Microcystis aeruginosa PCC 7820	Aquatic	N.I.	-	Microviridin 1706	1707.8	[46]
Planktothrix rubescens NIVA-CYA 98	Aquatic	Mesotrophic	+	Microviridin	1971.8	[33]
Microcystis sp.	Aquatic	Mesotrophic	-	Microviridin 1667 Microviridin 1684 Microviridin 1699 Microviridin 1777	1668.6 1695.8 1699.8 1778.8	[42]
Chroococcidiopsis sp. CENA 353	Leaf Surface	N.I.	-	N.I.	N.I.	[45]

Table 2. Cont.

Species/Genera	Isolation Source	Trophic State	Sequenced Genome	Microviridins	Mass (Da)	Ref.
Desmonostoc sp. CENA365	Leaf Surface	N.I.	-	N.I.	N.I.	[45]
Nostocaceae CENA358	Leaf Surface	N.I.	-	N.I.	N.I.	[45]
Nostocaceae CENA376	Leaf Surface	N.I.	-	N.I.	N.I	[45]

N.I.: not informed.

The genus *Microcystis* was the first to be described in the literature as a cyanobacteria producer of microviridins. This peptide was isolated from the bloom-forming *M. viridis* (NIES-102) on Kasumigaura Lake by Ishitsuka et al. (1990) [21]. This new oligopeptide demonstrated a noncanonical structure and was named microviridin by the name of the viridis species. In addition, other microviridins from the cyanobacteria of the genus *Microcystis* have been identified as microviridin B, C, L, SD1684, SD1634, SD1652, LH1667, 1777, O and M. Each of these microviridins has a considerable inhibition for at least one serine protease, such as elastase or trypsin [21,23,27,29–31].

An in-situ diversity investigation of the *Microcystis* communities present in lakes located around and in the city of Berlin, Germany demonstrated that 20% of 165 colonies analyzed were capable of producing microviridin. These cyanobacteria were present in almost all investigated areas. The majority of the microviridins producers also synthesized microcystins and cyanopeptolins. The coproduction of microviridin-aeruginosins and -microginins was rarely reported among the strains, being present in only 4% and 2%, respectively. The metabolomic profile of the peptides can be utilized to distinguish *Microcystis* strains with elevated morphological similarity whose visualization in the light microscope is not sufficient to differentiate them [42].

Martins and collaborators [43] isolated strains of cyanobacteria *M. aeruginosa* from a large range of lakes, rivers and reservoirs in Portugal. These strains were examined for the presence of secondary metabolites, such as aeruginosins, microviridins and microcystins. In this analysis, 47 strains from different sites were isolated among the identified peptides; microcystin was the most recurrent, appearing in 26 strains, and microviridins were contained in only three. The results of the analysis of the coproduction showed that the strains that produced microviridins did not produce microcystins. In another study, Walker et al [44] isolated the microviridin-producing strains of the *Planktothrix* genus from Maxsee in Germany incapable of producing microcystins.

In a study accomplished by Andreote [45], the purpose of which was to obtain information on the cyanobacterial community present in the phyllosphere of native plants from the Atlantic Forest, identified 40 cyanobacterial strains belonging to the genera *Nostocaceae*, *Desmontosc* and *Chroococcidiopsis* as microviridin producers obtained from *Merostachys neesii* (bamboo), *Euterpe edulis* (palmeira jacura), *Guapira opposita* and *Garcinia gardneriana*.

Andreote [45] was the pioneer in the identification of these peptides in the *Desmontosc* and *Chroococcidiopsis* genera. To identify the presence of this peptide in the strains, PCR amplifications of the *mdnA*, *mdnB* and *mdnC* genes were performed, which were related to the biosynthetic pathways of the microviridins. The strains *Nostocaceae* sp. CENA358 and CENA376, *Desmonostoc* sp. CENA365 and *Chroococcidiopsis* sp. CENA353 demonstrated the presence of these genes. Other strains lacked at least one of these genes, which did not rule out the synthesis of this peptide by these microorganisms due to the primers utilized that were constructed for strains of *Microcystis*, causing low-amplification performances, which implies that they might have more strains producing microviridins or possessing a biosynthetic cluster [45].

Eleven cyanopeptides from four different groups were reported from samples of cyanobacterial bloom in the Salto Grande reservoir, located in the State of São Paulo,

Brazil, including the microviridin variant 1706. Cyanopeptides such as aeroguniosins, microcystins and cyanopeptolin were also detected. The morphological research showed that the bulk of the population of cyanobacteria belonged to the genus *Microcystis* [46].

Variants of microviridins were characterized in two cyanobacteria isolated from Brazilian reservoirs. *R. fernadoii* strain 28 was obtained from the Furnas Reservoir, which is situated in the southeastern region of Brazil and is described as an oligo-to-mesotrophic aquatic environment that receives organic matter contributions from domestic, farming and agriculture wastewaters. The *R. fernadoii* 86 strain was identified in an urban eutrophic reservoir located in the city of Belo Horizonte, Brazil, which suffers a great impact from domestic pollution, industrial sewage. A total of twelve peptides were found in the two strains. In the *R. fernadoii* 28 strain, a microviridin MV-1709 was found, and, in the strain *R. fernadoii* 86, two microviridins were reported, MV-1707 and MV-1739. Along with microviridins, peptides such as microcystins, cyanopeptolin and an unidentified peptide were also detected [47].

6. Microviridin Ecology

Microviridins play a significant ecological function as antifeeding agents against cyanobacterial natural predators. This activity is correlated with their ability to inhibit proteolytic enzymes (Figure 9). The first study to explain this mechanism was performed by Rohrlack et al. (2014) [48]. A previous work, however, had already indicated microviridins as an agent capable of causing the interrupting the feeding of *Daphnia* microcrustacean via enzymatic inhibition. This ability can partly explain the dominance of these microorganisms in some habitats, including those with a high population density of *Daphnia* [49]. In a similar way, protease inhibitors are produced by terrestrial plants to protect against herbivores. Metatranscriptomic analyses of the Kranji Eutrophic Reservoir, located in Singapore, revealed important information on the functional dynamics between different bacterial phyla, including cyanobacteria, which were dominant microorganisms, especially those belonging to the *Microcystis* genus. The microviridin transcripts were found in high quantities, along with those involved in the buoyancy and photosynthetic operation. The highest peak of the gene expression related to microviridin biosynthesis was observed when the population of *Daphnia* moved from the mesopelagic zone to the epipelagic zone, corroborating its antipredator activity [49].

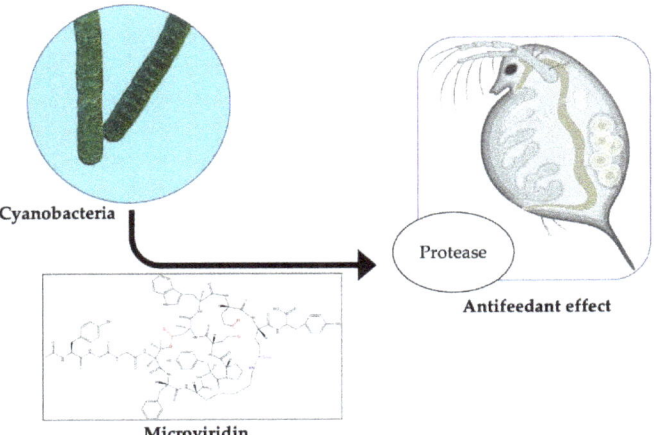

Figure 9. Ecological role of microviridins as antifeedant against the microcrustacean *Daphnia*.

Kaebernick et al. (2001) [50] compared the feeding inhibition of *Daphnia galeata* and *D. pulicaria* by a microcystin-producing *Microcystis* (MRD) and a microcystin-deficient

Microcystis (MRC), and it has been realized that this hepatotoxin is not associated with the ingestion rate reduction in both planktonic grazers. However, this metabolite was responsible for causing both species to decrease their survival rates. Before the death provoked by this hepatotoxin, these microcrustaceans remained immobile in the bottom of the vial and shifted only when the surrounding area suffered disturbances. In addition, the filter legs and antenna were momentarily paused, and the midgut was disrupted.

The same authors [50] described further effects of *Microcystis* strain UWOCC MRC ingestion by *D. galeata* and *D. pulicaria*. These microcrustaceans had a dysfunction in the peritrophic membrane. This membrane acts as a barrier formed by the chitin–protein complex created by the midgut cells. The consumption of *Microcystis* made this organ more enervated, as a result of which, food transport was impaired, resulting in particle aggregation in this region and in the digestive diverticula. The ingestion of these cells also disturbed the molting process. The old integument was not entirely separate from the *Daphnia* body, attached to the legs and filter antennas, and strongly hindered the ability of these species to swim and feed themselves. Individuals subjected to these conditions were more likely to die of malnutrition within two days. It was also confirmed that the freshly developed integument remained soft both in the presence of the old integument and after its mechanical removal. Under field conditions, these affected species would become easy prey to predators, since they would not be able to flee to any shelter.

The typical chitin–protein complex occurs in both structures (peritrophic membrane and integument), indicating that the reported effects were probably caused by the same bioactive compound in which the microviridin variant was cogitated. By its ability to inhibit the serine protease, this oligopeptide could be preventing the tyrosine conversion into dihydroxyphenylalanine (DOPA) and its subsequent transformation into dopamine by the enzyme DOPA decarboxylase [51]. Dopamine is involved in the cross-linkage of orthoquinones, which results in the cuticle sclerotization [52]. A complementary process was proposed by Rohrlack et al. (2003) [48]. According to this mechanism, *Daphnia*'s death was associated with incomplete protein digestion, which resulted in an important amino acid deficiency for tegument development and other structures. Ingestion of the strain of *Microcystis* UWOCC CBS, a producer of microviridin J, causes the same activity in the molting process of *D. pulicaria*. However, several additional findings have been made. Particles derived from food suspensions were found on the entire surface of the *Daphnia* body. This dysfunction was possibly due to the secretion of body fluids. Deformation on the freshly generated tegument has become more intense as the effort to eradicate it by these animals has increased. The same phenomenon was visualized when only the purified microviridin J was added.

Czarnecki et al. (2006) [53] detected eight microviridins distributed in three *Microcystis* strains (HUB08B03, HUB11G02 and HUB19B05) with ability to inhibit trypsin-like activity in the planktonic crustacean *Daphnia*. In addition to microviridins, other classes of protease inhibitors, such as some cyanopeptolins, were found in the extract obtained from these cyanobacteria. This ability of unique cyanobacterium or different cyanobacteria from the same genus can generate a variety of combinations of different oligopeptides with distinct proteolytic targets and inhibitory activity. This feature acts as an evolutionary barrier, preventing the adaptation process among zooplankton population.

Microviridin toxicity was also accessed in the fairy shrimp *Thamnocephalus platyurus*, which belonged to order Anostraca. In the course of searching for natural products with cytotoxicity property, Sieber et al. (2019) [32] detected in the extract of *M. aeruginosa* strain EAWAG 127 deleterious activity against this microcrustacean (LD_{50} = 0.43 mg.mL^{-1}). A metabologenomic approach revealed the presence of two novel microviridins: microviridin 1777 and microviridin O. The former showed a LD_{50} value of 95 µM for *Thamnocephalus platyurus*. This activity was ascribed to the strong capacity of this peptide in inhibiting elastase and chymotrypsin activity with an IC_{50} of 160 nM and 100 nM, respectively.

In addition to Cyanobacteria having a low susceptibility to a zooplankton attack, these microorganisms are also the target of various pathogenic bacteria and fungi that play an important role in controlling their growth [54,55]. True zoosporic fungi, commonly known as chytrids, are among the most pathogenic organisms capable of causing a significant number of deaths in the cyanobacterial community [56]. The success of this pathogen in infecting these photosynthetic microorganisms can be attributed to the development of chemotactic zoospores and the presence of rhizoids, which are capable of locating the target and used to extract the nutritional contents, respectively. Oligopeptides produced by cyanobacteria with an inhibitory activity against a predator's key enzymes is a great defense mechanism. The comparison between the cyanobacterial strain *P. agardhii* CYA126/8 with its mutants, each one with a type of disability in producing microcystins, anabaenopeptins or/and microviridins, was conclusive to defining the protective role of these metabolites. The wild strain when incubated with the chytrid strain was unaffected, while all mutant strains were infected, including those non-microviridin-producing strains [57].

Chytrides are a rich source of protease used as a mechanism to digest their hosts. Microviridins and anabaenopeptins can target these enzymes, reducing the virulence of these fungi. The vast variety of microviridins, as well as other oligopeptides, is a major obstacle in the process of the adaptation of these parasites. On the basis of the literature, the protection mechanism referred to above appears to be constitutive, since these substances typically form an oversaturated or saturated solution in the cytoplasm [57]. Microviridin was also found in bacteria belonging to the microbiome of the plant *Populus*. Unlike the lanthipeptides that are widely distributed among the member of this community, microviridins were restricted only to the genus *Chryseobacterium*, being present in 16 out of the 18 sequenced bacteria. Its role in this microbiome is not clear. A gene cluster for microviridin in this genus showed from one to four precursor peptides belonging to class I [20]. Different from cyanobacterial microviridin, the core peptide was composed of 18 amino acid residues. Only half of the microviridin clusters analyzed had a N-acetyltransferase gene. A resistant gene presence in the majority of the microviridin clusters suggested that this oligopeptide could have antibacterial properties, conferring a protection to plants against pathogenic microorganisms [58].

Other features given to microviridins are related to their allelochemical properties. Cyanobacteria produce a variety of proteases that are essential to different processes, including nutrient absorption, protein activation, unfolded or aggregated protein removal, photoacclimation and stress response [59]. Ghosh et al. (2008) [60] demonstrated that a cyanobacterial oligopeptide with the partial structure of a microviridin affected the proteolysis in *M. aeruginosa* PCC 7806, strongly inhibiting its capacity to degrade N-alpha-benzoyl-DL-Arg-p-nitroanilide (BApNA). The authors' hypothesis was that microviridin-producing *Microcystis* colonies could form an aggregate that could eventually develop as a bloom and suppress the growth of competing organisms by targeting critical functions that rely on protease activity. Another possibility is that microviridins will have a significant role to play in stress conditions by self-regulating the protease activity among cyanobacterial cells and thus enhancing their survival rates [60].

Some microviridins are not easily detected in environmental samples, since they may be rapidly degraded by other bacteria. *M. viridis* has its microviridin A content totally consumed when transferred to a nonaxenic medium [21]. The aquatic bacterium *Sphingomonas* sp. B-9, firstly isolated for its microcystin-degradation ability, has hydrolytic enzymes capable of degrading different cyclopeptides, including microviridin I. The degradation of this peptide by this bacterium is very slow, lasting around 48 h to reduce 50% of its initial content. This process occurs in two steps. Initially, the residue at the C-terminal region is removed, and, subsequently, the molecule undergoes a linearization step [61].

7. Regulation

Environmental factors play an important role in the regulation of the synthesis of oligopeptides, as they can increase the growth rate and, consequently, the production of these metabolites. In certain cases, however, the best conditions for growth did not lead to the most desirable conditions for their production [62]. Microcystin was the key subject of these studies [63]. Stress situations can alter the cell's physiological state and act as trigger for increasing the construction of these molecules. Nitrogen and phosphorus bioavailability are among the most nutritional factors investigated in cyanobacterial behaviors [64,65]. Both are involved in protein synthesis and in the energy dynamic. Due to anthropic actions, these elements have become more abundant in the aquatic environment [66].

Other parameters, such as temperature, pH and light intensity, have also been investigated and challenge many scientists [67,68]. An assessment of the combined effect of different environmental elements on the development of cyanopeptides can provide a link between field research and laboratory research. Any of these variables can be associated. As the culture reaches the stationary phase, the quantity of nutrients decreases, as well as the light availability among cells, thereby reducing their growth rate.

One method used by Rohrlack et al. (2007) [67] to individually determine the light impact was to track and maintain a constant nutrient load in the medium. This technique was used to analyze the production of microviridin I by *P. agardhii* strain PT2. The quantity of cell-bound microviridin I expressed in units per biovolume decreased until the eighth day. This behavior reversed when the light availability began to decline. Nitrogen and phosphate reduction also led to a decrease in the production of this microviridin. A similar trend was reported for microcystins and anabaenopeptins. Some authors strongly believe that many of these oligopeptides play the same ecological function. The loss of one can have, as a consequence, the enhanced production of another, unaffecting the cyanobacterial growth [69,70].

The influence of light intensities was also evaluated by Pereira et al. (2012) [47] on the profiles of toxic and nontoxic oligopeptides obtained from two strains of the cyanobacterium: *R. fernandoii* 28 and 86. In the course of the experiment, they employed three different irradiances, which were classified as low (25 μMol.m^{-2}.s^{-1}), medium (65 μMol.m^{-2}.s^{-1}) and high (95 μMol.m^{-2}.s^{-1}). Different from other oligopeptides investigated in this study, such as microcystins and cyanopeptolins, microviridins were not encountered in all growth conditions. Microviridin 1709 production reached the maximum amount when the cells of strain 28 were exposed to a medium light intensity, while microviridin 1707, identified in strain 86, was detected solely at low light conditions.

Ferreira et al. (2006) [71] evaluated the combination of different light intensities, nutritional contents, temperatures and growth phases on the oligopeptide production in distinct strains of *Microcystis* and *Aphanizomenon*, including microviridins. This protease inhibitor was detected solely in the *Microcystis* strain RST9501. In the absence of nitrate and phosphate, this peptide was produced in higher quantities. In the majority of the cases, the intracellular fraction was responsible for over 80% of the total microviridin pool. At the same nutritional conditions, an atypical behavior was found when the cells were cultivated at 20 °C. In this condition, the intracellular microviridin concentration diminished to 60%.

The cell-to-cell communication is also a factor to be considered in peptide production. When this mechanism is dependent on cell density, it is called quorum sensing. Nealson and Hastings (1979) [72] were pioneers in studying this phenomenon in the Gammaproteobacterium *Vibrio fischeri*. These two scientists were capable of demonstrating that the enzyme luciferase, whose role is to transform chemical energy into light energy, was expressed only at a high cell density, having its production controlled by autoinducer signaling molecules [72]. The most known autoinducers described are the acylated homoserine lactones [73]. The aquatic environment has a natural tendency to dilute the metabolites released by microorganisms. For this reason, some authors believe that oligopeptide production is regulated by quorum sensing [74]. There is little knowledge about this mechanism in cyanobacteria. During a bloom episode, the cyanobacterial population increased significantly, creating a favorable environment for quorum sensing. In this type of situation, the high cell density augments the concentration of signaling molecules in the environment [75].

To evaluate the quorum sensing effect on oligopeptide production, Pereira et al. [74] grew the cyanobacteria in a semicontinuous culture system. Hence, the biomass level and nutritional content were maintained constant. The growth rates of high and low cell density cultures were similar. Microviridin production was detected only in a low cell density culture of *R. fernandoii* (strain R28). In contrast, the microviridins N3-N9 in *N. punctiforme* PCC73102 had their synthesis optimized under high cell density conditions [19].

The cyanobacterial lifestyle may also have an effect on its oligopeptide content. Some cyanobacteria are typically located on the water and sediment surface. There are also those with a biphasic lifestyle, where they migrate to the top during the summer and to the bottom during the winter [76]. A comparative genomics of the genus *Planktothrix* with different lifestyles performed by Pancrace et al. (2016) [77] demonstrated that all planktonic strains investigated harbored the microviridin gene cluster. In contrast, in the benthic *Planktothrix*, this gene cluster was absent, with the exception of *Planktothrix* sp. PCC 11201, which is phylogenetically closer to free-living *Planktothrix*.

8. Application of Microviridins

Proteases play an important role in the regulation of biological processes in all living organisms by controlling the maintenance, recovery, development and modification of tissues, which may be beneficial or harmful. They may modulate protein–protein interactions that create bioactive molecules involved in DNA replication and transcription [78]. In plants, these enzymes lead to the maturation and degradation of a series of unique proteins relevant to the environmental condition and the stage of growth [79]. Thus, molecules with inhibitory activity against these enzymes have an immense biotechnological potential with a multitude of applications (Figure 10).

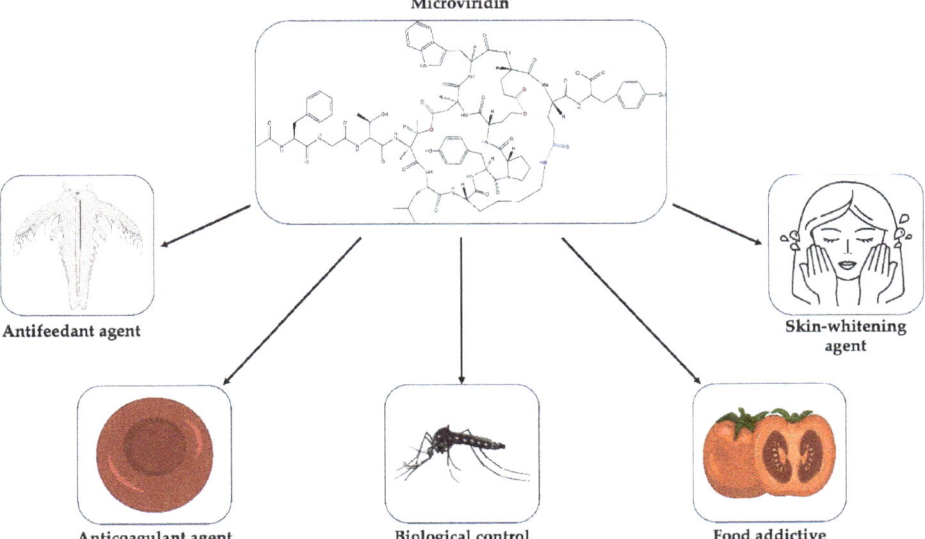

Figure 10. Potential applications of microviridins.

Tyrosinase is a multifunctional and metalloenzyme widely distributed among plants, microorganisms and animals, where it plays a key role in the development of melanin [80]. The excessive synthesis of this photoprotective pigment may lead to a condition known as hyperpigmentation, which may lead to an esthetic problem where one part of the skin is more pigmented than the other [81]. In addition, this disorder has been linked to many diseases, such as skin cancer and Parkinson's disease [82]. Molecules with the capacity to interfere with the catalytic activity of tyrosinase have been extensively studied as a skin-whitening agent. They can also be used as food additives, reducing the browning process of mushrooms and fruits caused by tyrosinase [83]. Some of these commercially available compounds exhibit low stability and safety [84]. Among the microviridins reported in the literature, microviridin A was demonstrated to be tyrosinase inhibitor. However, its action mechanism is not clear, and information regarding its toxicity to human cells has never been accessed (Table 3) [21]

Table 3. Inhibitory activities of microviridins.

Microviridin	Inhibitory Activity (IC_{50})							Reference
	Tyrosinase	Elastase	Trypsin	Chymotrypsin	Thrombin	Plasmin	Papain	
A	0.33 mM *	ND	ND	ND	ND	ND	ND	[21]
B	ND	25.5 nM	33.7 µM	1.45 µM	>58.1 µM	>58.1 µM	ND	[23]
C	ND	47.9 nM	18.2 µM	2.8 µM	>57.1 µM	>57.1 µM	ND	[23]
D	ND	388.5 nM	>55.5 µM	665.9 nM	>55.5 µM	>55.5 µM	>55.5 µM	[24]
E	ND	360.1 nM	>60 µM	660.3 nM	>60 µM	>60 µM	>60 µM	[24]
F	ND	3.4 µM	>59.5 µM	>59.5 µM	>59.5 µM	>59.5 µM	>59.5 µM	[24]
G	ND	10.5 nM	>55.4 µM	775.6 nM	>55.4 µM	>55.4 µM	>55.4 µM	[25]
H	ND	16.9 nM	>54.4 µM	1.6 µM	>54.4 µM	>54.4 µM	>54.4 µM	[25]
I	ND	192.7 nM	14.9 µM	12.3 µM	>56.7 µM	ND	ND	[26]
J	ND	>5.9 µM	20–90 µM	1.7 µM	ND	ND	ND	[27]
L	ND	>58 µM	42 µM	58 µM	ND	ND	ND	[31]
1777	ND	160 nM	>10 µM	100 nM	ND	ND	ND	[32]
SD1684	ND	ND	Inactive	Inactive	ND	ND	ND	[29]
SD1634	ND	ND	8.2 µM	15.7 µM	ND	ND	ND	[29]
SD1652	ND	ND	Inactive	Inactive	ND	ND	ND	[29]
LH1667	ND	20 nM	>45.5 µM	2.8 µM	ND	ND	ND	[30]

* IC_{50} not defined. ND, not determined.

The mechanism of coagulation is regulated by proteases. Serine protease inhibitors therefore function as essential regulators in this pathway, such as proteins in the serpin superfamily. Malfunctioning of one of these elements can lead to coagulation disorders. Excessive blood clotting can lead to a disorder known as thrombosis, where the blood flow is blocked by thrombus [85]. Thrombin is one the major target of anticoagulant drugs, since it acts in the conversion of soluble fibrinogen into insoluble filamentous of fibrins, which, together with platelets, are responsible for a hemostatic plug formation, impeding the bleeding. The thrombin inhibition by microviridin B is superior to the positive control Leupeptin, possessing an EC_{50} (half maximal effective concentration) value equal to 4.58 µM. This value was inferior than that encountered for Micropeptin K139, a serine protease also detected in cyanobacteria. In contrast, microviridins D-F do not affect thrombin activity, most likely due to the absence of an indole motif, which is encountered in microviridin B, suggesting its role as a recognition motif for thrombin [86].

Human neutrophil elastase is a proteolytic enzyme that belongs to the serum protein family of chymotrypsin-like. This highly active enzyme has revealed a wide substrate specificity and is one of the few proteases capable of degrading the extracellular matrix protein elastin, resulting in the enzyme's name [87]. The elastase overactivity is involved in tissue destruction and inflammation characteristic of various diseases, such as chronic obstructive hereditary emphysema, pulmonary disease, cystic fibrosis, adult respiratory distress syndrome and ischemic-reperfusion injury [88]. Pharmaceuticals already use elastase inhibitors for the treatment of diseases related to this enzyme, such as the drug Sivelastat, which has been cogitated in the treatment of COVID-19 [89].

A study by Masahiro Murakami et al. (1997) [25] evaluated the elastase inhibitory effect of some microviridins, synthesized by the cyanobacterium *Nostoc insulare* (NIES-26). The results of the analysis showed two new peptides, microviridin G and microviridin H. In the experiment, both IC_{50} were compared with the values of other microviridins already described in the literature. Microviridin A showed no inhibitory effect on elastase; microviridins D and F had the weakest values for inhibiting this enzyme. Microviridins G and H had the best results, followed by microviridins B and C, respectively. After the work of Murakami et al. [25], three new microviridins were described as elastase inhibitors: I, LH1667 and 1777 (Table 3) [26,30,32].

Proteases are also essential for the growth of insects, such as in the larval and adult stages, where they are present in the intestine and play an important role in digestion [90]. For example, silkworms, near the final stage of their metamorphosis, produce cocoonase, a serine protease capable of hydrolyzing silk protein, which enables the adult moth to emerge [91]. During the embryony phase, proteases digest egg-specific proteins, such as vitellin, for the amino acid release, which are utilized as a nitrogen source [92]. Serine protease can also confer protection against predation. The South American Saturniid caterpillars belonging to the genus *Lonomia* harbor in their hemolymph a toxic protease that some mammals who come in contact with can have, as a consequence, bleeding disorders [93]. Nowadays, various studies have focused on the search for a protease inhibitor whose target are proteases produced by insects involved in disease transmission, such as the *Aedes aegypti*, one of the largest vectors of arboviruses, being responsible for the propagation of the dengue virus, yellow fever, zika virus and chikungunya fever [94].

Microviridins have already shown to be good inhibitors of enzymes present in microcrustaceans intestines, such as those of the genus *Daphnia* and *Thamnocephalus* [32,50]. For instance, in the presence of microviridins B, C, I, J, L and SD1652, the enzyme trypsin has its activity negatively affected [23,26,27,29,31] (Table 3). They act by inhibiting enzymes that are closely related to the diet of these crustaceans. In insects, many of these serine proteases are located in the intestines as well [95], sharing similar functions. Two of these serine proteases are trypsin and chymotrypsin, well-known targets of some microviridins (Table 3).

Plants have served as a great heterology expression system for bioactive peptides. Hilder et al. (1987) [96] were the first to use these organisms to express serine protease inhibitors with the potential to kill predatory larvae insects. There is a considerable number of works employing plants as hosts of ribosomally synthesized and post-translationally modified peptides [97–99]. Plant-based microviridins have promises for future applications, since they can replace the use of pesticides to help control insect pests with low costs and low environmental impacts. Furthermore, they can be easily purified with a high yield, retaining full activity.

One of the bottlenecks for microviridin production and the evaluation in cyanobacteria is a low yield of this peptide. Several extraction approaches in different genus of this phylum demonstrated that these organisms are not well-suited for industrial applications when considering both the time and volume of the cultivations. A heterologous expression in *E. coli* demonstrated to be an efficient method for microviridin biosynthesis resulted in a yield of 60 °C 70 mg of microviridin L per 100 g of dried cells after five hours of cultivation. In comparison, about 0.87 mg.g^{-1} of microviridin A was obtained from *Microcystis viridis* (NIES-102) by a cultivation period of 10 °C for 14 days. In filamentous cyanobacteria, this yield was even lower, with a production of 9.1 mg.g^{-1} of microviridin E after the same period of incubation of *Planktothrix* in 400 L [21,25,31].

However, the problems related to microorganism cultivation, heterologous expression and laborious purification can still be tackled, and techniques have been developed to overcome these barriers in order to explore the diversity of the microviridins. As a consequence, the development of microviridins obtained from environmental DNA can be accomplished by the synthesis of the solid-phase peptide of the core peptide coupling with MdnC and -B enzymes fused to the leader peptide in the N-terminal. This chemoenzymatic approach allows an in vitro production of a fully processed microviridin, demonstrating the efficiency during production of different variants of this peptide [34]. Another approach for microviridin production in vitro is to provide the LP in trans for both MdnB and -C, also achieving a tricyclic microviridin J [36].

Another important feature for the biotechnological application of microviridin is its binding affinity to serine proteases. Microviridin J demonstrated a K_D value of 0.68 µM from its interaction with trypsin. This mode of inhibition is similar to a cyclic depsipeptide A90720A produced by a nonribosomal peptide synthetase [34,37]. However, the NRPS pathways are not well-susceptible to genetic engineering compared to RiPPs. Thus, in addition to the possibility of genetic modifications, the microviridin biosynthetic cluster is smaller than NRPS, facilitating a heterologous expression [37].

The crystallography structure of trypsin bound to N-acetylated tricyclic microviridin J (PDB codes: 4KTU and 4KTS; pH 6.5 and 8.5, respectively) has been determined to better understand the relationship between the microviridin structure and its enzymatic target (Figure 11). It was therefore possible to observe that the N-terminal of microviridin J was flexible and bound to the hydrophobic surface of trypsin [100]. As far as the catalytic domain is concerned, both crystallized structures showed the interface as a substrate-like trypsin-binding motif. The threonine residue at position 4 of microviridin J interacts with Leu99 at the S2 pocket through its methyl group. At the S1 pocket, Asp189 coordinates the side chain of arginine at position 5, which is located between the residues making ester and amide bonds. A van der Waals contact by the aliphatic region of Lys6 of microviridin is made with the disulfide bond between Cys43 and Cys58 of the S1' subsite. Finally, the C-terminal of microviridin J, Ser9-Trp14, stabilizes a helical structure of trypsin by the intramolecular covalent linkages of this inhibitor. The interaction between these two structures showed a K_D value of 0.68 µM, which is similar to the NRPS cyanobacterial inhibitor A90720A [100].

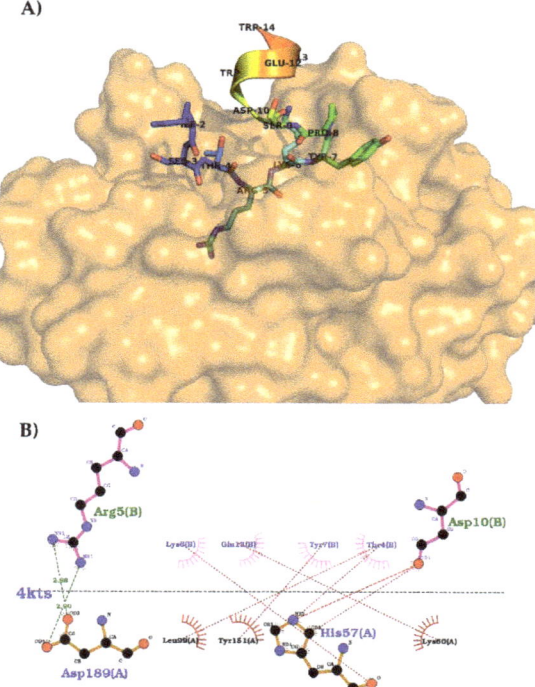

Figure 11. Interaction between microviridin J and trypsin at pH 8.5 (Protein Data Bank (PDB) code: 4KTS). (**A**) 3D representation of the interaction. (**B**) 2D view of the major interaction between microviridin J and trypsin. Hydrogen bonds are in green, while the hydrophobic interactions are in red.

As far as the Ser-His-Asp triad of trypsin is concerned, these three residues are located in the direction of the Arg5 carbonyl of microviridin. However, the peptide bond between Arg5 and Lys6 was not affected, suggesting that the rings and the compact structure of microviridin J neutralize the cleavage of this tricyclic structure [100].

According to the crystallized structures, it could be concluded that position 5 of the microviridins is essential to its inhibitory activity due to the interaction of the trypsin triad. This hypothesis supports the mutagenesis approach to the modification of residue 5 of microviridin L, which modified both the specificity and the inhibitory activity against different proteases. The wild-type microviridin L has its most potent inhibition against subtilisin (IC$_{50}$ = 5.8 µMol.L^{-1}); however, the replacement of Phe5 for other amino acids changed this activity. The F5L mutant improved the elastase inhibition; in comparison, F5R increased its inhibition toward trypsin. The F5Y variant shifted its activity against chymotrypsin, and F5M had an IC$_{50}$ = 0.09 µMol.L^{-1} toward subtilisin. In contrast, the exchange of amino acids at positions 7, 9 and 11 did not boost the inhibitory activity at the same scale, nor did any inhibition cease [20,100].

The G2A variant coupled with the shift in position 5 of microviridin J not only enhanced the post-translational modification performances but, also, increased the inhibitory function. The positive charged residues of Arg and Lys at position 5 had superior activity towards subtilisin and trypsin, while the latter was the only variant with a low micromolar activity against plasmin [100]. Similar findings were also observed with microviridin B variants L5R and L5K [38]. In addition, the hydrophobic residues of Leu and Val also demonstrated the inhibition of subtilisin and inhibition of elastase inhibitory activity, with minor variations compared to the single mutants at position 5 [100]. As a result, the amino acids at position 5 of the microviridins have shown great potential to be the focus for therapeutic development, with the goal of enhancing and defining the inhibitory action of microviridins by different synthetic chemical techniques.

9. Final Considerations

Microviridins are one of the largest oligopeptides present in cyanobacteria. While they were firstly identified in this community of microorganisms, the genomic approach has revealed gene clusters for these metabolites in bacteria belonging to another phyla. Their production is affected by abiotic and biotic factors such as temperature, pH, nutritional content and quorum sensing. This latter is poorly explored in cyanobacteria and can act as a powerful tool in the control of these microorganisms in the environment. Due to their protease inhibitory property, microviridins can be utilized for various purposes, such as an anticoagulant and as whitening agent, as well as in the control of disease vectors.

One of the greatest bottlenecks to the commercial application of microviridins is the low yield and the absence of information about their use in humans and animals. The former issue can be mitigated with the utilization of a heterologous expression system, which has well-described in the literature for this oligopeptide, mainly in the model organism *E. coli*. Others approaches would be the in vitro chemoenzymatic synthesis or the variations in the culture conditions, which could serve as an elicitor, leading to an upregulation of the metabolite. The strong inducible insertion of the promoter may make this process less laborious. In relation to health risks, further studies are required to better develop the inhibitory mechanism of microviridins, as well as their toxicity to humans. However, since they are a ribosomally synthesized and post-translationally modified peptide, they possess a certain plasticity for engineering that can reduce their risks and increase their specificity. The bulk of the cyanobacterial gene cluster remains undiscovered. The ability of these photosynthetic microorganisms to generate biomolecules is greater than was assumed before the genome age. Future studies will disclose new microviridins, as well as knowledge on their biological significance.

Author Contributions: Conceptualization, S.C.d.A., P.R.M., L.P.X. and A.V.S. Investigation, S.C.d.A., P.R.M. and G.M.S. Writing—original draft preparation, S.C.d.A., P.R.M., J.d.S.P.N. and G.M.S. Writing—review and editing, S.C.d.A., P.R.M., A.V.S. and L.P.X. Supervision, E.C.G., A.V.S. and L.P.X. All authors have read and agreed to the published version of the manuscript.

Funding: This study was financed in part by Coordenação de Aperfeiçoamento de Pessoal de Nível Superior—Brasil (CAPES)—Finance Code 001 and Fundação Amazônia Paraense de Amparo a Estudos e Pesquisas (FAPESPA)—03/2019.

Acknowledgments: The authors would like to thank Pró-Reitoria de Pesquisa e Pós-Graduação da Universidade Federal do Pará (PROPESP/UFPA).

Conflicts of Interest: The authors declare no conflict of interest.

References

1. Kulasooriya, S. Cyanobacteria: Pioneers of Planet Earth. *Ceylon J. Sci.* **2012**, *40*, 71.
2. Vijay, D.; Akhtar, M.; Hess, W. Genetic and metabolic advances in the engineering of cyanobacteria. *Curr. Opin. Biotechnol.* **2019**, *59*, 150–156. [PubMed]
3. Singh, P.K.; Rai, S.; Pandey, S.; Agrawal, C.; Shrivastava, A.K.; Kumar, S.; Rai, L.C. Cadmium and UV-B induced changes in proteome and some biochemical attributes of Anabaena sp. PCC7120. *Phykos* **2012**, *42*, 39–50.
4. Koch, R.; Kupczok, A.; Stucken, K.; Ilhan, J.; Hammerschmidt, K.; Dagan, T. Plasticity first: Molecular signatures of a complex morphological trait in filamentous cyanobacteria. *BMC Evol. Biol.* **2017**, *17*, 1–11.
5. Abed, R.; Dobretsov, S.; Sudesh, K. Applications of cyanobacteria in biotechnology. *J. Appl. Microbiol.* **2009**, *106*, 1–12.
6. Blin, K.; Pascal Andreu, V.; de los Santos, E.L.C.; Del Carratore, F.; Lee, S.Y.; Medema, M.H.; Weber, T. The antiSMASH database version 2: A comprehensive resource on secondary metabolite biosynthetic gene clusters. *Nucleic Acids Res.* **2019**, *47*, 625–630.
7. Wang, H.; Fewer, D.; Sivonen, K. Genome mining demonstrates the widespread occurrence of gene clusters encoding bacteriocins in cyanobacteria. *PLoS ONE* **2011**, *6*, 22384.
8. Fidor, A.; Konkel, R.; Mazur-Marzec, H. Bioactive peptides produced by cyanobacteria of the genus *Nostoc*: A review. *Marine Drugs* **2019**, *17*, 561.
9. Kehr, J.; Picchi, D.; Dittmann, E. Natural product biosynthesis in cyanobacteria: A treasure trove of unique enzymes. *Beilstein J. Org. Chem.* **2011**, *7*, 1622–1635.
10. Li, B.; Sher, D.; Kelly, L.; Shi, Y.; Huang, K.; Knerr, P.J.; Van Der Donk, W.A. Catalytic promiscuity in the biosynthesis of cyclic peptide secondary metabolites in planktonic marine cyanobacteria. *Proc. Natl. Acad. Sci. USA* **2010**, *107*, 10430–10435.
11. Martins, J.; Vasconcelos, V. Cyanobactins from cyanobacteria: Current genetic and chemical state of knowledge. *Marine Drugs* **2015**, *13*, 6910–6946. [PubMed]
12. Arnison, P.G.; Bibb, M.J.; Bierbaum, G.; Bowers, A.A.; Bugni, T.S.; Bulaj, G.; Camarero, J.A.; Campopiano, D.J.; Challis, G.L.; Clardy, J.; et al. Ribosomally synthesized and post-translationally modified peptide natural products: Overview and recommendations for a universal nomenclature. *Nat. Prod. Rep.* **2014**, *30*, 108–160.
13. Paz-Yepes, J.; Brahamsha, B.; Palenik, B. Role of a Microcin-C-like biosynthetic gene cluster in allelopathic interactions in marine *Synechococcus*. *Proc. Natl. Acad. Sci. USA* **2013**, *110*, 12030–12035. [PubMed]
14. Ziemert, N.; Ishida, K.; Liaimer, A.; Hertweck, C.; Dittmann, E. Ribosomal synthesis of tricyclic depsipeptides in bloom-forming cyanobacteria. *Angew. Chem. Int. Ed.* **2008**, *47*, 7756–7759.
15. Philmus, B.; Christiansen, G.; Yoshida, W.; Hemscheidt, T. Post-translational modification in microviridin biosynthesis. *ChemBioChem* **2008**, *9*, 3066–3073.
16. Lee, H.; Park, Y.; Kim, S. Enzymatic Cross-Linking of Side Chains Generates a Modified Peptide with Four Hairpin-like Bicyclic Repeats. *Biochemistry* **2017**, *56*, 4927–4930.
17. Moore, B.S. Extending the biosynthetic repertoire in ribosomal peptide assembly. *Angew. Chem. Int. Ed.* **2008**, *47*, 9386–9388.
18. Ziemert, N. Identification and Characterization of Ribosomal Biosynthesis Pathways of Two Cyclic Peptides from Cyanobacteria. Ph.D. Thesis, Faculty of Mathematics and Natural Sciences, Humboldt-Universität zu Berlin, Berlin, Germany, 2009. Available online: https://edoc.hu-berlin.de/handle/18452/16681 (accessed on 10 July 2020).
19. Dehm, D.; Krumbholz, J.; Baunach, M.; Wiebach, V.; Hinricht, K.; Guljamow, A.; Tabuchi, T.; Jenke-Kodama, H.; Sussmuth, R.D.; Dittmann, E. Unlocking the spatial control of secondary metabolism uncovers hidden natural product diversity in *Nostoc punctiforme*. *ACS Chem. Biol.* **2019**, *14*, 1271–1279.
20. Ahmed, M.; Reyna-González, E.; Schmid, B.; Wiebach, V.; Süssmuth, R.D.; Dittmann, E.; Fewer, D.P. Phylogenomic analysis of the microviridin biosynthetic pathway coupled with targeted chemo-enzymatic synthesis yields potent protease inhibitors. *ACS Chem. Biol.* **2017**, *12*, 1538–1546.
21. Ishitsuka, M.O.; Kusumi, T.; Kakisawa, H.; Kaya, K.; Watanabe, M.M. Microviridin: A Novel Tricyclic Depsipeptide from the Toxic Cyanobacterium *Microcystis viridis*. *J. Am. Chem. Soc.* **1990**, *112*, 8180–8182.
22. Zolghadri, S.; Bahrami, A.; Hassan Khan, M.T.; Munoz-Munoz, J.; Garcia-Molina, F.; Garcia-Canovas, F.; Saboury, A.A. A comprehensive review on tyrosinase inhibitors. *J. Enzyme Inhib. Med. Chem.* **2019**, *34*, 279–309. [CrossRef] [PubMed]
23. Okino, T.; Matsuda, H.; Murakami, M.; Yamaguchi, K. New microviridins, elastase inhibitors from the blue-green alga *Microcystis aeruginosa*. *Tetrahedron* **1995**, *51*, 10679–10686. [CrossRef]
24. Shin, H.; Murakami, M.; Matsuda, H.; Yamaguchi, K. Microviridins D-F, serine protease inhibitors from the cyanobacterium *Oscillatoria agardhii* (NIES-204). *Tetrahedron* **1996**, *52*, 8159–8168. [CrossRef]

25. Murakami, M.; Sun, Q.; Ishida, K.; Matsuda, H.; Okino, T.; Yamaguchi, K. Microviridins, elastase inhibitors from the cyanobacterium *Nostoc minutum* (NIES-26). *Phytochemistry* **1997**, *45*, 1197–1202. [CrossRef]
26. Fujii, K.; Sivonen, K.; Naganawa, E.; Harada, K. Non-toxic peptides from toxic cyanobacteria, *Oscillatoria agardhii*. *Tetrahedron* **2000**, *56*, 725–733. [CrossRef]
27. Rohrlack, T.; Christoffersen, K.; Hansen, P.E.; Zhang, W.; Czarnecki, O.; Henning, M.; Fastner, J.; Erhard, M.; Neilan, B.A.; Kaebernick, M. Isolation, characterization, and quantitative analysis of microviridin J, a new *Microcystis* metabolite toxic to *Daphnia*. *J. Chem. Ecol.* **2003**, *29*, 1757–1770. [CrossRef]
28. Funk, M.; Van Der Donk, W. Ribosomal Natural Products, Tailored to Fit. *Acc. Chem. Res.* **2017**, *50*, 1577–1586. [CrossRef]
29. Reshef, V.; Carmeli, S. New microviridins from a water bloom of the cyanobacterium *Microcystis aeruginosa*. *Tetrahedron* **2006**, *62*, 7361–7369. [CrossRef]
30. Vegman, M.; Carmeli, S. Three aeruginosins and a microviridin from a bloom assembly of *Microcystis* spp. collected from a fishpond near Kibbutz Lehavot HaBashan, Israel. *Tetrahedron* **2014**, *70*, 6817–6824. [CrossRef]
31. Ziemert, N.; Ishida, K.; Weiz, A.; Hertweck, C.; Dittmann, E. Exploiting the natural diversity of microviridin gene clusters for discovery of novel tricyclic depsipeptides. *Appl. Environ. Microbiol.* **2010**, *76*, 3568–3574. [CrossRef]
32. Sieber, S.; Grendelmeier, S.; Harris, L.; Mitchell, D.; Gademann, K. Microviridin 1777: A Toxic Chymotrypsin Inhibitor Discovered by a Metabologenomic Approach. *J. Nat. Prod.* **2020**, *83*, 438–446. [CrossRef] [PubMed]
33. Rounge, T.; Rohrlack, T.; Nederbragt, A.; Kristensen, T.; Jakobsen, K. A genome-wide analysis of nonribosomal peptide synthetase gene clusters and their peptides in a *Planktothrix rubescens* strain. *BMC Genom.* **2009**, *10*, 396. [CrossRef] [PubMed]
34. Lee, H.; Choi, M.; Park, J.; Roh, H.; Kim, S. Genome Mining Reveals High Topological Diversity of ω-Ester-Containing Peptides and Divergent Evolution of ATP-Grasp Macrocyclases. *J. Am. Chem. Soc.* **2020**, *142*, 3013–3023. [CrossRef] [PubMed]
35. Philmus, B.; Guerrette, J.; Hemscheidt, T. Substrate specificity and scope of MvdD, a GRASP-like ligase from the microviridin biosynthetic gene cluster. *ACS Chem. Biol.* **2009**, *4*, 429–434. [CrossRef]
36. Li, K.; Condurso, H.; Li, G.; Ding, Y.; Bruner, S. Structural basis for precursor protein-directed ribosomal peptide macrocyclization. *Nat. Chem. Biol.* **2016**, *12*, 973–979. [CrossRef]
37. Weiz, A.R.; Ishida, K.; Makower, K.; Ziemert, N.; Hertweck, C.; Dittmann, E. Leader peptide and a membrane protein scaffold guide the biosynthesis of the tricyclic peptide microviridin. *Chem. Biol.* **2011**, *18*, 1413–1421. [CrossRef]
38. Reyna-González, E.; Schmid, B.; Petras, D.; Süssmuth, R.; Dittmann, E. Leader Peptide-Free *In Vitro* Reconstitution of Microviridin Biosynthesis Enables Design of Synthetic Protease-Targeted Libraries. *Angew. Chem. Int. Ed.* **2016**, *55*, 9398–9401. [CrossRef]
39. Zhang, Y.; Li, K.; Yang, G.; McBride, J.L.; Bruner, S.D.; Ding, Y. A distributive peptide cyclase processes multiple microviridin core peptides within a single polypeptide substrate. *Nat. Commun.* **2018**, *9*, 1–10. [CrossRef]
40. Hemscheidt, T.K. Chapter Two—Microviridin Biosynthesisin. In *Methods in Enzymology*; Academic Press Inc.: Cambridge, MA, USA, 2012; Volume 516, pp. 25–35.
41. Gatte-Picchi, D.; Weiz, A.; Ishida, K.; Hertweck, C.; Dittmann, E. Functional analysis of environmental DNA-derived microviridins provides new insights into the diversity of the tricyclic peptide family. *Appl. Environ. Microbiol.* **2014**, *80*, 1380–1387. [CrossRef]
42. Welker, M.; Brunke, M.; Preussel, K.; Lippert, I.; von Döhren, H. Diversity and distribution of *Microcystis* (cyanobacteria) oligopeptide chemotypes from natural communities studies by single-colony mass spectrometry. *Microbiology* **2004**, *150*, 1785–1796. [CrossRef]
43. Martins, J.; Saker, M.; Moreira, C.; Welker, M.; Fastner, J.; Vasconcelos, V. Peptide diversity in strains of the cyanobacterium *Microcystis aeruginosa* isolated from Portuguese water supplies. *Appl. Environ. Microbiol.* **2009**, *82*, 951–961. [CrossRef] [PubMed]
44. Welker, M.; Christiansen, G.; von Döhren, H. Diversity of coexisting *Planktothrix* (cyanobacteria) chemotypes deduced by mass spectral analysis of microystins and other oligopeptides. *Arch. Microbiol.* **2005**, *182*, 288–298. [CrossRef] [PubMed]
45. Andreote, A.P.D. Filosfera da Mata Atlântica: Isolamento e Sistemática de Cianobactérias, Bioprospecção e Caracterização da Comunidade Diazotrófica. Ph.D. Thesis, Centro de Energia Nuclear na Agricultura, São Paulo, Brazil, 2014. Available online: www.teses.usp.br (accessed on 10 September 2020).
46. Sandonato, B.B.; Santos, V.G.; Luizete, M.F.; Bronzel, J.L., Jr.; Eberlin, M.N.; Milagre, H.M.S. MALDI Imaging Mass Spectrometry of Fresh Water Cyanobacteria: Spatial Distribution of Toxins and Other Metabolites. *J. Braz. Chem. Soc.* **2017**, *28*, 521–528. [CrossRef]
47. Pereira, D.; Pimenta, A.; Giani, A. Profiles of toxic and non-toxic oligopeptides of *Radiocystis fernandoi* (Cyanobacteria) exposed to three different light intensities. *Microbiol. Res.* **2012**, *167*, 413–421. [CrossRef]
48. Rohrlack, T.; Christiansen, G.; Kurmayer, R. Putative antiparasite defensive system involving ribosomal and nonribosomal oligopeptides in cyanobacteria of the genus *Planktothrix*. *Appl. Environ. Microbiol.* **2014**, *79*, 2642–2647. [CrossRef]
49. Penn, K.; Wang, J.; Fernando, S.; Thompson, J. Secondary metabolite gene expression and interplay of bacterial functions in a tropical freshwater cyanobacterial bloom. *ISME J.* **2014**, *8*, 1866–1878. [CrossRef]
50. Kaebernick, M.; Rohrlack, T.; Christoffersen, K.; Neilan, B. A spontaneous mutant of microcystin biosynthesis: Genetic characterization and effect on *Daphnia*. *Environ. Microbiol.* **2001**, *3*, 669–679. [CrossRef]
51. Arakane, Y.; Noh, M.Y.; Asano, T.; Kramer, K.J. Tyrosine Metabolism for Insect Cuticle Pigmentation and Sclerotization. In *Extracellular Composite Matrices in Arthropods*; Cohen, E., Moussian, B., Eds.; Springer: Cham, Switzerland, 2016.
52. Weiss, L.C.; Leese, F.; Laforsch, C.; Tollrian, R. Dopamine is a key regulator in the signalling pathway underlying predator-induced defences in *Daphnia*. *Proc. R. Soc. B Biol. Sci.* **2015**, *282*, 20151440. [CrossRef]

53. Czarnecki, O.; Henning, M.; Lippert, I.; Welker, M. Identification of peptide metabolites of *Microcystis* (Cyanobacteria) that inhibit trypsin-like activity in planktonic herbivorous *Daphnia* (Cladocera). *Environ. Microbiol.* **2006**, *8*, 77–87. [CrossRef]
54. Mohamed, Z.; Hashem, M.; Alamri, S. Growth inhibition of the cyanobacterium *Microcystis aeruginosa* and degradation of its microcystin toxins by the fungus *Trichoderma citrinoviride*. *Toxicon* **2014**, *86*, 51–58. [CrossRef]
55. Meyer, M.; Bigalke, A.; Kaulfuß, A.; Pohnert, G. Strategies and ecological roles of algicidal bacteria. *FEMS Microbiol. Rev.* **2017**, *41*, 880–899. [CrossRef] [PubMed]
56. Gerphagnon, M.; Colombet, J.; Latour, D.; Sime-Ngando, T. Spatial and temporal changes of parasitic chytrids of cyanobacteria. *Sci. Rep.* **2017**, *7*, 1–9. [CrossRef] [PubMed]
57. Sŕnstebŕ, J.; Rohrlack, T. Possible implications of Chytrid parasitism for population subdivision in freshwater cyanobacteria of the genus *Planktothrix*. *Appl. Environ. Microbiol.* **2011**, *77*, 1344–1351.
58. Blair, P.; Land, M.; Piatek, M.; Jacobson, D.; Lu, T.; Doktycz, M.; Pelletier, D. Exploration of the Biosynthetic Potential of the *Populus* Microbiome. *mSystems* **2018**, *7*, 1–17.
59. Dagnino, D.; de Abreu, D.; de Aquino, J.C. Growth of nutrient-replete *Microcystis* PCC 7806 cultures is inhibited by an extracellular signal produced by chlorotic cultures. *Environ. Microbiol.* **2006**, *8*, 30–36. [CrossRef]
60. Ghosh, S.; Bagchi, D.; Bagchi, S.N. Proteolytic activity in *Microcystis aeruginosa* PCC7806 is inhibited by a trypsin-inhibitory cyanobacterial peptide with a partial structure of microviridin. *J. Appl. Phycol.* **2008**, *20*, 1045–1052. [CrossRef]
61. Kato, H.; Imanishi, S.; Tsuji, K.; Harada, K. Microbial degradation of cyanobacterial cyclic peptides. *Water Res.* **2007**, *41*, 1754–1762. [CrossRef]
62. Raksajit, W.; Satchasataporn, K.; Lehto, K.; Mäenpää, P.; Incharoensakdi, A. Enhancement of hydrogen production by the filamentous non-heterocystous cyanobacterium *Arthrospira* sp. PCC 8005. *Int. J. Hydrog. Energy* **2012**, *37*, 18791–18797. [CrossRef]
63. Omidi, A.; Esterhuizen-Londt, M.; Pflugmacher, S. Still challenging: The ecological function of the cyanobacterial toxin microcystin–What we know so far. *Toxin Rev.* **2018**, *37*, 87–105. [CrossRef]
64. Xu, Q.; Yang, L.; Yang, W.; Bai, Y.; Hou, P.; Zhao, J.; Zhou, L.; Zuo, Z. Volatile organic compounds released from *Microcystis flos-aquae* under nitrogen sources and their toxic effects on *Chlorella vulgaris*. *Ecotoxicol. Environ. Saf.* **2017**, *135*, 191–200. [CrossRef]
65. Zuo, Z.; Yang, L.; Chen, S.; Ye, C.; Han, Y.; Wang, S.; Ma, Y. Effects of nitrogen nutrients on the volatile organic compound emissions from *Microcystis aeruginosa*. *Ecotoxicol. Environ. Saf.* **2018**, *161*, 214–220. [CrossRef] [PubMed]
66. Huisman, J.; Codd, G.; Paerl, H.; Ibelings, B.; Verspagen, J.; Visser, P. Cyanobacterial blooms. *Nat. Rev. Microbiol.* **2018**, *16*, 471–483. [CrossRef] [PubMed]
67. Rohrlack, T.; Utkilen, H. Effects of nutrient and light availability on production of bioactive anabaenopeptins and microviridin by the cyanobacterium *Planktothrix agardhii*. *Hydrobiologia* **2007**, *583*, 231–240. [CrossRef]
68. Hameed, S.; Lawton, L.; Edwards, C.; Khan, A.; Farooq, U.; Khan, F. Effects of temperature and salinity on the production of cell biomass, chlorophyll-a and intra- and extracellular nodularins (NOD) and nodulopeptin 901 produced by *Nodularia spumigena* KAC 66. *J. Appl. Phycol.* **2017**, *29*, 1801–1810. [CrossRef]
69. Repka, S.; Koivula, M.; Harjunpä, V.; Rouhiainen, L.; Sivonen, K. Effects of Phosphate and Light on Growth of and Bioactive Peptide Production by the Cyanobacterium Anabaena Strain 90 and Its Anabaenopeptilide Mutant. *Appl. Environ. Microbiol.* **2004**, *70*, 4551–4560. [CrossRef] [PubMed]
70. Briand, E.; Bormans, M.; Gugger, M.; Dorrestein, P.; Gerwick, W. Changes in secondary metabolic profiles of *Microcystis aeruginosa* strains in response to intraspecific interactions. *Environ. Microbiol.* **2016**, *18*, 384–400. [CrossRef]
71. Ferreira, A. Peptides in Cyanobacteria under Different Environmental Conditions. Ph.D. Thesis, Technische Universität Berlin, Berlin, Germany, 2006; pp. 1–120.
72. Nealson, K.; Hastings, W. Bacterial bioluminescence: Its control and ecological significance. *Microbiol. Rev.* **1979**, *43*, 496–518. [CrossRef]
73. Fuqua, C.; Greenberg, E. Listening in on bacteria: Acyl-homoserine lactone signalling. *Nat. Rev. Mol. Cell Biol.* **2002**, *3*, 685–695. [CrossRef]
74. Pereira, D. Quorum Sensing em Cianobactérias. Ph.D. Thesis, Universidade Federal de Minas Gerais, Belo Horizonte, Brazil, 2014; pp. 1–110.
75. Luc Rolland, J.; Stien, D.; Sanchez-Ferandin, S.; Lami, R. Quorum sensing and quorum quenching in the phycosphere of phytoplankton: A case of chemical interactions in ecology. *J. Chem. Ecol.* **2016**, *42*, 1201–1211. [CrossRef]
76. Sánchez-Baracaldo, P. Origin of marine planktonic cyanobacteria. *Sci. Rep.* **2015**, *5*, 14–17. [CrossRef]
77. Pancrace, C.; Barny, M.; Ueoka, R.; Calteau, A.; Scalvenzi, T.; Pédron, J.; Barbe, V.; Piel, J.; Humbert, J. Insights into the *Planktothrix* genus: Genomic and metabolic comparison of benthic and planktic strains. *Sci. Rep.* **2017**, *7*, 1–10. [CrossRef] [PubMed]
78. López-Otín, C.; Bond, J. Proteases: Multifunctional enzymes in life and disease. *J. Biol.* **2008**, *283*, 30433–30437. [CrossRef] [PubMed]
79. García-Lorenzo, M.; Sjödin, A.; Jansson, S.; Funk, C. Protease gene families in *Populus* and *Arabidopsis*. *BMC Plant. Biol.* **2006**, *6*, 1–24. [CrossRef] [PubMed]
80. Chang, T.-S. An Updated Review of Tyrosinase Inhibitors. *Int. J. Mol. Sci.* **2009**, *10*, 2440–2475. [CrossRef] [PubMed]
81. Brenner, M.; Hearing, V. The Protective Role of Melanin Against UV Damage in Human Skin. *Photochem. Photobiol.* **2008**, *84*, 539–549. [CrossRef]

82. Carballo-Carbajal, I.; Laguna, A.; Romero-Gímenez, J.; Cuadros, T.; Bové, J.; Martinez-Vicente, M.; Gonzalez-Sepulveda, M.; Parent, A.; Penuelas, N.; Torra, A.; et al. Brain tyrosinase overexpression implicates age-dependent neuromelanin production in Parkinson's disease pathogenesis. *Nat. Commun.* **2018**, *10*, 1–19. [CrossRef]
83. Pillaiyar, T.; Manickam, M.; Namasivayam, V. Skin whitening agents: Medicinal chemistry perspective of tyrosinase inhibitors. *J. Enzyme Inhib. Med. Chem.* **2017**, *32*, 403–425. [CrossRef]
84. Tan, S.; Sim, C.; Goh, C. Hydroquinone-induced exogenous ochronosis in Chinese—Two case reports and a review. *Int. J. Dermatol.* **2008**, *47*, 639–640. [CrossRef]
85. Owens, A.; MacKman, N. Microparticles in hemostasis and thrombosis. *Circ. Res.* **2011**, *108*, 1284–1297. [CrossRef]
86. Anas, A.; Mori, A.; Tone, M.; Naruse, C.; Nakajima, A.; Asukabe, H.; Takaya, Y.; Imanish, S.; Nishizawa, T.; Shirai, M.; et al. FVIIa-sTF and thrombin inhibitory activities of compounds isolated from *Microcystis aeruginosa* K-139. *Marine Drugs* **2017**, *15*, 275. [CrossRef]
87. Von Nussbaum, F.; Li, V. Neutrophil elastase inhibitors for the treatment of (cardio)pulmonary diseases: Into clinical testing with pre-adaptive pharmacophores. *Bioorg. Med. Chem. Lett.* **2015**, *25*, 4370–4381. [CrossRef] [PubMed]
88. Korkmaz, B.; Horwitz, M.S.; Jenne, D.E.; Gauthier, F. Neutrophil elastase, proteinase 3, and cathepsin G as therapeutic targets in human diseases. *Pharmacol. Rev.* **2010**, *62*, 726–759. [CrossRef] [PubMed]
89. Sahebnasagh, A.; Saghafi, F.; Safdari, M.; Khataminia, M.; Sadremomtaz, A.; Ghaleno, H.R.; Bagheri, M.; Bagheri, M.S.; Habtemariam, S.; Avan, R. Neutrophil Elastase Inhibitor (Sivelestat), may be a Promising Therapeutic Option for Management of Acute Lung Injury/Acute Respiratory Distress Syndrome or Disseminated Intravascular Coagulation in COVID-19. *Authorea Prepr.* **2020**. [CrossRef]
90. Kanost, M.R.; Clem, J.R. Insect Proteases. In *Reference Module in Life Sciences*; Elsevier: Amsterdam, The Netherlands, 2017; pp. 1–16.
91. Kafatos, F. The Cocoonase zymogen cells of silk moths: A model of terminal cell differentiation for specific protein synthesis. *Curr. Top. Dev. Biol.* **1972**, *5*, 125–191.
92. Sojka, D.; Francischetti, I.; Calvo, E.; Kotsyfakis, M. Cysteine Proteases from Bloodfeeding Arthropod Ectoparasites. *Adv. Exp. Med. Biol.* **2011**, *712*, 171–191.
93. Pinto, A.; Silva, K.; Guimarães, J. Proteases from *Lonomia obliqua* venomous secretions: Comparison of procoagulant, fibrin(ogen)olytic and amidolytic activities. *Toxicon* **2006**, *47*, 113–121. [CrossRef] [PubMed]
94. Soares, T. Molecular Studies of Trypsin-like Enzymes Present in Midgut of *Aedes aegypti* larvae. Master's Thesis, Universidade Federal de São Paulo, UNIFESP, Sao Paulo, Brazil, 2009.
95. Terra, W.; Ferreira, C. Insect digestive enzymes: Properties, compartmentalization and function. *Comp. Biochem. Physiol. B. Biochem. Mol. Biol.* **1994**, *109*, 1–62. [CrossRef]
96. Hilder, V.; Gatehouse, A.; Sheerman, S.; Barker, R.; Boulter, D. A novel mechanism of insect resistance engineered into tobacco. *Nature* **1987**, *330*, 160–163. [CrossRef]
97. Rooney, W.M.; Grinter, R.W.; Correia, A.; Parkhill, J.; Walker, D.C.; Milner, J.J. Engineering bacteriocin-mediated resistance against the plant pathogen *Pseudomonas syringae*. *Plant Biotechnol. J.* **2020**, *18*, 1296–1306. [CrossRef]
98. Di, R.; Blechl, A.; Dill-Macky, R.; Tortora, A.; Tumer, N.E. Expression of a truncated form of yeast ribosomal protein L3 in transgenic wheat improves resistance to *Fusarium* head blight. *Plant Sci.* **2010**, *178*, 374–380. [CrossRef]
99. Liang, X.; Liu, Y.; Xie, L.; Liu, X.; Wei, Y.; Zhou, X.; Zhang, S. A ribosomal protein AgRPS3aE from halophilic *Aspergillus glaucus* confers salt tolerance in heterologous organisms. *Int. J. Mol. Sci.* **2015**, *16*, 3058–3070. [CrossRef] [PubMed]
100. Weiz, A.R.; Ishida, K.; Quitterer, F.; Meyer, S.; Kehr, J.-C.; Muller, K.M.; Groll, M.; Hertweck, C.; Dittmann, E. Harnessing the evolvability of tricyclic microviridins to dissect protease-inhibitor interactions. *Angew. Chem. Int. Ed.* **2014**, *53*, 3735–3738. [CrossRef] [PubMed]

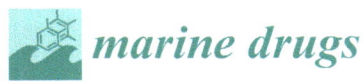

Article

Nostoc edaphicum CCNP1411 from the Baltic Sea—A New Producer of Nostocyclopeptides

Anna Fidor [1], Michał Grabski [2], Jan Gawor [3], Robert Gromadka [3], Grzegorz Węgrzyn [2] and Hanna Mazur-Marzec [1,*]

[1] Division of Marine Biotechnology, Faculty of Oceanography and Geography, University of Gdańsk, Marszałka J. Piłsudskiego 46, PL-81378 Gdynia, Poland; anna.fidor@phdstud.ug.edu.pl
[2] Department of Molecular Biology, University of Gdansk, Wita Stwosza 59, 80-308 Gdansk, Poland; michal.grabski@phdstud.ug.edu.pl (M.G.); grzegorz.wegrzyn@biol.ug.edu.pl (G.W.)
[3] DNA Sequencing and Oligonucleotide Synthesis Laboratory, Polish Academy of Sciences, Institute of Biochemistry and Biophysics, 02-106 Warsaw, Poland; gaworj@ibb.waw.pl (J.G.); robert@ibb.waw.pl (R.G.)
* Correspondence: hanna.mazur-marzec@ug.edu.pl; Tel.: +48-58-523-66-21 or +48-609-419-132

Received: 31 July 2020; Accepted: 25 August 2020; Published: 26 August 2020

Abstract: Nostocyclopeptides (Ncps) constitute a small class of nonribosomal peptides, exclusively produced by cyanobacteria of the genus *Nostoc*. The peptides inhibit the organic anion transporters, OATP1B3 and OATP1B1, and prevent the transport of the toxic microcystins and nodularin into hepatocytes. So far, only three structural analogues, Ncp-A1, Ncp-A2 and Ncp-M1, and their linear forms were identified in *Nostoc* strains as naturally produced cyanometabolites. In the current work, the whole genome sequence of the new Ncps producer, *N. edaphicum* CCNP1411 from the Baltic Sea, has been determined. The genome consists of the circular chromosome (7,733,505 bps) and five circular plasmids (from 44.5 kb to 264.8 kb). The nostocyclopeptide biosynthetic gene cluster (located between positions 7,609,981–7,643,289 bps of the chromosome) has been identified and characterized *in silico*. The LC-MS/MS analyzes of *N. edaphicum* CCNP1411 cell extracts prepared in aqueous methanol revealed several products of the genes. Besides the known peptides, Ncp-A1 and Ncp-A2, six other compounds putatively characterized as new noctocyclopeptide analogues were detected. This includes Ncp-E1 and E2 and their linear forms (Ncp-E1-L and E2-L), a cyclic Ncp-E3 and a linear Ncp-E4-L. Regardless of the extraction conditions, the cell contents of the linear nostocyclopeptides were found to be higher than the cyclic ones, suggesting a slow rate of the macrocyclization process.

Keywords: cyanobacteria; nostocyclopeptides; *Nostoc*; *ncp* gene cluster; nonribosomal peptide synthetase

1. Introduction

Secondary metabolites produced by cyanobacteria of the genus *Nostoc* (Nostocales) are characterized by a high variety of structures and biological activities [1–6]. On the basis of chemical structure, these compounds are mainly classified to peptides, polyketides, lipids, polysaccharides and alkaloids [7]. Abundantly produced cyanopeptides with anticancer, antimicrobial, antiviral and enzyme-inhibiting activity, have attracted attention of many research groups [6,8–12]. Some of the metabolites, such as nostocyclopeptides (Ncps) or cryptophycins are exclusively produced by the cyanobacteria of the genus *Nostoc* (Figure 1A). Ncps constitute a small class of nonribosomal peptides. Thus far, only three analogues of the compounds and their linear forms have been discovered. This includes Ncp-A1 and Ncp-A2 detected in *Nostoc* sp. ATCC53789 isolated from a lichen collected at Arron Island in Scotland [13]. The same peptides were detected in *Nostoc* sp. ASN_M, isolated from soil samples of paddy fields in the Golestan province in Iran [14] and in *Nostoc* strains from liverwort *Blasia pusilla* L. collected in Northern Norway [15]. A different analogue, Ncp-M1, was found in *Nostoc* sp. XSPORK 13A, the cyanobacterium living in symbiosis with gastropod from shallow seawaters at the Cape of Porkkala (Baltic Sea) [16].

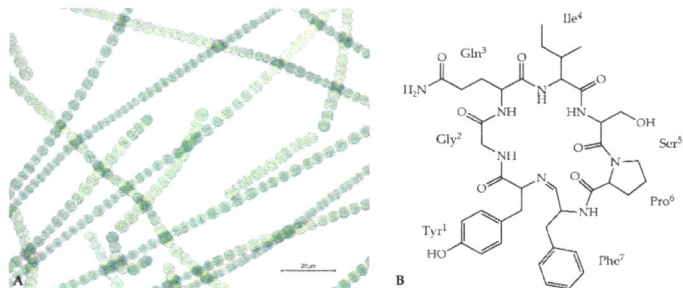

Figure 1. *Nostoc edaphicum* CCNP1411 (**A**) and the proposed chemical structure of Ncp-E1 (**B**).

Ncps are composed of seven residues and a unique imino linkage formed between C-terminal aldehyde and an *N*-terminal amine group of the conserved Tyr^1 (Figure 1B) [13,16]. The presence of modified amino acid residues, e.g., 4-methylproline, homoserine and D-configured glutamine, indicated the nonribosomal biosynthetic pathway of the molecules. Genetic analysis of *Nostoc* sp. ATCC53789 revealed the presence of the 33-kb Ncp gene cluster composed of two genes, *ncpA* and *ncpB*, encoding NcpA1-A3 and NcpB1-B4 modules. These proteins catalyze the activation and incorporation of Tyr, Gly, Gln, Ile and Ser into the Ncp structure [17]. They show high similarity to NosE and NosF which take part in the biosynthesis of nostopeptolides in *Nostoc* sp. GSV224 [18]. The *ncpFGCDE* fragment of the Ncp gene cluster is involved in the synthesis of MePro (*ncpCDE*), transport (*ncpF*) and proteolysis (*ncpG*) of the peptides. The characteristic features of the Ncp enzymatic complex in *Nostoc* sp. ATCC53789 is the presence of the epimerase domain (NcpA3) responsible for D-configuration of glutamine, and the unique reductase domain at C-terminal end of NcpB which catalyze the reductive release of a linear peptide aldehyde [19,20].

The activity of Ncps have been explored [13] and their potential as antitoxins, inhibiting the transport of hepatotoxic microcystin-LR and nodularin into the rat hepatocytes through the organic anion transporter polypeptides OATP1B1/1B3 was revealed [21]. As OATP1B3 is overexpressed in some malignant tumors (e.g., colon carcinomas) [22], Ncps, as inhibitors of this transporter protein, are suggested to be promising lead compounds for new drug development.

In our previous studies, *Nostoc edaphicum* CCNP1411 (Figure 1A) from the Baltic Sea was found to be a rich source of cyanopeptolins, the nonribosomal peptides with potent inhibitory activity against serine proteases [6]. In the current work, the potential of the strain to produce other bioactive metabolites was explored. The whole-genome sequence of *N. edaphicum* CCNP1411 has been determined, and the nostocyclopeptide biosynthetic gene cluster has been identified in the strain and characterized in silico for the first time. Furthermore, the new products of the Ncp gene cluster have been detected and their structures have been characterized by LC-MS/MS.

2. Results and Discussion

2.1. Analysis of N. edaphicum CCNP1411 Genome

Total DNA has been isolated from *N. edaphicum* CCNP1411, and the whole genome sequence has been determined. Identified replicons of *N. edaphicum* CCNP1411 genome consist of the circular chromosome of 7,733,505 bps, and five circular plasmids (Table 1). Within the total size of 8,316,316 bps genome (chromosome and plasmids, Figure 2), we have distinguished, according to annotation, the total number of 6957 genes from which 6458 potentially code for proteins (CDSs), 415 are classified as pseudo-genes and 84 are coding for non-translatable RNA molecules. Pseudo-genes can be divided into subcategories due to the shift in the coding frame (180), internal stop codons (77), incomplete sequence (228), or occurrence of multiple problems (63). Genes coding for functional RNAs consist of those encoding ribosomal (rRNA) (9), transporting (tRNA) (71) and regulatory noncoding (ncRNA) (4), all embedded on the chromosome. Out of total coding and pseudo-genes sequences (6873), the vast majority (5846) initiates with the ATG start codon, while GTG and TTG occur less frequently (561 and 217 times, respectively). The frequencies of stop codons were set out as follows: TAA (3455), TAG (1750), TGA (1526). Coding and pseudo-genes sequences are distributed almost equally on the leading and complementary strand, including 3408 and 3465 sequences, respectively.

Table 1. Composition and coverage of *N. edaphicum* CCNP1411 genome.

Replicon	Accession Number	Length (bp)	Topology	G+C Content (%)	Coverage (x) Nanopore Data	Coverage (x) Illumina Data
pNe_1	CP054693.1	44,503	Circular	42.3	115.5	244.8
pNe_2	CP054694.1	99,098	Circular	40.2	168.4	135.3
pNe_3	CP054695.1	120,515	Circular	41.3	256.4	177.1
pNe_4	CP054696.1	53,840	Circular	41.6	102.4	211.5
pNe_5	CP054697.1	264,855	Circular	41.0	226.3	160.7
chr	CP054698.1	7,733,505	Circular	41.6	160.7	116.9

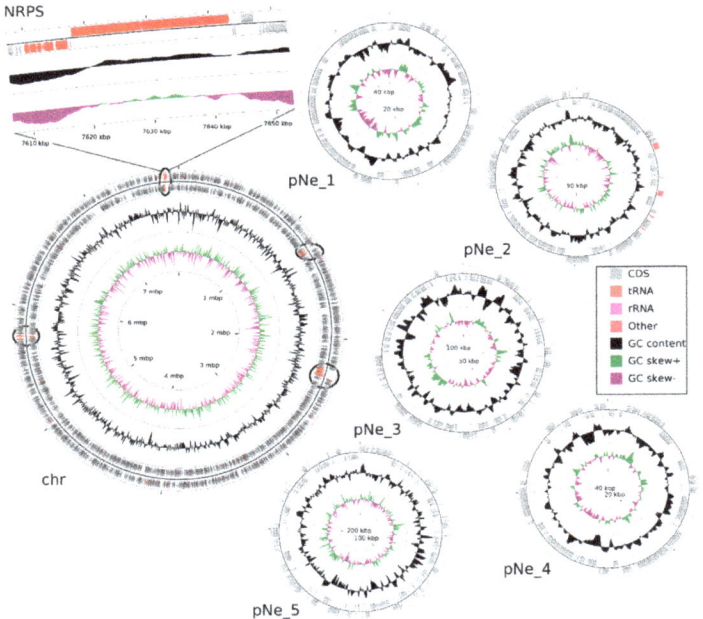

Figure 2. Map of the *N. edaphicum* CCNP1411 genome where chromosome (chr) and five plasmids (pNe_1–5) are presented. The ORFs are indicated with grey arrows split into two rings outermost showing ORFs on direct strand and inner showing complementary strand ORFs. The middle circle shows GC content (black) and the innermost circle shows GC skew (green and purple). Genes for putative NRPS/PKS are marked on the chromosome in their proper position (red within a black circle), with closeup on NRPS in position 7,609,981–7,643,289 putatively coding for Ncp biosynthetic gene cluster.

2.2. Non-Ribosomal Peptide Synthetase (NRPS) Gene Cluster of Nostocyclopeptides

Having the whole genome sequence of *N. edaphicum* CCNP1411, we have analyzed in detail the non-ribosomal peptide synthetase (NRPS) cluster, containing potential genes coding for enzymes involved in the synthesis of nostocyclopeptides. To establish correct spans for non-ribosomal peptide synthetases, 35 complete nucleotide sequence clusters derived from *Cyanobacteria* phylum were aligned resulting in hits scattered around positions 2,287,143–2,323,617 and 7,609,981–7,643,289 within the *N. edaphicum* CCNP1411 chromosome (7.7 Mbp) (Figure 2). This method of characterization presented the overall similarity of selected spans to micropeptin (cyanopeptolin) biosynthetic gene cluster [23] and nostocyclopeptide biosynthetic gene cluster [17], respectively. To confirm these results, the antiSMASH analysis was employed resulting in confirmation of previously defined NRPS spans and adding two more regions 1,213,069–1,258,319 and 5,735,625–5,780,238, to small extent (12% and 30%, respectively) similar to anabaenopeptin gene cluster [24]. For the purpose of this study, we focused on putative nostocyclopeptide producing non-ribosomal peptide synthetase. Annotation of the selected region revealed nine putative open reading frames (ORFs), transcribed in reverse (7) and forward (2) direction. The identified cluster was arranged in a similar fashion to AY167420.1 (nostocyclopeptide biosynthetic gene cluster from *Nostoc sp.* ATCC 53789), with the exception of two ORFs (>170 bp), intersecting operon (*ncpFGCDE*) putatively encoding proteins involved in MePro assembly, efflux and hydrolysis of products of the second putative operon *ncpAB* (Figure 3).

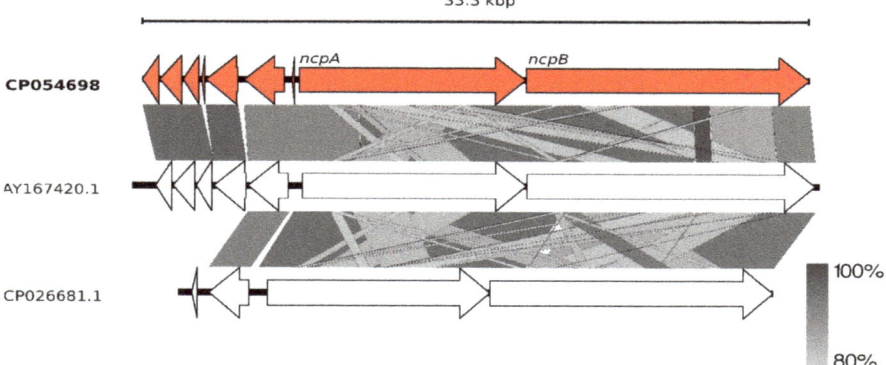

Figure 3. Schematic alignment of genes coding for putative non-ribosomal peptide synthetase from *N. edaphicum* CCNP1411 (red) and two related Ncp-producing synthetases AY167420.1 and CP026681.1 (white). The grey bar in the lower right corner shows the identity percentage associated with color of the bars connecting homologous regions. The analysis was conducted at the nucleotide level.

Two sequences ORF1 (HUN01_34350) (837 bp) and ORF2 (HUN01_34355) (1107 bp) embedded on 3′ end of nostocyclopeptide gene cluster resemble *nosF* and *nosE* genes, found in the nostopeptolide (*nos*) gene cluster [18] with 96% nucleotide sequence identities in both instances, putatively encoding for zinc-dependent long-chain dehydrogenase and a Δ1-pyrroline-5-carboxylic acid reductase. Further upstream, there is an ORF3 (HUN01_34360) (798 bp) of 98% homology to unknown gene from AF204805.2 gene cluster, suggested previously to be involved in 4-methylproline biosynthesis [17,25], due to close proximity of downstream genes encompassing this reaction, but no experimental evidence was presented. Alignment of the sequence of this putative protein have shown a sequence homology, to some extent, to 4′-phosphopantetheinyl transferase, crucial for PCP aminoacyl substrate binding (Figure 4) [26]. Moreover, partially present adenylate-forming domain within ORF4 (HUN01_34365) (165 bp) belongs to the acyl- and aryl- CoA ligases family, and may putatively engage substrate for post-translational modification of the PCP domain. Facing the same direction, an ORF5 (HUN01_34370)

(1605 bp)-bearing putative domain classified as transpeptidase superfamily DD-carboxypeptidase and ORF6 (HUN01_34375) (2010 bp) homologous to ABC transporter ATP-binding protein/permease may be engaged in *ncpAB* peptide product transport [27]. Neither the ORF7 (HUN01_34780) Shine–Delgarno (SD) sequence upfront translation start codon could be assigned nor the TA-like signal ~12 nucleotides upstream could be found.

```
WP_000986023.1    1  -------MAILGLCTDIVEIARI----------------EAVIARSGDRLARRV--LSDN
ORF3             61  DCYQNVNPKIERICITVFEYNRISKAAYFQAVERTTKLRDCIMAASFNPLERLMVKIREC

WP_000986023.1   36  EWAIWKTHHQPV----------------RFLAKRFAVKEAAAKAFGTGIRNGLAFNQFEVF
ORF3            121  TGATVRIASEPLYGSYYAGLIRKIEQGTQLHIDYAPLEQSKWEIGTVIYQ-LSWNLYLKF

WP_000986023.1   81  N-DELCKPRL--RLW--GEALKLAEKLGVANMHVTLADE---RHYACATVTIES------
ORF3            180  SPNNHCQTRIYDRQWQPGDDQYKLDSYGYGDTVIADADAIAFQPYVGDVFTFNTRNFHIV
```

Figure 4. Structure-based sequence alignment of 4'-phosphopantetheinyl transferase and partial ORF3. Amino-acids highlighted in black color indicate conserved residues, whereas those in grey color indicate conservative mutations.

The main part of the Ncp biosynthetic gene cluster is located on the forward strand comprising two large genes which nucleotide sequences are homologous over 80% to *ncpA* and *ncpB* subunits of the *ncp* cluster in *Nostoc* sp. ATCC53789 [17]. Both these genes code for proteins consisting of repetitive modules incorporating single residue into elongating peptide. ORF 8 (HUN01_34785) (11,334 bp) encompasses three of these modules, whereas ORF 9 (HUN01_34380) (14,157 bp) encodes four modules. The core of one NRPS module consists of three succeeding domains: condensation (C), adenylation (A) and peptidyl carrier protein (PCP). Moreover, adjacent to coding spans of extreme modules, two tailoring domains were found within ORF8 and ORF9 genes (Figure 5).

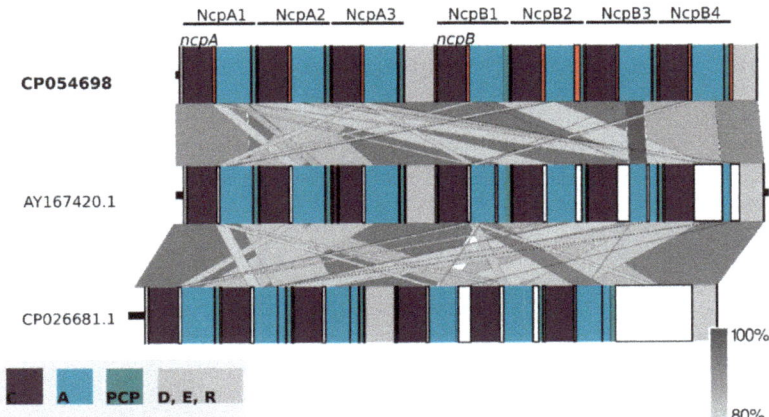

Figure 5. Schematic representation of conserved domains within *ncpA* and *ncpB* coding nucleotide sequences. They are composed of repetitive modules condensation (C), adenylation (A) and peptidyl carrier protein (PCP) domains adjacent to delineating docking, epimerization and reductase domains aligned with two related synthetases AY167420.1 and CP026681.1. The analysis was conducted at the nucleotide level.

Alignment of nucleotide sequences to the *ncpAB* operon revealed major differences in consecutive NcpB3 and NcpB4 modules. Utilizing the selected spans conjoined with conserved domain search allowed us to distinguish and compare C, A and PCP amino-acid sequences (Figure 6). Intrinsic modules of NRPS, with an exception of NcpB3 adenylation domain sequence, were found homologous above 91%, whereas extremes have shown the biggest composition differences ranging from 13–15% to 24% in the NcpB4 adenylation domain (Figure 6).

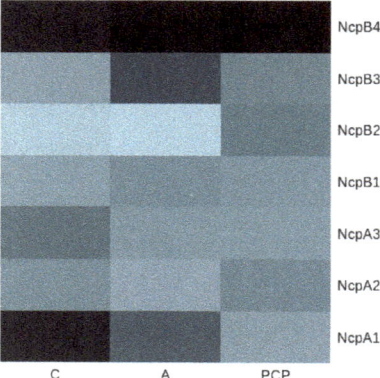

Figure 6. Heatmap of the highest (light blue) and lowest (black) percentage of similarities between NcpA and NcpB domains in *N. edaphicum* CCNP1411 and ATCC53789; values scaled by rows. The analysis was conducted at the amino acid level.

The determination of the whole genome sequence of *N. edaphicum* CCNP1411 allowed us to perform analyses of genes coding for enzymes involved in the synthesis of nostocyclopeptides. The general analysis demonstrated homology of the NRPS/PKS clusters of *N. edaphicum* CCNP1411 to systems occurring in other cyanobacteria, however, with some differences. The non-ribosomal consensus code [28,29] allowed to recognize and predict the substrate specificities of NRPS adenylation domains: tyrosine (NcpA1), glycine (NcpA2), glutamine (NcpA3) for NcpA and isoleucine/valine (NcpB1) serine (NcpB2) 4-methylproline/proline (NcpB3) phenyloalanine/leucin/tyrosine (NcpB4) for NcpB (Table 2). This prediction was found to be in line with the structures of the Ncps detected in *N. edaphicum* CCNP1411.

Table 2. Characterization of substrate binding pocket amino acid residues adenylation domains of NcpA and NcpB modules based on gramicidin S synthetase (GrsA) phenylalanine activating domain. Residues in brackets mark inconsistency with AY167420.1 residues.

NRPS Module	Adenylation Domain Residue Position									Proposed Substrate
	235	236	239	278	299	301	322	330	331	
NcpA1	D	A	S	T	[I]	A	A	V	C	Tyr
NcpA2	D	I	L	Q	L	G	L	I	W	Gly
NcpA3	D	A	W	Q	F	G	L	I	D	Gln
NcpB1	D	A	F	F	L	G	V	T	F	Ile/Val
NcpB2	D	V	W	H	I	S	L	I	D	Ser
NcpB3	D	V	Q	[F]	I	A	H	V	A	Pro/MePro
NcpB4	D	A	W	[T]	I	G	[A]	V	C	Phe/Tyr/Leu

To devolve elongating product onto subsequent condensation domain, the studied synthetase utilizes PCP domains, subunits responsible for thiolation of nascent peptide intermediates, where post-transcriptional modification of conserved serine residue shifts the state of the domain from inactive *holo* to active *apo*. Modification of this residue is related to PPTase which transfers a covalently-bound 4′-phosphopantetheine arm of CoA onto the PCP active site, enabling peptide intermediates to bind as reactive thioesters. Case residue which undergoes a nucleophilic attack by the hydroxyl group was conserved in every module within the PCP domain predicted at the front of the second helix [30].

The stand-alone docking domain (D) (7,617,812–7,617,964 bp) found on N-terminus of NcpA may be an essential component mediating interactions, recognition and specific association within NRPS subunits. The potential acceptor domain, based on sequence homology of conserved residues to C-terminal communication-mediating donor domains (COM), was found at the NcpB4 PCP domain second helix, encompassing conserved serine residue within potential binding sequence [31]. Moreover, this communication-mediating domain may putatively bind to C-terminus of NcpB3 and NcpB4 condensation (C) domains based on conserved motif LLEGIV, found by sequence homology to last five amino-acids of C-terminal docking domains residues, key for their interactions [32]. Within the same β-hairpin, a group of charged residues (ExxxxxKxR) putatively determines the binding affinity of the N-terminal domain [33].

Two tailoring domains encoded at the 5′ ends of *ncpA* and *ncpB* genes were classified as epimerization (E) (7,627,742–7,629,043 bp) domain and reductase (R) (7,642,183–7,643,238 bp) domain, accordingly. Epimerization domain catalyzes the conversion of L-amino acids to D-amino acids, a reaction coherent with D-stereochemistry of the peptide glutamine residue, where His of the conserved HHxxxDG motif and Glu from the upstream EGHGRE motif raceB comprise an epimerisation reaction active site [34]. Homologous HHxxxDG conserved motif sequence is found in condensation domains (C), where a similar reaction is catalyzed within peptide bond formation, putatively by the second His residue [35]. As in *ncp* cluster [17], module NcpA1 motif includes degenerate sequences in two positions HQIVGDL with leucine instead of phenylalanine residue at the start of the helix. The second histidine site-directed mutagenesis abolished enzymatic activity which might suggest that NcpA1 condensation domain is inactive [36].

Reductase domain (R) found at the C-terminus of NRPS was classified as oxidoreductase. Despite 15% discrepancy in domain composition compared to NcpB core catalytic triad Thr-Tyr-Lys and Rossmann-fold, a NAD (P) H nucleotide-binding motif GxxGxxG positions were not affected. The mechanism driving this chain release utilizes NAD (P) H cofactor for redox reaction of the final moiety of the nascent peptide to aldehyde or alcohol [37,38].

2.3. Structure Characterization of Ncps Produced by N. edaphicum CCNP1411

Thus far, only three Ncps, Ncp-A1, A2 and M1, and their linear aldehydes were isolated as pure natural products of *Nostoc* strains [13,16]. Ncp-A3, with MePhe in the C-terminal position, was obtained through aberrant biosynthesis in the *Nostoc* sp. ATCC53789 culture supplemented with MePhe [13]. The linear aldehydes of Ncp-A1 and Ncp-A2, with Pro instead of MePro, were chemically synthesized and used to study the Ncps epimerization and macrocyclization equilibria [19,20]. In our work, ten Ncps, differing mainly in position 4 and 7, were detected by LC-MS/MS in the *N. edaphicum* CCNP1411 cell extract (Table 3, Figure 1, Figure 7, Figure 8 and Figure S1–S7). These include five cyclic structures, four linear Ncp aldehydes, and one linear hexapeptide Ncp. The putative structures of the six peptides, which were found to be naturally produced by *Nostoc* for the first time, are marked in Table 3 in bold (Ncp-E1, Ncp-E1-L, Ncp-E2, Ncp-E2-L, Ncp-E3 and Ncp-E4-L).

Table 3. The putative structures of nostocyclopeptides (Ncps) detected in the crude extract of *N. edaphicum* CCNP1411 and the structure of Ncp-M1 identified in *Nostoc* sp. XSPORK 13 A [16]. The new analogues are marked in bold and the peptides detected in trace amounts are marked with [T]. The variable residues in position 4 and 7 are marked in blue.

Compound	Structure	m/z [M+H]+ Cyclic	m/z [M+H]+ Linear–COH	Retention Time [min]
Ncp-A1	cyclo[Tyr+Gly+Gln+Ile+Ser+MePro+Leu]	757		7.1
Ncp-A1-L	Tyr+Gly+Gln+Ile+Ser+MePro+Leu		775	5.8
Ncp-A2	cyclo[Tyr+Gly+Gln+Ile+Ser+MePro+Phe]	791		6.0
Ncp-A2-L	Tyr+Gly+Gln+Ile+Ser+MePro+Phe		809	5.6
Ncp-E1	**cyclo[Tyr+Gly+Gln+Ile+Ser+Pro+Phe]**	777 [T]		7.2
Ncp-E1-L	**Tyr+Gly+Gln+Ile+Ser+Pro+Phe**		795	5.7
Ncp-E2	**cyclo[Tyr+Gly+Gln+Ile+Ser+Pro+Leu]**	743 [T]		6.3
Ncp-E2-L	**Tyr+Gly+Gln+Ile+Ser+Pro+Leu**		761	5.1
Ncp-E3	**cyclo[Tyr+Gly+Gln+Val+Ser+MePro+Leu]**	743 [T]		7.0
* **Ncp-E4-L**	**[Tyr+Gly+Gln+Ile+Ser+MePro]**		677 [T]	6.0
** Ncp-M1	cyclo[Tyr+Tyr+HSe+Pro+Val+MePro+Tyr]		882	27.5

* Ncp-E4-L is the only linear Ncps analogue with carboxyl group in C-terminus. ** Identified in *Nostoc* sp. XSPORK [16].

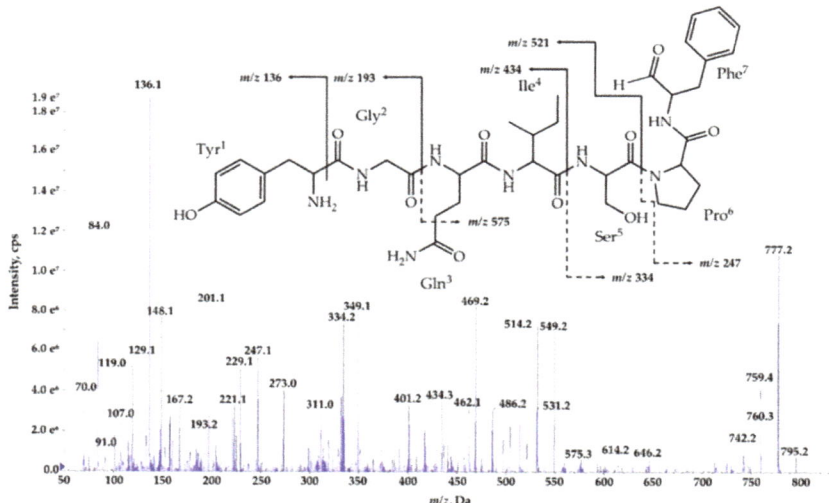

Figure 7. Postulated structure and enhanced product ion mass spectrum of the linear aldehyde nostocyclopeptide **Ncp-E1-L**; Tyr+Gly+Gln+Ile+Ser+Pro+Phe characterized based on the following fragment ions: m/z 795 [M+H]; 777 [M+H−H$_2$O]; 759 [M+H−2H$_2$O]; 646 [M+H − Phe]; 614 [M+H − Tyr−H$_2$O]; 575 [M+H−(Tyr+Gly)]; 549 [Tyr+Gly+Gln+Ile+Ser+H]; 531 [Tyr+Gly+Gln+Ile+Ser+H−H$_2$O]; 462 [Tyr+Gly+Gln+Ile+H]; 349 [Tyr+Gly+Gln+H]; 334 [Ser+Pro+Phe+2H]; 247 [Phe+Pro+H]; 229 [Phe+Pro+H]; 201 [Phe+Pro+H − CO]; 148 [Tyr−NH$_2$]; 136 Tyr immonium; 129, 101 (immonium), 84 Gln; 70 Pro immonium.

The process of *de novo* structure elucidation was performed manually, based mainly on a series of b and y fragment ions produced by a cleavage of the peptide bonds (Figures 7–9, Figures S1–S7), and on the presence of immonium ions (e.g., m/z 70 for Pro, 84 for MePro, 136 for Tyr) in the product ion mass spectra of the peptides. The process of structure characterization was additionally supported by the previously published MS/MS spectra of Ncps [14]. The fragment ions that derived from the two amino acids in C-terminus usually belonged to the most intensive ions in the spectra and in this study they facilitated the structure characterization. For example, in the product ion mass spectrum of Ncp-A1

(Figure S1) and Ncp-E3 (Figure S7), ions at *m/z* 209 [MePro+Leu+H] and *m/z* 181 [MePro+Leu+H−CO] were present, while in the spectrum of Ncp-E2 (Figure S5) with Pro (instead MePro), the corresponding ions at 14 unit lower *m/z* values, i.e., 195 and 167 were observed. The spectra of the linear Ncps contained the intensive Tyr immonium ion at *m/z* 136. Based on the previously determined structures of Ncp-A1 and Ncp-A2 [13], we assumed that in Ncp-E2, the amino acids in position 4 and 7, are Ile and Leu, respectively (Table 3; Figure S5). These two amino acids are difficult to distinguish by MS. Definitely, the NMR analyses are required to confirm the structures of the Ncps. The presence of Val in position 4, instead of Ile, distinguishes the Ncp-E3 from other Ncps produced by *N. edaphicum* CCNP1411. As it was previously reported [17], and also confirmed in this study, the predicted substrates of the NcpB1 protein encoded by *ncpB* and involved in the incorporation of the residue in position 4 are Ile/Leu and Val. However, the domain preferentially activates Ile, which explains why only traces of Val-containing Ncps were detected in *N. edaphicum* CCNP1411 (Table 3).

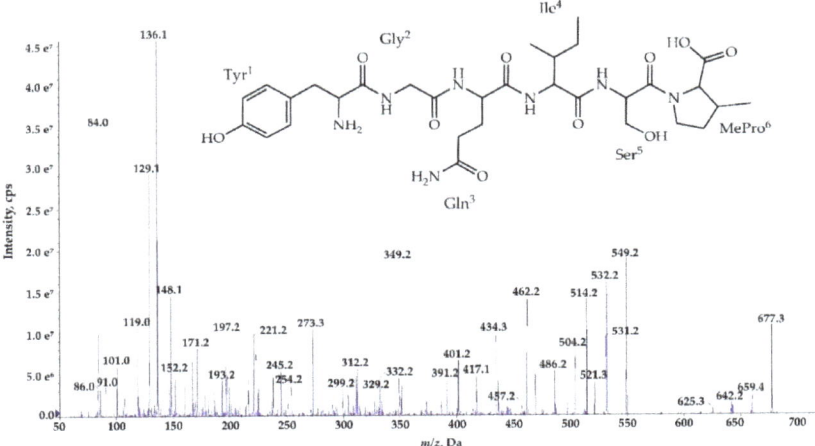

Figure 8. Postulated tructure and enhanced product ion mass spectrum of a linear nostocyclopeptide Ncp-E4-L [Tyr+Gly+Gln+Ile+Ser+MePro] characterized based on the following fragment ions: *m/z* 677 [M+H]; 659 [M+H−H$_2$O]; 642 [M+H−H$_2$O−NH$_3$]; 549 [Tyr+Gly+Gln+Ile+Ser+H]; 531 [Tyr+Gly+Gln+Ile+Ser+H−H$_2$O]; 521 [Tyr+Gly+Gln+Ile+Ser+H−CO]; 462 [Tyr+Gly+Gln+Ile+H]; 434 [Tyr+Gly+Gln+Ile+H−CO]; 349 [Tyr+Gly+Gln+H]; 329 [Gln+Ile+Ser+H]; 312 [Ile+Ser+MePro+H]; 221 [Tyr+Gly+H]; 193 [Tyr+Gly+H−CO]; 148 [Tyr−NH$_2$]; 136 Tyr immonium; 86 Ile immonium; 84, 101 (immonium), 129 Gln; 84 MePro immonium.

Methylated Pro (MePro) in position 6 is quite conserved. MePro is a rare non-proteinogenic amino acid biosynthesized from Leu through the activity of the zinc-dependent long chain dehydrogenases and Δ^1-pyrroline-5-carboxylic acid (P5C) reductase homologue encoded by the gene cassette *ncpCDE* [17,18,25]. The genes involved in the biosynthesis of MePro were found in 30 of the 116 tested cyanobacterial strains, majority (80%) of which belonged to the genus *Nostoc* [39]. The new Ncp-E1 and Ncp-E2, detected at trace amounts, are the only Ncps produced by *N. edaphicum* CCNP1411 which contain Pro (Table 3). The presence of *m/z* 84 ion in the fragmentation spectra of the two Ncps complicated the process of *de novo* structure elucidation. This ion corresponds to the immonium ion of MePro and could indicate the presence of this residue. However, the two ions *m/z* 101 and 129, which together with ion at *m/z* 84, are characteristic of Gln, suggested the presence of this amino acid in Ncp-E1 and Ncp-E2. The detailed characterization of Ncp fragmentation pathways is presented in Figures 7–9 and in Supplementary Materials (Figures S1–S7).

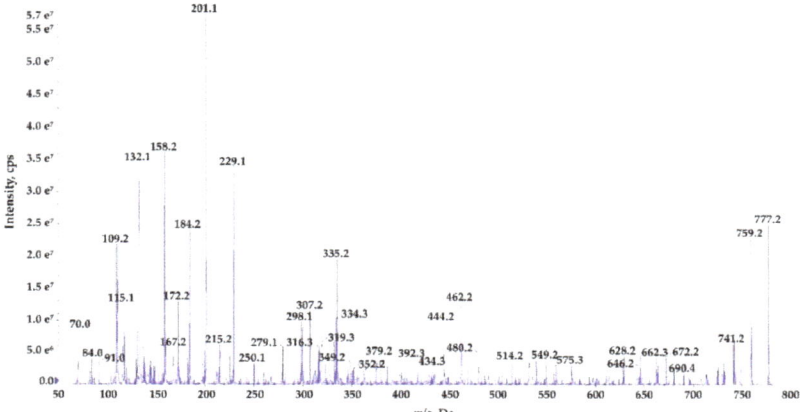

Figure 9. Enhanced product ion mass spectrum of the cyclic nostocyclopeptide **Ncp-E1** with putative structure cyclo[Tyr+Gly+Gln+Ile+Ser+Pro+Phe] characterised based on the following fragment ions: *m/z* 777 [M+H]; 759 [M+H−H$_2$O]; 741 [M+H−2H$_2$O]; 690 [M+H−Ser]; 672 [M+H−Ser−H$_2$O]; 662 [M+H−Pro−H$_2$O]; 646 [M+H−Phe]; 628 [M+H−Phe−H$_2$O]; 575 [M+H−(Ser+Pro)−H$_2$O]; 549 [Tyr+Gly+Glu+Ile+Ser+H]; 480 [Phe+Tyr+Gly+Gln+H]; 462 [Tyr+Gly+Gln+Ile+H]; 444 [Tyr+Gly+Gln+Ile+H−H$_2$O]; 434 [Tyr+Gly+Gln+Ile+H−CO]; 392 [Pro+Phe+Tyr+H]; 352 [Phe+Tyr+Gly+H]; 335 [Phe+Tyr+Gly+H−H$_2$O]; 316 [Ser+Pro+Phe+H]; 307 [Phe+Tyr+Gly+H−H$_2$O -CO]; 298 [Ile+Ser+Pro+H]; 229 [Phe+Pro+H]; 201 [Phe+Pro+H−CO]; 158 [Gly+Gln+H−CO]; 132 Phe; 70 Pro immonium. Structure of the peptide is presented in Figure 1.

In addition to the heptapeptide Ncps, *N. edaphicum* CCNP1411 produces a small amount of the linear hexapeptide, Ncp-E4-L, whose putative structure is Tyr+Gly+Gln+Ile$^+$Ser+MePro (Table 3, Figure 9). This Ncp was detected only when higher biomass of *Nostoc* was extracted. As the proposed amino acids sequence in this molecule is the same as the sequence of the first six residues in Ncp-A1 and Ncp-A2, the hexapeptide can be a precursor of the two Ncps. The other option is that the cell concentration of the Ncps is self-regulated and the Ncp-E4-L is released through proteolytic cleavage of the final products. This hypothesis could be verified when the role of the Ncps for the producer is discovered. In the *ncp* gene cluster, the presence of *ncpG* encoding the NcpG peptidase, with high homology to enzymes hydrolyzing D-amino acid-containing peptides was revealed by Becker et al. [17] and also confirmed in this study. Therefore, the in-cell degradation of Ncps by the NcpG peptidase is possible, but it probably proceeds at D-Gln and gives other products than Ncp-E4-L.

2.4. Production of Ncps by N. edaphicum CCNP1411

Apart from the structural analysis, we also made attempts to determine the relative amounts of the individual Ncps produced by *N. edaphicum* CCNP1411. To exclude the effect of the extraction procedure on the amounts of the detected peptides, different solvents and pH were applied. As the process of Ncp linearization during long storage of the freeze-dried material was suggested [16], both the fresh and lyophilized biomasses were analyzed. Regardless of the extraction procedure, Ncp-A2-L with Phe in C-terminus was always found to be the main Ncp analogue (Figure 10A–D). In addition, when MePro and Pro-containing peptide were compared separately, the peak intensity of the linear Ncps with Phe in C-terminus (i.e., Ncp-A2-L and Ncp-E1-L) was higher than the Ncps with Leu. These results might indicate preferential incorporation of Phe into the synthesized peptide chain.

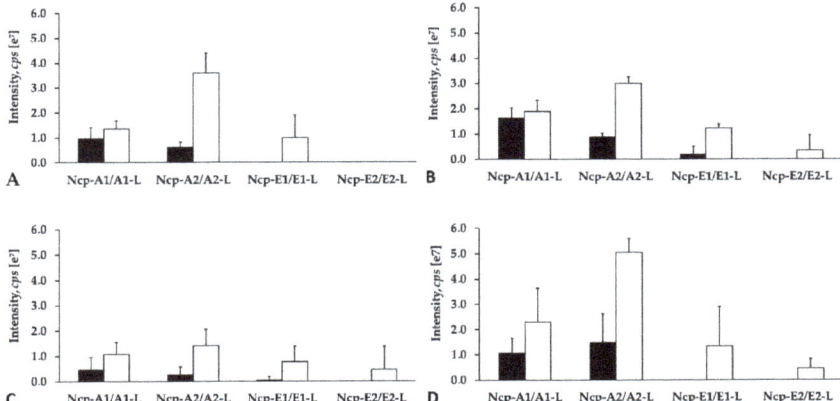

Figure 10. Relative cell contents of nostocyclopeptides extracted from 10 mg of lyophilized (**A,B,D**) or 500 mg fresh (**C**) biomass of *N. edaphicum* CCNP1411 with MilliQ water (**A**), 50% methanol in water (**B**), and 20% methanol in water (**C,D**). The cell content was expressed as peak intensity in LC-MS/MS chromatogram.

The study also showed that the cell contents of the linear Ncps are higher than the cyclic ones. (Figure 10A–D and Figure S8). The release of Ncps from the synthetase as linear aldehydes is catalyzed by a reductase domain, located in the C-terminal part of the NcpB [17]. This reductive release triggers the spontaneous, and enzyme independent, macrocyclization of the linear peptide [19,20]. The reaction leads to the formation of a stable imino bond between the C-terminal aldehyde and the N-terminal amine group of Tyr [19,20]. In *N. edaphicum* CCNP1411 cells, depending on the Ncp analogue, the analyzed material (fresh or lyophilized) and extraction solvent, the cyclic Ncps constituted from even less than 10% (Ncp-A2, fresh biomass) to over 90% of the linear peptide (Figure 10A–D and Figure S8). In case of Ncp-A1, with MePro-Leu in C-terminus, the contribution of the cyclic form was always most significant, and at pH 8 it reached up to 91.7% of the linear peptide aldehyde (Ncp-A1-L) (Figure 10A–D and Figure S8). The cyclic analogues, Ncp-E1 and Ncp-E3 were produced in trace amounts and their spectra were sporadically recorded. It was proven that the macrocyclization process of Ncps is determined by the geometry of the linear peptide aldehyde and the conformation of D-Gln and Gly is crucial for the folding and formation of the imino bond [19]. As these two residues are present in all detected Ncps, then, probably other elements of the structure affect the cyclization process, as well. We hypothesize that due to the steric hindrances, the cyclization of Ncp-A1 with Leu in C-terminal position is easier than the cyclization of Ncp-A2 with Phe. As a consequence, the proportion of the cyclic Leu-containing Ncp-A1 to the linear form of the peptide is higher.

Thus far, Ncps synthesis was reported in few *Nostoc* strains, and the structural diversity of the peptides was found to be low. Other classes of NRPs were detected in cyanobacteria representing different orders and genera, and within one class of the peptides numerous analogues were detected. For example, the number of naturally produced cyclic heptapeptide microcystins (MCs), is over 270 [40,41] and in one cyanobacterial strains even 47 MCs analogues were detected [40]. Cyanopeptolins are produced by many cyanobacterial taxa and so far more than 190 structural analogues of the peptides have been discovered [41]. In this work, cyanopeptolin gene cluster was identified in *N. edaphicum* CCNP1411 and thirteen products of the genes were previously reported [6]. These peptides contain seven amino acids and a short fatty acid chain, and only one element of the structure, 3-amino-6-hydroxy-2-piperidone (Ahp), is conserved [6]. The structural diversity of NRPs is generated by frequent genetic recombination events and point mutations in the NRP gene cluster. The changes in gene sequences affect the structure and substrate specificity of the encoded enzymes. The tailoring enzymes can further modify the product, leading to even higher diversity of the synthetized peptides [42]. In case of Ncps, both the number of the producing organisms and the structural diversity of the peptides are limited. Ncp-M1 from *Nostoc* living in symbiosis with gastropod [16] is the only Ncp with structure distinctly different from Ncp-A1, Ncp-A2 and other Ncps described in this work.

The diversity within one class of bioactive metabolites offers a good opportunity for structure-activity relationship studies, without the need to synthesize the variants. The studies are of paramount importance when the efficacy and safety of a drug candidate are optimized. Therefore, in our future work, when sufficient quantities of pure Ncps are isolated, the activity of individual analogues against different cellular targets will be tested and compared, in order to select the lead compound for further studies.

3. Materials and Methods

3.1. Isolation, Purification and Culturing of Nostoc CCNP1411

Nostoc strain CCNP1411 was isolated in 2010 from the Gulf of Gdańsk, southern Baltic Sea, by Dr. Justyna Kobos. Based on the 16S rRNA sequence (GenBank accession number KJ161445) and morphological features, such as the shape of trichomes, cell size (4.56 ± 0.30 µm wide and 4.12 ± 0.72 µm long) and lack of akinetes [43,44], the strain was classified to *N. edaphicum* species. Purification of the strain was carried out by multiple transfers to a liquid and solid (1% bacterial agar) Z8 medium supplemented with NaCl to obtain the salinity of 7.3 [45]. To establish the strain as a monoculture, free from accompanying heterotrophic bacteria, a third-generation cephalosporin, ceftriaxone (100 µg/mL) (Pol-Aura, Olsztyn, Poland) was used. In addition, the purity of the culture was regularly tested by inoculation on LA agar (solid LB medium with 1.5% agar) [46] and on agar Columbia +5% sheep blood (BTL Ltd. Łódź, Poland), a highly nutritious medium, recommended for fastidious bacteria. Cyanobacteria cultures were grown in liquid Z8 medium (100 mL) at 22 ± 1 °C, continuous light of 5–10 µmol photons $m^{-2}\ s^{-1}$. After three weeks of growth, the cyanobacterial biomass was harvested by passing the culture through a nylon net (mesh size 25 µm) and then freeze-dried before further processing.

3.2. Isolation and Sequencing of Genomic DNA

Genomic DNA of *N. edaphicum* CCNP1411 was isolated using SDS/Phenol method as described previously [47,48]. DNA quality control was performed by measuring the absorbance at 260/230 nm, template concentration was determined using Qubit fluorimeter (Thermo Fisher Scientific, Waltham, MA, USA), and DNA integrity was analyzed by 0.8% agarose gel electrophoresis and by PFGE using Biorad CHEF-III instrument (BioRad, Hercules, CA, USA).

Paired-end sequencing library was constructed using the NEB Ultra II FS Preparation Kit (New England Biolabs, Beverly, CA, USA) according to the manufacturer's instructions. The library was sequenced using an Illumina MiSeq platform (Illumina, San Diego, CA, USA) with 2 × 300 paired-end reads. Sequence quality metrics were assessed using FASTQC (http://www.bioinformatics.babraham.ac.uk/projects/fastqc/) [49].

The long reads were obtained using the GridION sequencer (Oxford Nanopore Technologies, Oxford, UK). Prior to long-read library preparation, genomic DNA was sheared into 30 kb fragments using 26 G needle followed by size selection on Bluepippin instrument (Sage Science, Beverly, MA, USA). DNA fragments above 20 kb were recovered using PAC30 kb cassette. 5 µg of recovered DNA was taken for 1D library construction using SQK-LSK109 kit and 0.5 µg of the final library was loaded into R9.4.1 flowcell and sequenced on MinION sequencer.

3.3. Genome Assembling

Raw nanopore data was basecalled using Guppy v3.2.2 (Oxford Nanopore Technologies, Oxford, UK). After quality filtering using NanoFilt [50] and residual adapter removal using Porechop (https://github.com/rrwick/Porechop), the obtained dataset was quality checked using NanoPlot [50]. Long nanopore reads were then assembled using Flye v2.6 [51]. Flye assembled contigs were further polished using Illumina sequencing reads and Unicycler_polish pipeline (https://github.com/rrwick/Unicycler).

3.4. Genome and NRPS Alignment

Genome assembly was annotated using the NCBI Prokaryotic Genome Annotation Pipeline [52] with the assistance of prokka [53] refine annotation, with additionally curated database comprised of sequences selected by Nostocales order from NCBI non-redundant and refseq_genomes (280 positions) databases, enriched by 35 NRPS/PKS clusters selected by cyanobacteria phylum. To create circular maps of *N. edaphicum* CCNP1411 genome, the CGView Comparison Tool [54] was engaged with additional GC skew and GC content analyses.

Selected span for potential NRPS cluster was confirmed with BLASTn, BLASTp [55] and antiSMASH [56]. ORFs start codons within a putative cluster were verified by the presence of ribosome binding sites, 4–12 nucleotides upstream of the start codon. Schematic comparison of ORF BLASTn from relative synthetases, AY167420.1 and CP026681.1, was visualized by EasyFig program (http://mjsull.github.io/Easyfig/files.html). Annotated regions of NRPS span were subjected for NCBI Conserved Domain Database search [57] with a set e-value threshold (10^{-3}), determining evolutionarily-conserved protein domains and motifs against CDD v3.18 database. Recognized motifs were selected using samtools v.1.9 and were subjected for protein structure and function prediction by I-TASSER [58], and results were confirmed with literature reports, PKS/NRPS Analysis Web-site prediction [59] and reevaluated using MEGAX suite [60]. Amino-acid sequence was visualized by BOXSHADE 3.2 program (https://embnet.vital-it.ch/software/BOX_form.html). Determination of domain ligand binding and active sites was achieved using COFACTOR and COACH part of I-TASSER analyses confirmed by MUSCLE amino acid alignment from MEGA X.

3.5. Data Deposition

Genomic sequences generated and analyzed in this study were deposited in the GenBank database under BioProject number: PRJNA638531.

3.6. Extraction and LC-MS/MS Analysis

For LC-MS/MS analyses of Ncps, the lyophilized (10 mg DW) biomass of *N. edaphicum* CCNP1411 was homogenized by grinding with mortar and pestle, and extracted in 1 mL of milliQ water, 20% methanol (pH 3.5, 6.0 and 8.0) and 50% methanol in water. The pH was adjusted with 0.5 M HCl and 1.0 M NaOH. In addition, the fresh material (500 mg FW) was extracted in 20% methanol in water. The samples were vortexed for 15 min and centrifuged at 14,000 rpm for 10 min, at 4 °C. The collected supernatants were directly analyzed by LC-MS/MS system.

The LC-MS/MS was carried out on an Agilent 1200 HPLC (Agilent Technologies, Waldbronn, Germany) coupled to a hybrid triple quadrupole/linear ion trap mass spectrometer QTRAP5500 (Applied Biosystems MDS Sciex, Concord, ON, Canada). The separation was achieved on a Zorbax Eclipse XDB-C18 column (4.6 mm ID × 150 mm, 5 μm; Agilent Technologies, Santa Clara, CA, USA). The extract components were separated by gradient elution from 10% to 100% B (acetonitrile with 0.1% formic acid) over 25 min, at a flow rate of 0.6 mL/min. As solvent A, 5% acetonitrile in MilliQ water with 0.1% formic acid was used. The mass spectrometer was operated in positive mode, with turbo ion source (5.5 kV; 550 °C). An information-dependent acquisition method at the following settings was used: for ions within the *m/z* range 500–1100 and signal intensity above the threshold of 500,000 cps the MS/MS spectra were acquired within the m/z range 50–1000, at a collision energy of 60 eV and declustering potential of 80 eV. Data were acquired with the Analyst ® Sofware (version 1.7 Applied Biosystems, Concord, ON, Canada).

4. Conclusions

Genes coding for subunits of the non-ribosomal peptide synthetase, in nostocyclopeptide-producing *N. edaphicum* CCNP1411, revealed differences in nucleotide compositions, compared to the previously described *ncp* cluster of *Nostoc* sp. ATCC53789. Although the analysis of fragments of genes coding for active sites and ligand binding sites of the conserved protein domains derived from *N. edaphicum* CCNP1411 and *Nostoc* sp. ATCC53789 indicated identical amino-acid compositions, residues within adenylation domains and substrate binding sites were different between compared sequences. This finding may highlight sites prone to mutations within regions accounted for structure and substrate stability. Analysis of *ncp* gene products in *N. edaphicum* CCNP1411 led to the detection of new nostocyclopeptide analogues. However, modifications in their structure were minor and limited to three positions of the heptapeptides. Although the naturally produced nostocyclopeptides were previously described as cyclic structures, in *N. edaphicum* CCNP1411 they are mainly present as linear peptide aldehydes, indicating a slow cyclization process.

Supplementary Materials: The following are available online at http://www.mdpi.com/1660-3397/18/9/442/s1. Figure S1: Structure and enhanced product ion mass spectrum of the cyclic nostocyclopeptide Ncp-A1 cyclo [Tyr+Gly+Gln+Ile+Ser+MePro+Leu] identified based on the following fragment ions: m/z 757 [M+H]; 739 [M+H−H$_2$O]; 729 [M+H−CO]; 721 [M+H−2H$_2$O]; 628 [M+H−MePro−H$_2$O]; 626 [M+H−Ile−H$_2$O]; 594 [M+H−Tyr]; 549 [Tyr+Gly+Gln+Ile+Ser+H]; 541 [M+H−(Ser+MePro)−H$_2$O]; 446 [M+H−(Ile+Ser+MePro)]; 428 [M+H−(Ile+Ser+MePro)−H$_2$O]; 386 [Gly+Gln+Ile+Ser+H]; 372 [MePro+Leu+Tyr+H]; 300 [Leu+Tyr+Gly+H−H$_2$O]; 209 [MePro+Leu+H]; 181 [MePro+Leu+H−CO]; 86−Ile/Leu immonium; 84 MePro immonium, Figure S2: Structure and enhanced product ion mass spectrum of the linear peptide aldehyde Ncp-A1-L (linear aldehyde of Ncp-A1) Tyr+Gly+Gln+Ile+Ser+MePro+Leu identified based on the following fragment ions: m/z 775 [M+H]; 757 [M+H − H$_2$O]; 739 [M+H−2H$_2$O]; 660 [M+H−Leu]; 549 [Tyr+Gly+Gln+Ile+Ser+H]; 531 [Tyr+Gly+Gln+Ile+Ser+H−H$_2$O]; 521 [Tyr+Gly+Gln+Ile+Ser+H−CO]; 532 [M+H−(MePro+Leu)−H$_2$O]; 462 [Tyr+Gly+Gln+Ile+H]; 434 [Tyr+Gly+Gln+Ile+H−CO]; 386 [Gly+Gln+Ile+Ser+H]; 349 [Tyr+Gly+Gln+H]; 301 [Gln+Ile+Ser+H−CO]; 227 [MePro+Leu+H]; 221 [Tyr+Gly+H]; 209 [MePro+Leu+H−H$_2$O]; 181 [MePro+Ile+H−H$_2$O−CO]; 148 [Tyr−NH$_2$]; 136 Tyr immonium; 86−Ile/Leu immonium; 84, 101 (immonium),129 Gln; 84 MePro immonium, Figure S3: Structure and enhanced product ion mass spectrum of the cyclic nostocyclopeptide Ncp-A2 cyclo[Tyr+Gly+Gln+Ile+Ser+MePro+Phe] identified based on the following fragment ions: m/z 791 [M+H]; 773 [M+H−H$_2$O]; 763 [M+H−CO]; 755 [M+H−2H$_2$O]; 745 [M+H−CO−H$_2$O]; 678 [M+H−Ile]; 628 [M+H−Tyr]; 593 [M+H−(Ser+MePro)]; 549 [Tyr+Gly+Gln+Ile+Ser+H]; 531 [Tyr+Gly+Gln+Ile+Ser+H−H$_2$O]; 480 [M+H−(Ile+Ser+MePro)]; 462 [Tyr+Gly+Gln+Ile+H]; 406 [MePro+Phe+Tyr+H]; 379 [MePro+Phe+Tyr+H−CO]; 349 [Tyr+Gly+Gln+H]; 335 [Phe+Tyr+Gly+H−H$_2$O]; 312 [Ile+Ser+MePro+H]; 307 [Phe+Tyr+Gly+H−H$_2$O−CO]; 243 [MePro+Phe+H]; 215 [MePro+Phe+H−CO]; 158 [Gly+Gln+H−CO]; 132 Phe; 84 MePro immonium, Figure S4: Structure and enhanced product ion mass spectrum of the linear nostocyclopeptide aldehyde Ncp-A2-L (linear aldehyde of Ncp-A2) Tyr+Gly+Gln+Ile+Ser+MePro+Phe identified based on the following fragment ions: m/z 809 [M+H]; 791 [M+H− H$_2$O]; 773 [M+H−2H$_2$O]; 763 [M+H−CO−H$_2$O]; 660 [M+H−Phe]; 628 [M+H−Tyr−H$_2$O]; 549 [Tyr+Gly+Gln+Ile+Ser+H]; 531 [M+H−(MePro+Phe)−H$_2$O]; 462 [Tyr+Gly+Gln+Ile+H]; 434 [Tyr+Gly+Gln+Ile+H−CO]; 312 [Ile+Ser+MePro+H]; 261 [MePro+Phe+H]; 243 [MePro+Phe+H − H$_2$O]; 221 [Tyr+Gly+H], 193 [Tyr+Gly+ H−CO]; 148 [Tyr−NH$_2$]; 136 Tyr immonium; 84, 101 (immonium), 129 Gln; 84 MePro immonium, Figure S5: Proposed structure and enhanced product ion mass spectrum of cyclic nostocyclopeptide Ncp-E2 cyclo[Tyr+Gly+Gln+Ile+Ser+Pro+Leu] characterized based on the following fragment ions: m/z 743 [M+H]; 725 [M+H−H$_2$O]; 715 [M+H−CO]; 707 [M+H−2H$_2$O]; 697 [M+H − H$_2$O−CO]; 656 [M+H−Ser]; 638 [M+H−Ser−H$_2$O]; 628 [M+H−Ser−CO]; 612 [M+H−Ile−H$_2$O]; 549 [Tyr+Gly+Gln+Ile+Ser+H]; 541 [M+H−(Ser+Pro)−H$_2$O]; 531 [Tyr+Gly+Gln+Ile+Ser+H−H$_2$O]; 428 [M+H−(Ile+Ser+Pro)−H$_2$O]; 349 [Tyr+Gly+Gln+H]; 300 [Leu+Tyr+Gly+H−H$_2$O]; 195 [Pro+Leu+H]; 167 [Pro+Leu+H−CO]; 84 Gln; 70 Pro immonium, Figure S6: Proposed structure and enhanced product ion mass spectrum of the linear nostocyclopeptide aldehyde Ncp-E2-L (linear aldehyde of Ncp-E2) with general structure Tyr+Gly+Gln+Ile+Ser+Pro+Leu characterized based on the following fragment ions: m/z 761 [M+H]; 743 [M+H−H$_2$O]; 725 [M+H−2H$_2$O]; 549 [Tyr+Gly+Gln+Ile+Ser+H]; 532 [Tyr+Gly+Gln+Ile+Ser+H]; 462 [Tyr+Gly+Gln+Ile+H]; 349 [Tyr+Gly+Gln+H]; 434 [Tyr+Gly+Gln+Ile+H−CO]; 300 [Ser+Pro+Leu+H]; 221 [Tyr+Gly+H]; 213 [Pro+Leu+H]; 195 [Pro+Leu+H−H$_2$O]; 148 [Tyr−NH$_2$]; 136 Tyr immonium; 84, 101 (immonium), 129 Gln; 70 Pro immonium, Figure S7: Proposed structure and enhanced product ion mass spectrum of cyclic nostocyclopeptide Ncp-E3 cyclo[Tyr+Gly+Gln+Val+Ser+MePro+Leu] characterized based on the following fragment ions: m/z 743 [M+H]; 725 [M+H−H$_2$O]; 715 [M+H−CO]; 707 [M+H − 2H$_2$O]; 697 [M+H−H$_2$O−CO];

645 [M+H−Val]; 580 [M+H−Tyr]; 527 [M+H−(Ser+MePro)−H$_2$O]; 428 [M+H−(Val+Ser+MePro)−H$_2$O]; 410 [M+H−(Val+Ser+MePro)−2H$_2$O]; 372 [Gly+Gln+Val+Ser+H]; 344 [Gly+Gln+Val+Ser+H−CO]; 300 [Leu+Tyr+Gly+H−H$_2$O]; 233 [Leu+Tyr+H−CO]; 209 [MePro+Leu+H]; 181 [MePro−Leu+H−CO]; 84 MePro immonium; 72 Val immonium, Figure S8: Relative contents of nostocyclopeptides extracted from 10 mg of lyophilized biomass of N. edaphicum CCNP1411 with 20% MeOH of different pH (3.5, 6 and 8)

Author Contributions: Conceptualization, H.M.-M. and G.W.; methodology, H.M.-M. and G.W.; software, M.G., J.G. and R.G.; validation, M.G., J.G. and R.G.; formal analysis, A.F. and M.G.; investigation, A.F. and M.G.; resources, data curation, M.G., H.M.-M., J.G. and R.G.; writing—original draft preparation, A.F. and M.G.; writing—review and editing, A.F., M.G., H.M.-M. and G.W.; visualization, A.F. and M.G.; supervision, H.M.-M. and G.W.; project administration, H.M.-M.; funding acquisition, H.M.-M. All authors have read and agreed to the published version of the manuscript.

Funding: This research was funded by the National Science Centre in Poland 2016/21/B/NZ9/02304.

Conflicts of Interest: The authors declare no conflict of interest.

References

1. Moore, R. Cyclic peptides and depsipeptides from cyanobacteria: A review. *J. Ind. Microbiol.* **1996**, *16*, 134–143. [CrossRef] [PubMed]
2. Golakoti, T.; Ogino, J.; Heltzel, C.; Le Husebo, T.; Jensen, C.; Larsen, L.; Patterson, G.; Moore, R.; Mooberry, S.; Corbett, T.; et al. Structure determination, conformational analysis, chemical stability studies, and antitumor evaluation of the cryptophycins. Isolation of new 18 analogs from *Nostoc* sp. strain GSV 224. *J. Am. Chem. Soc.* **1995**, *117*, 12030–12049. [CrossRef]
3. Boyd, M.; Gustafson, K.; McMahon, J.; Shoemaker, R.; O'Keefe, B.; Mori, T.; Gulakowski, R.; Wu, L.; Rivera, M.; Laurencot, C.; et al. Discovery of cyanovirin-N, a novel human immunodeficiency virus-inactivating protein that binds viral surface envelope glycoprotein gp120: Potential applications to microbicide development. *Antimicrob. Agents Chemother.* **1997**, *41*, 1521–1530. [CrossRef]
4. Ploutno, A.; Carmeli, S. Nostocyclyne A, a novel antimicrobial cyclophane from the cyanobacterium *Nostoc* sp. *J. Nat. Prod.* **2000**, *63*, 1524–1526. [CrossRef]
5. El-Sheekh, M.; Osman, M.; Dyan, M.; Amer, M. Production and characterization of antimicrobial active substance from the cyanobacterium *Nostoc muscorum*. *Environ. Toxicol. Pharmacol.* **2006**, *21*, 42–50. [CrossRef] [PubMed]
6. Mazur-Marzec, H.; Fidor, A.; Cegłowska, M.; Wieczerzak, E.; Kropidłowska, M.; Goua, M.; Macaskill, J.; Edwards, C. Cyanopeptolins with trypsin and chymotrypsin inhibitory activity from the cyanobacterium *Nostoc edaphicum* CCNP1411. *Mar. Drugs* **2018**, *16*, 220. [CrossRef] [PubMed]
7. Řezanka, T.; Dor, I.; Dembitsky, V. Fatty acid composition of six freshwater wild cyanobacterial species. *Folia Microbiol.* **2003**, *48*, 71–75. [CrossRef]
8. Schwartz, R.; Hirsch, C.; Sesin, D.; Flor, J.; Chartrain, M.; Fromtling, R.; Harris, G.; Salvatore, M.; Liesch, J.; Yudin, K. Pharmaceuticals from cultured algae. *J. Ind. Microbiol.* **1990**, *5*, 113–124. [CrossRef]
9. Gustafson, K.; Sowder, R.; Henderson, L.; Cardellina, J.; McMahon, J.; Rajamani, U.; Pannell, L.; Boyd, M. Isolation, primary sequence determination, and disulfide bond structure of cyanovirin-N, an anti-HIV (Human Immunodeficiency Virus) protein from the cyanobacterium *Nostoc ellipsosporum*. *Biochem. Biophys. Res. Commun.* **1997**, *238*, 223–228. [CrossRef]
10. Okino, T.; Qi, S.; Matsuda, H.; Murakami, M.; Yamaguchi, K. Nostopeptins A and B, elastase inhibitors from the cyanobacterium *Nostoc minutum*. *J. Nat. Prod.* **1997**, *60*, 158–161. [CrossRef]
11. Kaya, K.; Sano, T.; Beattie, K.; Codd, G. Nostocyclin, a novel 3-amino-6-hydroxy-2-piperidone containing cyclic depsipeptide from the cyanobacterium *Nostoc* sp. *Tetrahedron Lett.* **1996**, *37*, 6725–6728. [CrossRef]
12. Mehner, C.; Müller, D.; Kehraus, S.; Hautmann, S.; Gütschow, M.; König, G. New peptolides from the cyanobacterium *Nostoc insulare* as selective and potent inhibitors of human leukocyte elastase. *ChemBioChem* **2008**, *9*, 2692–2703. [CrossRef] [PubMed]
13. Golakoti, T.; Yoshida, W.; Chaganty, S.; Moore, R. Isolation and structure determination of nostocyclopeptides A1 and A2 from the terrestrial cyanobacterium *Nostoc* sp. ATCC53789. *J. Nat. Prod.* **2001**, *64*, 54–59. [CrossRef] [PubMed]
14. Nowruzi, B.; Khavari-Nejad, R.; Sivonen, K.; Kazemi, B.; Najafi, F.; Nejadsattari, T. Indentification and toxigenic potential of *Nostoc* sp. *Algae* **2012**, *27*, 303–313. [CrossRef]

15. Liaimer, A.; Jensen, J.; Dittmann, E. A genetic and chemical perspective on symbiotic recruitment of cyanobacteria of the genus *Nostoc* into the host plant *Blasia pusilla* L. *Front. Microbiol.* **2016**, *7*, 1963. [CrossRef] [PubMed]
16. Jokela, J.; Herfindal, L.; Wahlsten, M.; Permi, P.; Selheim, F.; Vasconçelos, V.; Døskeland, S.; Sivonen, K. A novel cyanobacterial nostocyklopeptide is a potent antitoxin against Microcystis. *ChemBioChem* **2010**, *11*, 1594–1599. [CrossRef]
17. Becker, J.; Moore, R.; Moore, B. Cloning, sequencing, and biochemical characterization of the nostocycyclopeptide biosynthetic gene cluster: Molecular basis for imine macrocyclization. *Gene* **2004**, *325*, 35–42. [CrossRef]
18. Hoffmann, D.; Hevel, J.; Moore, R.; Moore, B. Sequence analysis and biochemical characterization of the nostopeptolide A biosynthetic gene cluster from *Nostoc* sp. GSV224. *Gene* **2003**, *311*, 171–180. [CrossRef]
19. Kopp, F.; Mahlet, C.; Grünewald, J.; Marahiel, M. Peptide macrocyclization: The reductase of the nostocyclopeptide synthetase triggers the self-assembly of a macrocyclic imine. *J. Am. Chem. Soc.* **2006**, *128*, 16478–16479. [CrossRef]
20. Enck, S.; Kopp, F.; Marahiel, M.; Geyer, A. The entropy balance of nostocyclopeptide macrocyclization analysed by NMR spectroscopy. *ChemBioChem* **2008**, *9*, 2597–2601. [CrossRef]
21. Herfindal, L.; Myhren, L.; Kleppe, R.; Krakstad, C.; Selheim, F.; Jokela, J.; Sivonen, K.; Døskeland, S. Nostocyclopeptide-M1: A potent, nontoxic inhibitor of the hepatocyte drug trasporters OATP1B3 and OATP1B1. *Mol. Pharm.* **2011**, *8*, 360–367. [CrossRef]
22. Lee, W.; Belkhiri, A.; Lockhart, A.; Merchant, N.; Glaeser, H.; Harris, E.; Washington, M.; Brunt, E.; Zaika, A.; Kim, R.; et al. Overexpression of OATP1B3 confers apoptotic resistance in colon cancer. *Cancer Res.* **2008**, *68*, 10315–10323. [CrossRef] [PubMed]
23. Nishizawa, T.; Ueda, A.; Nakano, T.; Nishizawa, A.; Miura, T.; Asayama, M.; Fuji, K.; Harada, K.; Shirai, M. Characterization of the locus of genes encoding enzymes producing heptadepsipeptide micropeptin in the unicellular cyanobacterium Microcystis. *J. Biochem.* **2011**, *149*, 475–485. [CrossRef] [PubMed]
24. Rouhiainen, L.; Jokela, J.; Fewer, D.; Urmann, M.; Sivonen, K. Two alternative starter modules for the non-ribosomal biosynthesis of specific anabaenopeptin variants in *Anabaena* (cyanobacteria). *Chem. Biol.* **2010**, *17*, 265–273. [CrossRef] [PubMed]
25. Luesch, H.; Hoffmann, D.; Hevel, J.; Becker, J.; Golakoti, T.; Moore, R. Biosynthesis of 4-Methylproline in Cyanobacteria: Cloning of *nosE* and *nosF* and biochemical characterization of the encoded dehydrogenase and reductase activities. *J. Org. Chem.* **2003**, *68*, 83–91. [CrossRef] [PubMed]
26. Lambalot, R.; Walsh, C. Cloning, Overproduction, and Characterization of the *Escherichia coli* Holo-acyl Carrier Protein Synthase. *J. Biol. Chem.* **1995**, *270*, 24658–24661. [CrossRef]
27. Marchler-Bauer, A.; Derbyshire, M.; Gonzales, N.; Lu, S.; Chitsaz, F.; Geer, L.; Geer, R.; He, J.; Gwadz, M.; Hurwitz, D.; et al. CDD: NCBI's conserved domain database. *Nucleic Acids Res.* **2015**, *43*, d222–d226. [CrossRef]
28. Stachelhaus, T.; Mootz, H.; Marahiel, M. The specificity-conferring code of adenylation domains in nonribosomal peptide synthetases. *Chem. Biol.* **1999**, *6*, 493–505. [CrossRef]
29. Challis, G.; Ravel, J.; Townsend, C. Predictive, structure-based model of amino acid recognition by nonribosomal peptide synthetase adenylation domains. *Chem. Biol.* **2000**, *7*, 211–224. [CrossRef]
30. Stein, T.; Vater, J.; Kruft, V.; Otto, A.; Wittmann-Liebold, B.; Franke, P.; Panico, M.; McDowell, R.; Morris, H. The multiple carrier model of nonribosomal peptide biosynthesis at modular multienzymatic templates. *J. Biol. Chem.* **1996**, *271*, 15428–15435. [CrossRef]
31. Dehling, E.; Volkmann, G.; Matern, J.; Dörner, W.; Alfermann, J.; Diecker, J.; Mootz, H. Mapping of the Communication-Mediating Interface in Nonribosomal Peptide Synthetases Using a Genetically Encoded Photocrosslinker Supports an Upside-Down Helix-Hand Motif. *J. Mol. Biol.* **2016**, *428*, 4345–4360. [CrossRef]
32. Hacker, C.; Cai, X.; Kegler, C.; Zhao, L.; Weickhmann, K.; Wurm, J.; Bode, H.; Wöhnert, J. Structure-based redesign of docking domain interactions modulates the product spectrum of a rhabdopeptide-synthesizing NRPS. *Nat. Commun.* **2018**, *9*, 4366. [CrossRef]
33. Richter, C.; Nietlispach, D.; Broadhurst, R.; Weissman, K. Multienzyme docking in hybrid megasynthetases. *Nat. Chem. Biol.* **2008**, *4*, 75–81. [CrossRef] [PubMed]

34. Haese, A.; Schubert, M.; Herrmann, M.; Zocher, R. Molecular characterization of the enniatin synthetase gene encoding a multifunctional enzyme catalysing N-methyldepsipeptide formation in *Fusarium scirpi*. *Mol. Biol.* **1993**, *7*, 905–914. [CrossRef]
35. Marahiel, M.; Stachelhaus, T.; Mootz, H. Modular peptide synthetases involved in nonribosomal peptide synthesis. *Chem. Rev.* **1997**, *97*, 2651–2674. [CrossRef]
36. Chang, C.; Lohman, J.; Huang, T.; Michalska, K.; Bigelow, L.; Rudolf, J.; Jędrzejczak, R.; Yan, X.; Ma, M.; Babnigg, G.; et al. Structural Insights into the Free-Standing Condensation Enzyme SgcC5 Catalyzing Ester-Bond Formation in the Biosynthesis of the Enediyne Antitumor Antibiotic C-1027. *Biochemistry* **2018**, *57*, 3278–3288. [CrossRef]
37. Du, L.; Lou, L. PKS and NRPS release mechanisms. *Nat. Prod. Rep.* **2010**, *27*, 255–278. [CrossRef] [PubMed]
38. Koketsu, K.; Minami, A.; Watanabe, K.; Oguri, H.; Oikawa, H. Pictet-Spenglerase involved in tetrahydroisoquinoline antibiotic biosynthesis. *Curr. Opin. Chem. Biol.* **2012**, *16*, 142–149. [CrossRef] [PubMed]
39. Liu, L.; Jokela, J.; Herfindal, L.; Wahlsten, M.; Sinkkonen, J.; Permi, P.; Fewer, D.; Døskeland, S.; Sivonen, K. 4-Methylproline guided natural product discovery: Co-occurrence of a 4-hydroxy- and 4-methtylprolines in nostoweipeptins and nostopeptolides. *ACS Chem. Biol.* **2014**, *9*, 2646–2655. [CrossRef]
40. Bouaïcha, N.; Miles, C.; Beach, D.; Labidi, Z.; Djabri, A.; Benayache, N.; Nguyen-Quang, T. Structural diversity, characterization and toxicology of microcystins. *Toxins* **2019**, *11*, 714. [CrossRef]
41. Jones, M.; Pinto, E.; Torres, M.; Dörr, F.; Mazur-Marzec, H.; Szubert, K.; Tartaglione, L.; Dell'Aversano, C.; Miles, C.; Beach, D.; et al. Comprehensive database of secondary metabolites from cyanobacteria. *BioRxiv* **2020**. [CrossRef]
42. Meyer, S.; Kehr, J.; Mainz, A.; Dehm, D.; Petras, D.; Süssmuth, R.; Dittmann, E. Biochemical dissection of the natural diversification of microcystin provides lessons for synthetic biology of NRPS. *Cell. Chem. Biol.* **2016**, *23*, 462–471. [CrossRef] [PubMed]
43. Kondratyeva, N.V. Novyi vyd synio-zelenykh vodorostey—*Nostoc edaphicum* sp. n. [A new species of blue-green algae—*Nostoc edapicum* sp. n. *Ukr. Bot. J.* **1962**, *19*, 58–65.
44. Komárek, J. *Süsswasserflora von Mitteleuropa. Cyanoprokaryota: 3rd Part: Heterocystous Genera*; Springer Spectrum: Berlin/Heidelberg, Germany, 2013; Volume 19, pp. 1–1130.
45. Kotai, J. *Instructions for Preparation of Modified Nutrient Solution Z8 for Algae*; Publication: B-11/69; Norwegian Institute for Water Research: Oslo, Norway, 1972; p. 5.
46. Bertani, G. Studies on lysogenesis. I. The mode of phage liberation by lysogenic *Escherichia Coli*. *J. Bacteriol.* **1951**, *62*, 293–300. [CrossRef] [PubMed]
47. Nowak, R.; Jastrzębski, J.; Kuśmirek, W.; Sałamatin, R.; Rydzanicz, M.; Sobczyk-Kopcioł, A.; Sulima-Celińska, A.; Paukszto, Ł.; Makowaczenko, K.; Płoski, R.; et al. Hybrid de novo whole genome assembly and annotation of the model tapeworm *Hymenolepis diminuta*. *Sci. Data* **2019**, *6*, 302. [CrossRef]
48. Wilson, K. Preparation of genomic DNA from bacteria. In *Current Protocols in Molecular Biology*; Ausubel, R., Bent, R.E., Eds.; Kingston: Fountain Valley, CA, USA; Wiley & Sons: New York, NY, USA, 1987; pp. 2.10–2.12.
49. Andrews, S. Babraham Bioinformatics, FastQC—A Quality Control Application for High Throughput Sequence Data. 2010. Available online: http://www.bioinformatics.babraham.ac.uk/projects/fastqc/ (accessed on 11 February 2020).
50. De Coster, W.; D'Hert, S.; Schultz, D.; Cruts, M.; Van Broeckhoven, C. NanoPack: Visualizing and processing long–read sequencing data. *Bioinformatics* **2018**, *34*, 2666–2669. [CrossRef]
51. Kolmogorov, M.; Yuan, J.; Lin, Y.; Pevzner, P. Assembly of long, error–prone reads using repeat graphs. *Nat. Biotechnol.* **2019**, *37*, 540–546. [CrossRef]
52. Tatusova, T.; DiCuccio, M.; Badretdin, A.; Chetvernin, V.; Nawrocki, E.; Zaslavsky, L.; Lomsadze, A.; Pruitt, K.; Borodovsky, M.; Ostell, J. NCBI prokaryotic genome annotation pipeline. *Nucleic Acids Res.* **2016**, *44*, 6614–6624. [CrossRef]
53. Seemann, T. Prokka: Rapid prokaryotic genome annotation. *Bioinformatics* **2014**, *30*, 2068–2069. [CrossRef]
54. Grant, J.; Arantes, A.; Stothard, P. Comparing thousands of circular genomes using the CGView comparison tool. *BMC Genom.* **2012**, *13*, 202. [CrossRef]
55. Altschul, S.; Madden, T.; Schäffer, A.; Zhang, J.; Zhang, Z.; Miller, W.; Lipman, D. Gapped BLAST and PSI–BLAST: A new generation of protein database search programs. *Nucleic Acids Res.* **1997**, *25*, 3389–3402. [CrossRef] [PubMed]

56. Medema, M.; Blin, K.; Cimermanic, P.; de Jager, V.; Zakrzewski, P.; Fischbach, M.; Weber, T.; Takano, E.; Breitling, R. antiSMASH: Rapid identification, annotation and analysis of secondary metabolites biosynthesis gene clusters in bacterial and fungal genome sequences. *Nucleic Acids Res.* **2011**, *39*, w339–w346. [CrossRef]
57. Marchler-Bauer, A.; Lu, S.; Anderson, J.; Chitsaz, F.; Derbyshire, M.; DeWesse-Scott, C.; Fong, J.; Geer, L.; Geer, R.; Gonzales, N.; et al. CDD: A conserved database for the functional annotation of proteins. *Nucleic Acids Res.* **2011**, *39*, d225–d229. [CrossRef] [PubMed]
58. Yang, J.; Yan, R.; Roy, A.; Xu, D.; Poisson, J.; Zhang, Y. The I–TASSER Suite: Protein structure and function prediction. *Nat. Methods* **2015**, *12*, 7–8. [CrossRef] [PubMed]
59. Bachmann, B.; Ravel, J. Methods for in silico prediction of microbial polyketide and nonribosomal peptide biosynthetic pathways from DNA sequence data. *Methods Enzymol.* **2009**, *458*, 181–217.
60. Kumar, S.; Stecher, G.; Li, M.; Knyaz, C.; Tamura, K. MEGA X: Molecular Evolutionary Genetics Analysis across computing platforms. *Mol. Biol. Evol.* **2018**, *35*, 1547–1549. [CrossRef]

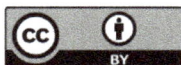

© 2020 by the authors. Licensee MDPI, Basel, Switzerland. This article is an open access article distributed under the terms and conditions of the Creative Commons Attribution (CC BY) license (http://creativecommons.org/licenses/by/4.0/).

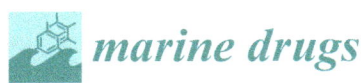

Article

Eighteen New Aeruginosamide Variants Produced by the Baltic Cyanobacterium *Limnoraphis* CCNP1324

Marta Cegłowska [1], Karolia Szubert [2], Ewa Wieczerzak [3], Alicja Kosakowska [1] and Hanna Mazur-Marzec [2],*

[1] Institute of Oceanology, Polish Academy of Sciences, Powstańców Warszawy 55, PL-81712 Sopot, Poland; mceglowska@iopan.pl (M.C.); akosak@iopan.gda.pl (A.K.)
[2] Division of Marine Biotechnology, Faculty of Oceanography and Geography, University of Gdańsk, Marszałka J. Piłsudskiego 46, PL-81378 Gdynia, Poland; karolina.szubert@phdstud.ug.edu.pl
[3] Department of Biomedical Chemistry, Faculty of Chemistry, University of Gdańsk, Wita Stwosza 63, PL-80308 Gdańsk, Poland; ewa.wieczerzak@ug.edu.pl
* Correspondence: hanna.mazur-marzec@ug.edu.pl

Received: 31 July 2020; Accepted: 25 August 2020; Published: 27 August 2020

Abstract: Cyanobactins are a large family of ribosomally synthesized and post-translationally modified cyanopeptides (RiPPs). Thus far, over a hundred cyanobactins have been detected in different free-living and symbiotic cyanobacteria. The majority of these peptides have a cyclic structure. The occurrence of linear cyanobactins, aeruginosamides and virenamide, has been reported sporadically and in few cyanobacterial taxa. In the current work, the production of cyanobactins by *Limnoraphis* sp. CCNP1324, isolated from the brackish water Baltic Sea, has been studied for the first time. In the strain, eighteen new aeruginosamide (AEG) variants have been detected. These compounds are characterized by the presence of prenyl and thiazole groups. A common element of AEGs produced by *Limnoraphis* sp. CCNP1324 is the sequence of the three C-terminal residues containing proline, pyrrolidine and methyl ester of thiazolidyne-4-carboxylic acid (Pro-Pyr-TzlCOOMe) or thiazolidyne-4-carboxylic acid (Pro-Pyr-TzlCOOH). The aeruginosamides with methylhomotyrosine (MeHTyr[1]) and with the unidentified N-terminal amino acids showed strong cytotoxic activity against human breast cancer cells (T47D).

Keywords: cyanobacteria; aeruginosamides; *Limnoraphis*; cytotoxicity

1. Introduction

Nonribosomal and ribosomal cyanobacterial peptides, with their structural diversity and modified amino acid moieties, constitute one of the most interesting and biotechnologically promising groups of marine natural products [1–5]. Ribosomally synthesized and post-translationally modified (RiPPs) cyanobactins constitute a large family of compounds containing from three to twenty amino acids [6–9]. The biosynthesis of these metabolites starts with the encoding of a precursor peptide that undergoes multiple cleavages leading to a release of a core peptide that is subjected to further enzymatic modifications. The structure of cyanobactins is characterized by the presence of heterocyclized amino acids, mainly cysteine (cyclized to thiazole or oxidized thiazoline), threonine and serine (cyclized to oxazole or oxazoline) [6,7,10]. Cyanobactins can also contain prenyl or, more rarely, geranyl groups. Other modifications include carboxylation of glutamine, hydroxylation of proline, valine or lysine, bromination of tryptophan, acetylation of tyrosine, epimerization or formation of disulfate bridge [7,10,11].

Some cyanobactins, such as comoramides, keenamide A, patellamides and vineramides, exhibit cytotoxic activity against several cancer cell lines [12–17]. Venturamides, another class of the peptides, had strong in vitro antimalarial activity against *Plasmodium falciparum* [18]. Cyanobactins have been also described as allelopathic agents. Nostocyclamide from *Nostoc* 31 inhibited the growth of cyanobacterial strains representing other genera *Anabaena*, *Synechococcus* and *Synechocystis*, diatom *Navicula minima* and chlorophyceae *Nannochloris coccoides* [19,20].

The first cyanobactins, ulicyclamide and ulithiacyclamide with cytotoxic activity, were isolated from a tunicate *Lissoclinum patella* from Palau, Western Caroline Islands [21]. It was later established that some cyanobactins were in fact produced by the ascidians symbiont, *Prochloron* spp. [22,23]. Thus far, over a hundred cyanobactins have been detected in different free-living and symbiotic cyanobacteria. Amongst others, these compounds have been found and chemically characterized in *Anabaena* (anacyclamides) [24], *Arthrospira* (arthrospiramides) [25], *Lyngbya* (aesturamides) [26], *Microcystis* (aerucyclamides, aeruginosamides, kawaguchipeptins, microcyclamide, microphycin) [15,27–30], *Scytonema* (scytodecamide) [31] and *Sphaerospermopsis* (sphaerocyclamides) [32]. Cyanobactin gene clusters were found in up to 30% of cyanobacteria representing *Prochloron*, *Anabaena*, *Microcystis*, *Arthrospira* and other genera [6–8,24,33,34].

Initially, cyanobactins were described as cyclic peptides. Lawton et al. [28] reported the production of a linear aeruginosamide by *M. aeruginosa* from bloom sample collected in Rutland Water reservoir (Scotland). This peptide contained the diisoprenylamine and the carboxylated thiazole moieties and was later called aeruginosamide A (AEG-A) [34]. Further studies revealed the presence of modified linear cyanobactins: aeruginosamides B and C in *Microcystis aeruginosa* PCC 9432 and a virenamide A in *Oscillatoria nigro-viridis* PCC 7112 [34].

In the current study, the potential of *Limnoraphis* to produce cyanobactins has been explored for the first time. The non-targeted liquid chromatography-tandem mass spectrometry (LC-MS/MS) analysis of extract and fractions from *Limnoraphis* sp. CCNP1324, isolated from the brackish water Baltic Sea, led to the detection of eighteen new aeruginosamide variants. In cell viability assays some of the aeruginosamides produced by *Limnoraphis* sp. CCNP1324 showed cytotoxic activity against human breast cancer cells (T47D).

2. Results and Discussion

The existing knowledge about the structural diversity of aeruginosamides and aeruginosamide-producing cyanobacteria is limited. To date, only three aeruginosamides have been detected [28,34] (Table 1), and no reports on cyanobactins or genes involved in their biosynthesis in cyanobacteria of *Limnoraphis* genus have been published. In our work, the production and structural diversity of cyanobactins produced by *Limnoraphis* sp. CCNP1324 from the Baltic Sea were studied. As a result, eighteen new structural analogues of the linear aeruginosamides were characterized.

Of the eighteen AEGs produced by *Limnoraphis* sp. CCNP1324, the cell-bound content of AEG707, estimated on the basis of chromatographic peak area, was the highest. Ten peptides were produced in trace amounts and were only detected when a larger portion of cyanobacterial biomass was used for the extraction (Table 1). The structure elucidation of AEGs was based on the mass fragmentation spectra with characteristic immonium ions (e.g., at m/z 70 (proline Pro), 86 (isoleucine Ile/leucine Leu), 120 (phenylalanine Phe), 134 (homophenylalanine Hph/N-methyl-phenylalanine N-MePhe), 136 (tyrosine Tyr), 164 (N-methyl-homotyrosine N-MeHTyr)) and a series of other fragment ions. In addition, the collected product ion spectra were compared with the previously published spectra of AEG-A [28], AEG-B and AEG-C [34].

Table 1. Postulated structures of aeruginosamides (AEGs) described thus far, and identified in *Limnoraphis* sp. CCNP1324.

Aeruginosamide AEG	m/z	Retention Time [min]	Relative Peak Area of Extracted Ion	AEG Chemical Structure	Reference
AEG-A	561	-	-	(Pre)$_2$+Ile+Val+Pyr+TzlCOOMe	[28]
571 [1],[2]	572	9.94	1.39 × 10^9	Tyr+Val+Pro+Pyr+TzlCOOMe	This study
AEG-B	575	-	-	Pre+Phe+Phe+Pyr+TzlCOOMe	[34]
595 [2]	596	5.12	T	187+Val+Pro+Pyr+TzlCOOMe	This study
603 [2]	604	9.74	T	Phe+Phe+Pro+Pyr+TzlCOOMe	This study
625 [1],[2]	626	4.61	6.82 × 10^8	Pre+Tyr+Val+Pro+Pyr+TzlCOOH	This study
639 [1],[2]	640	6.78	1.23 × 10^9	Pre+Tyr+Val+Pro+Pyr+TzlCOOMe	This study
657 [1],[2]	658	2.27	5.8 × 10^8	Pre+Phe+Phe+Pro+Pyr+TzlCOOH	This study
667 [2]	668	8.22	T	Pre+MeHTyr+Val+Pro+Pyr+TzlCOOMe	This study
671 [1],[2]	672	9.24	4.45 × 10^8	Pre+Phe+Phe+Pro+Pyr+TzlCOOMe	This study
AEG-C	674	-	-	Pre+Phe+Phe+Pro+Val+TzlCOOMe	[34]
681a [2]	682a	7.16	T	Pre+205+Val+Pro+Pyr+TzlCOOMe	This study
681b [2]	682b	11.78	T	225+Phe+Pro+Pyr+TzlCOOMe	This study
683 [2]	684	12.34	T	Pre+207+Val+Pro+Pyr+TzlCOOMe	This study
685 [2]	686	12.62	T	Pre+Phe+Hph/MePhe+Pro+Pyr+TzlCOOMe	This study
693 [1],[2]	694	9.10	2.85 × 10^9	(Pre)$_2$+Tyr+Val+Pro+Pyr+TzlCOOH	This study
705 [2]	706	8.73	T	(Pre)$_2$+Hph/MePhe+Val+Pro+Pyr+TzlCOOMe	This study
707 [1],[2]	708	9.76	8.69 × 10^9	(Pre)$_2$+Tyr+Val+Pro+Pyr+TzlCOOMe	This study
721 [1],[2]	722	10.12	1.89 × 10^8	(Pre)$_2$+Tyr+Ile/Leu+Pro+Pyr+TzlCOOMe	This study
735 [2]	736	11.26	T	Pre+225+Phe+Pro+Pyr+TzlCOOH	This study
749 [2]	750	11.50	T	Pre+225+Phe+Pro+Pyr+TzlCOOMe	This study

[1] Detected in the 10 mg extract. [2] Detected in the 20 g extract and flash fractions from CCNP1324. T traces of AEGs detected in 10 mg extract. Hph: homophenylalanine; MePhe: N-methy-phenylalanine; Ile/Leu: isoleucine/leucine; Phe: phenylalanine, Pre: prenyl group; Pro: proline; Pyr: pyrrolidine; Tyr: tyrosine; MeHTyr: N-methyl-homotyrosine; TzlCOOH: thiazolidyne-4-carboxylic acid; TzlCOOMe: methyl ester of thiazolidyne-4-carboxylic acid; Val: valine; 187, 205, 225: unknown residues.

Thiazole (Tzl) group, a characteristic element of numerous cyanobactins [6,7,25,35] was present in all AEGs produced by *Limnoraphis* sp. CCNP1324. In the fragmentation spectra, TzlCO gave a peak at *m/z* 112, while the ion at *m/z* 144 was indicative of methyl ester of thiazolidyne-4-carboxylic acid (TzlCOOMe) (Figures 1–3, Figures S1, S2, S5–S11 and S13). In the spectra of four AEGs, the ion at *m/z* 112 was present but instead of the *m/z* 144 ion, the ion at *m/z* 130 occurred, suggesting a modification in the ester group of TzlCOOMe. In the spectra of these peptides, instead of ions at *m/z* 213 (Pyr+TzlCOOMe) and *m/z* 310 (Pro+Pyr+TzlCOOMe), there were peaks at 14 units lower values, i.e., *m/z* 199 and 296. Pyr stands for pyrrolidine ring which constitutes a part of the proline structure. The 14-unit shift in the *m/z* value of the ions, compared to TzlCOOMe-containing peptides, and the ion at *m/z* 112 indicated the presence of thiazolidyne-4-carboxylic acid (TzlCOOH). Such modifications were observed in AEG625 (Figure 4), AEG657 (Figure S3), AEG693 (Figure 5) and AEG735 (Figure S12) (Table 1). The three C-terminal residues in aeruginosamides identified in CCNP1324, were found to be conserved. In other AEGs identified thus far the residues adjacent to TzlCOOMe were Val (valine)+Pyr [28], Phe+Pyr or Pro+Val [34] (Table 1).

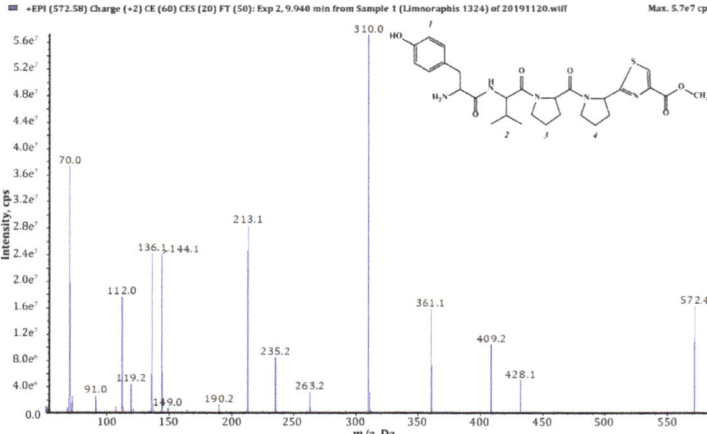

Figure 1. Chemical structure and enhanced product ion mass spectrum of aeruginosamide AEG571 Tyr+Val+Pro+Pyr+TzlCOOMe identified based on the following fragment ions: 572 [M+H], 428 [M+H−TzlCOOMe], 409 [Val+Pro+Pyr+TzlCOOMe], 361 [M+H−Pyr+TzlCOOMe], 310 [Pro+Pyr+TzlCOOMe+H], 263 [Tyr+Val+H], 235 [Tyr+Val+H−CO], 213 [Pyr+TzlCOOMe+H], 144 [TzlCOOMe], 136 Tyr immonium ion, 112 TzlCO, 70 Pro immonium ion.

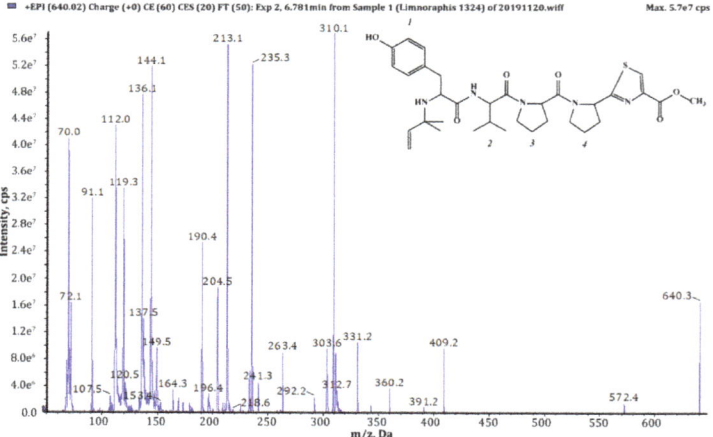

Figure 2. Chemical structure and enhanced product ion mass spectrum of aeruginosamide AEG639 Pre+Tyr+Val+Pro+Pyr+TzlCOOMe identified based on the following fragment ions: 640 [M+H], 572 [M+H−Pre], 409 [Val+Pro+Pyr+TzlCOOMe], 391 [Val+Pro+Pyr+TzlCOOMe−H_2O], 360 [Tyr+Val+Pro+H], 331 [Pre+Tyr+Val+H], 310 [Pro+Pyr+TzlCOOMe+H], 303 [Pre+Tyr+Val+H−CO], 263 [Tyr+Val+H], 235 [Tyr+Val+H−CO], 213 [Pyr+TzlCOOMe+H], 204 [Pre+Tyr+H−CO], 144 [TzlCOOMe], 136 Tyr immonium ion, 112 TzlCO, 72 Val immonium ion, 70 Pro immonium ion.

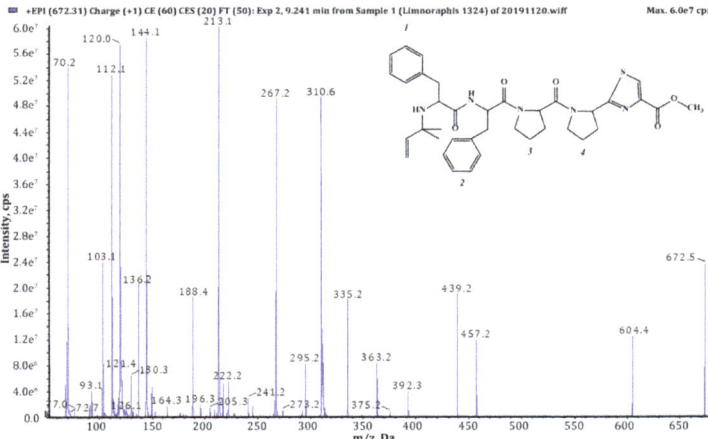

Figure 3. Chemical structure and enhanced product ion mass spectrum of aeruginosamide AEG671 Pre+Phe+Phe+Pro+Pyr+TzlCOOMe identified based on the following fragment ions: 672 [M+H], 604 [M+H–Pre], 457 [M+H–(Pre+Phe)], 439 [M+H–(Pre+Phe)–H$_2$O], 392 [Phe+Phe+Pro+H], 363 [Pre+Phe+Phe+H], 335 [Pre+Phe+Phe+H–CO], 310 [Pro+Pyr+TzlCOOMe+H], 295 [Phe+Phe+H], 267 [Phe+Phe+H–CO], 213 [Pyr+TzlCOOMe+H], 188 [Pre+Phe+H–CO], 144 [TzlOMe], 136 Tyr immonium ion, 120 Phe immonium ion; 112 TzlCO, 70 Pro immonium ion.

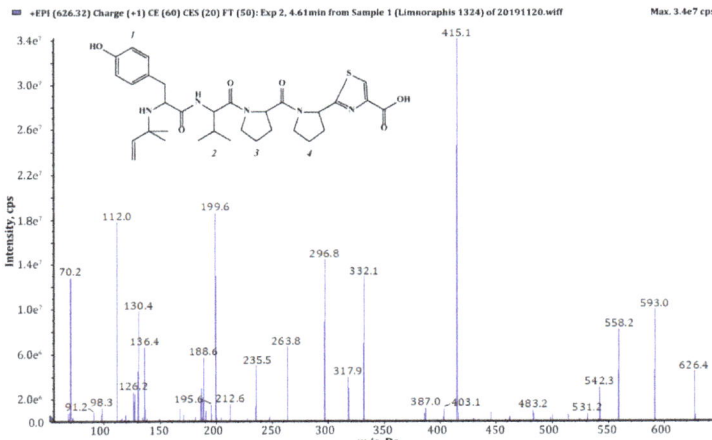

Figure 4. Chemical structure and enhanced product ion mass spectrum of aeruginosamide AEG625 Pre+Tyr+Val+Pro+Pyr+TzlCOOH identified based on the following fragment ions: 626 [M+H], 558 [M+H–Pre], 296 [Pro+Pyr+TzlCOOH+H], 263 [Tyr+Val+H], 332 [Tyr+Val+Pro+H–CO], 235 [Tyr+Val+H–CO], 199 [Pyr+TzlCOOH+H], 130 [TzlCOOH], 136 Tyr immonum ion, 112 TzlCO, 70 Pro immonium ion.

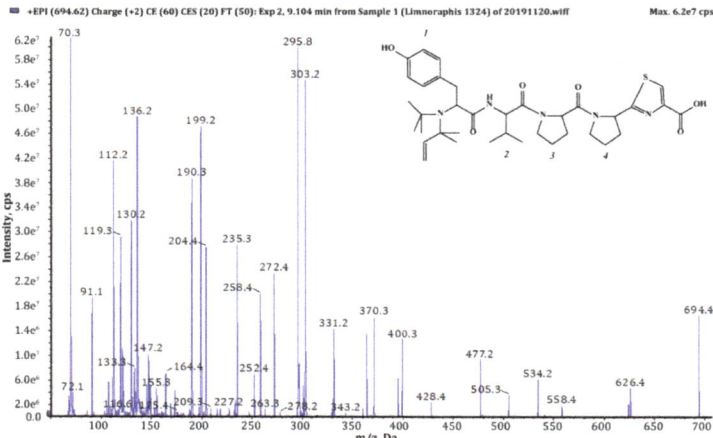

Figure 5. Chemical structure and enhanced product ion mass spectrum of aeruginosamide AEG693 (Pre)$_2$+ Tyr+Val+Pro+Pyr+TzlCOOH identified based on the following fragment ions: 694 [M+H], 626 [M+H–Pre], 558 [M+H–(Pre)$_2$], 477 [(Pre)$_2$+Tyr+Val+Pro+H–H$_2$O], 428 [Pre+Tyr+Val+Pro+H], 400 [Pre+Tyr+Val+Pro+H–CO], 370 [(Pre)$_2$+Tyr+Val+H–CO], 331 [Pre+Tyr+Val+H],303 [Pre+Tyr+Val+H–CO], 295 [Pro+Pyr+TzlCOOH+H], 272 [(Pre)$_2$+Tyr+H–CO], 235 [Tyr+Val+H–CO], 204 [Pre+Tyr+H–CO], 199 [Pyr+TzlCOOH+H], 130 [TzlOH], 136 Tyr immonium ion, 112 TzlCO, 72 Val immonium ion, 70 Pro immonium ion.

Tyr^1 was found to be the most frequent residue at the N-terminus and was present in six out of eighteen AEGs identified in this study. In other AEGs produced by *Limnoraphis* sp. CCNP1324, this position was occupied by MeHTyr^1, Phe^1 or Hph^1 (Table 1, Figures 1–5 and Figures S1–S13). In the case of six AEGs (m/z [M+H] 596, 682a, 682b, 684, 736 and 750) we were not able to fully elucidate the structure and identify the N-terminal residue. Based on the fragmentation spectrum it was concluded that the residues gave strong immonium ions at m/z 160, 178, 180 and 198 and their residue masses were 187, 205, 207 and 225 respectively. In previously described linear cyanobactins such as virenamide A–C, aeruginosamide B and C, and viridisamide A, Phe^1 was the most commonly identified N-terminal residue [12,34]. In other cyanobactins, position 1 was occupied by Ile [28,36] or Val [37]. The high residue masses of the unidentified amino acids and a frequent occurrence of aromatic amino acids at N-terminus of AEGs produced by *Limnoraphis* sp. indicated the presence of modified Tyr or Phe variants in this position. In some RiPPs, such as cyanobactins and microviridins, the presence of acetylated Tyr (AcTyr) was reported [11,38]. Based on the mass fragmentation spectrum, the presence of AcTyr^1 in AEG681a is also possible (Figure S5). The position 2 in AEGs produced by *Limnoraphis* sp. CCNP1324 was least conserved and occupied by both aliphatic and aromatic amino acids: Val, Ile, Phe and Hph/MePhe (Table 1, Figures 1–5 and Figures S1–S13).

Limnoraphis sp. CCNP1324 synthesizes aeruginosamides with two, one and no prenyl groups at N-terminus (Table 1, Figures 1–5 and Figures S1–S13). The presence of prenyl was confirmed by the loss of one or two 68-Da fragments from the pseudomolecular ion of the analyzed peptides. The differences in retention times between AEGs without and with prenyl group (Table 1), indicate that the former ones are not the products of in-source degradation. In other cyanobactins, the number of Pre groups also varied depending on the peptide. Doubly prenylated cyanobactin, virenamide A, was reported from *D. virens* [12], while monoprenylated AEG-B, AEG-C, viridisamide A [34] and virenamide B and C [12] were identified in *M. aeruginosa* PCC9432, *O. nigro viridis* PCC7112 and *D. virens*, respectively. Prenyl groups at both C- and N-terminus were found in muscoride A and B from *N. muscorum* IAM M-14, *Nostoc* sp. PCC7906 and *Nostoc* sp. UMCC0398 [36,37].

Due to the chromatographic behaviour of AEG671, which allowed for the isolation of the peptide (1 mg) as a pure compound, the structural analyses with application of Nuclear Magnetic Resonance (NMR) were possible. Unfortunately, under the chromatographic conditions used in the current study, the majority of the detected aeruginosamides were poorly separated. They occurred in the chromatograms as broad peaks or/and co-eluted with other components of *Limnoraphis* extract. The NMR analyses of the isolated AEG671 confirmed the correctness of structure elucidation performed based on the MS/MS fragmentation pattern of pseudomolecular ion. The ^{1}H NMR spectrum of the studied compound displayed a typical pattern of a peptide. The Correlation Spectroscopy COSY, Total Correlation Spectroscopy TOCSY and Heteronuclear Multiple Bond Correlation HMBC data (Figures S14–S19) allowed for the identification of the residues in AER671 as Dma (Dma = 1, 1-dimethylallyl), Phe, Phe, Pro, Pyr and TzlCOOMe (Table 2, Figure 6). Proton and carbon chemical shifts unambiguously showed that the prenyl group in the studied compound was in reverse prenyl, 1, 1-dimethylallyl form.

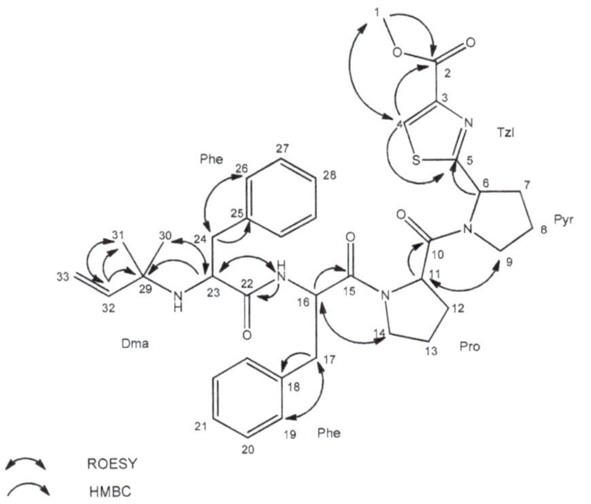

Figure 6. Key Rotation Frame Nuclear Overhauser Effect Spectroscopy ROESY and Heteronuclear Multiple Bond Coherence HMBC correlations for aeruginosamide AEG671.

The signals occurring in the aromatic region of the spectrum (δ_H 7.1–7.5 ppm) and the TOCSY interaction between 19 (26), 20 (27) and 21 (28) protons were indicative of the presence of two aromatic phenylalanine residues in the molecule. The existence of proline residue and pyrrolidine ring was confirmed by their characteristic spin systems in the TOCSY spectrum. HMBC correlation of proton 6 (δ_H 5.32 ppm) to thiazole carbon 5 (δ_C 173.4 ppm) confirmed the connection of Pyr to Tzl ring. The presence of methyl thiazole-carboxylate was shown by characteristic proton (δ_H 3.81 ppm) and carbon (δ_C 51.1 ppm) chemical shifts and HMBC correlation of methyl protons 1 (δ_H 3.81 ppm) to carbon 2 (δ_C 160.3 ppm), and by HMBC and Heteronuclear Single Quantum Correlation HSQC of proton 4 (δ_H 8.43 ppm) to carbons 2 (δ_C 160.3 ppm), 5 (δ_C 173.4 ppm), and 4 (δ_C 128.0 ppm).

Table 2. Nuclear Magnetic Resonance NMR Spectroscopic Data (500 MHz, dimethyl sulfoxide-d_6 DMSO-d_6) for aeruginosamide AEG371 (Dma-Phe-Phe-Pro-Pyr-Tzl-COOMe).

Residue	Position	δ_C, Type	δ_H (J in Hz)	ROESY [a]	HMBC [b]
Tzl-COOMe	1	51.1, CH_3	3.81, s	4	2
	2	160.3, C			
	3	144.5, C			
	4	128.0, CH	8.43, s	1	2, 5
	5	173.4, C			
Pyr	6	57.5, CH	5.32, dd (8.2, 2.4)		
	7	30.5, CH_2	2.05, m 2.27, m		5
	8	23.3, CH_2	1.87, m 1.96, m		
	9	45.9, CH_2	3.70, m	11	
	10	169.7, C			
Pro	11	56.7, CH	4.68, brs	9	10
	12	27.1, CH_2	1.81, m 2.20, m		
	13	23.7, CH_2	2.04, m		
	14	46.0, CH_2	3.50, m 3.66, m	16	
	15	168.2, C			
Phe	16	50.0, CH	4.77, brs	14	15, 18
	17	36.1, CH_2	2.76, dd (14.1, 8.8) 2.97, dd (14.1, 4.3)	19	15, 16, 18
	18	136.3, C			
	19	128.6, CH	7.11, d (7.1)	17	
	20	127.1, CH	7.23, m		
	21	125.3, CH	7.18, m		
	NH(1)		8.18, d (8.9)	23	22
Phe	22	173.3, C			
	23	57.1, CH	3.03, dd (9.0, 4.2)	30, NH(1)	29
	24	39.6, CH_2	2.35, dd (13.3, 9.0) 2.67, dd (13.3, 4.1)	26	22, 23, 25
	25	137.4, C			
	26	128.6, CH	7.11, d (7.1)	24	
	27	127.1, CH	7.23, m		
	28	125.4, CH	7.18, m		
	NH(2)				
Dma [c]	29	53.2, C			
	30	24.7, CH_3	0.79, s	23	
	31	26.6, CH_3	0.76, s	32	
	32	144.9, CH	5.26, dd (17.5, 10.7)	31	29, 31
	33	110.9, CH_2	4.72, m		

[a] ROESY Rotation Frame Nuclear Overhauser Effect Spectroscopy; [b] HMBC correlations are given from proton(s) stated to the indicated carbon atom; [c] Dma: 1,1-dimethylallyl.

Apart from reversed prenyl as present in AEG671, cyanobactins can also contain a forward prenylated N-terminus (e.g., AEG-A [28] and virenamide A [12]), as well as, a forward C-, and reverse prenylated N-terminus (muscoride A [36]) or forward prenylated both C- and N-termini (muscoride B [37]).

Protein prenylation is an important posttranslational modification which increases the lipophilicity and affinity of compounds for biological membranes [39–41]. Prenylation also increases the biological activity of natural products [42,43]. The cytotoxic activities of prenylated licoflavone C and isobavachinas from plants, as well as their non-prenylated analogues (apigenin, liquiritigenin), were examined against glioma (C6) and rat hepatoma (H4IIE) cells. The prenylated compounds showed pronounced cytotoxicity against both types of cells while their non-prenylated analogues were weakly active [42].

The activity of cyanobactins and cyanobactin-like peptides has been tested against bladder carcinoma (T24), colon adenocarcinoma (HT29), lung carcinoma (A549) and murine leukemia (P388) cell lines, proving the pharmacological potential of these compounds [12–17]. Cyanobactins also showed multidrug-resistance reversing activity [44].

The existing knowledge about the activity of aeruginosamides is scarce. To date, only mild cytotoxic effects of aeruginosamide A against human ovarian tumor (A2780) and human leukemia (K562) cells have been reported [28]. In our work, the cytotoxic activity of three chromatographically separated samples labelled as A, B and C, was tested against T47D cancer cells. The sample marked as A contained AEG671, sample B contained partially separated AEG681a and, in sample C, a mixture of AEG681a and AEG667 was present. After 24-h exposure, sample B containing partially separated AEG681a with unknown residue in position 1 (residue mass 205) reduced the relative cell viability to 4.2% ± 0.5% at 200 µg mL^{-1}. Sample C, containing a mixture of AEG681a and AEG667 (with MeHTyr^1), reduced the relative cell viability to 21% ± 1.2% at 200 µg mL^{-1}. These effects were dose dependent. No activity was observed for Phe^1 containing AEG671 present in sample A. Unfortunately, the cytotoxic peptides with the unidentified residues are produced by *Limnoraphis* sp. CCNP1324 in minute amounts (Table 1), which seriously restricts the ability to perform more detailed structural analyses with the application of NMR technique.

The vast structural diversity of AEGs, as well as the cytotoxic activity of some of the variants, create an opportunity for more detailed studies on the structure-activity relationship. Several cyanobacterial peptides are already in clinical or pre-clinical trials as potent anti-cancer agents [45]. The most successful was the development of Auristatine (brentuximab vedotin), a synthetic analogue of dolastatin 10 isolated from *Dolabella auricularia*, but actually produced by the cyanobacterium *Symploca* sp. [46]. This microtubule-impacting agent was approved by the Food and Drug Administration (FDA), and is globally used in the treatment of Hodgkin's lymphoma [47].

3. Materials and Methods

Limnoraphis sp. CCNP1324 was isolated from the Puck Bay in the Southern Baltic Sea (54.45 N, 18.30 E) by Dr. Justyna Kobos in 2012. The strain was obtained from the Culture Collection of Northern Poland (CCNP) at the University of Gdańsk and grown in F/2 medium (7 PSU), at 22 °C ± 0.5, with constant illumination (10 µM photons m^{-2} s^{-1}) provided by standard cool white fluorescent lamps.

3.1. Extraction and Isolation

Freeze-dried *Limnoraphis* CCNP1324 cells were homogenized using mortar and pestle. The ground cyanobacterial biomass (10 mg) was extracted with 75% methanol in MilliQ water (1 mL) by vortexing (5 min). The sample was then centrifuged (10,000× g; 15 min; 4 °C) and the content of aeruginosamides in the obtained supernatant was analyzed using LC-MS/MS.

For fractionation and isolation of aeruginosamides, the homogenized biomass (20 g) was extracted twice with 75% methanol in MilliQ water (2 × 500 mL) by vortexing (20 min). After centrifugation (4000× g; 15 min; 4 °C), the supernatants were combined and diluted with MilliQ water, so that the final concentration of MeOH in the extract was <10%. For flash and preparative chromatography a Shimadzu HPLC system model LC-20AP (Shimadzu, Canby, OR, USA) equipped with isocratic and binary pumps, a fraction collector and photodiode array detector (PDA) was used. PDA operated in a range from 190 nm to 500 nm and, during all chromatographic runs, the absorbance at 210 nm and 280 nm was recorded.

To perform flash chromatography, the aqueous methanol extract (MeOH < 10%) was loaded onto a preconditioned 120 g SNAP KP-C_{18}-HS cartridge (Biotage Uppsala, Sweden) using an isocratic pump, at a flow rate of 15 mL min^{-1}. Components of the extract were separated with a mixture of a mobile phase composed of MilliQ water (A_1) and 100% MeOH (B_1). The gradient started at 10% B_1 and went to 30% B_1 within 20 min. After 90 min, the content of B_1 increased to 70% and was kept at that level for 10 min before increasing to 100% B_1 within the next 30 min. The flow rate of the eluent was 20 mL m^{-1} and 50 mL fractions were collected.

AEGs-containing flash fractions, eluted with 86–93% B_1 (Prep1), and 58–68% B_1 (Prep2), were combined and concentrated in a centrifugal vacuum concentrator (MiVac, SP Scientific, Ipswich, UK). Dried samples (Prep1 and Prep2) were first solubilized using 0.6 mL of 60% MeOH, followed by 0.6 mL of 20% MeOH. After centrifugation, the supernatants were loaded onto a preparative column using the Rheodyne injector. The sample components were separated on a Jupiter Proteo C_{12} column (250 × 21.2 mm; 4 µm; 90 Å) (Phenomenex, Aschaffenburg, Germany) with a mobile phase composed of 5% acetonitrile in MilliQ water (A_2) and acetonitrile (B_2), both with the addition of 0.1% formic acid. During the separation process the flow rate was 20 mL m^{-1} and 4 mL fractions were collected.

In the case of fractions 86–93% (Prep1), the gradient started at 20% B_2, then went to 30% B_2 in 25 min, after 10 min B_2 reached 90%. After another 2 min, B_2 increased to 100% and was kept at that level for 13 min. Fractions eluted with 25–27% B_2 (vials 75–103) and containing an isolated single peak were pulled, vacuum concentrated and marked as sample A (1 mg). Fractions eluted with 23–25% B_2 (vials 40–74), which also corresponded to a single peak in HPLC-PDA chromatogram, were pulled, evaporated to dryness and marked as sample B (0.9 mg).

The preparative separation of flash fractions 58–68% B_1 (Prep2) started at 15% B_2 and went to 30% B_2 in 20 min, after 10 min B_2 reached 90%. After another 2 min, B_2 increased to 100% and was kept at that level for 8 min. Fractions eluted with 24–27% B_2 (with AEGs) were prepared as described above and subjected to further separation. In the subsequent run, the gradient started at 5% B_2 and went to 40% B_2 in 20 min, after 5 min B_2 reached 100% and was kept at that level for 5 min. Fractions eluted with 27–37% B_2, containing a single peak were pulled evaporated to dryness and marked as sample C (1.2 mg). The samples A, B and C were subjected to LC-MS/MS analyses and cytotoxicity assays. For sample A, the NMR analyses were additionally performed.

3.2. LC-MS/MS Analysis

The contents of cyanobacterial extracts, fractions and isolated compounds, were analyzed with the application of an Agilent 1200 (Agilent Technologies, Waldboronn, Germany) HPLC system coupled with a hybrid triple quadrupole/linear ion trap mass spectrometer (QTRAP5500, Applied Biosystems, Sciex, Concorde, ON, Canada). For peptide separation a Zorbax Eclipse XDB-C_{18} column (4.6 × 150 mm; 5 µm) (Agilent Technologies, Santa Clara, CA, USA) was used. The mobile phase was composed of a mixture of 5% acetonitrile in MilliQ water (A_2) and acetonitrile (B_2), both with the addition of 0.1% formic acid. A gradient elution at 0.6 mL min^{-1} was applied. The system operated in positive mode with a turbo ion spray (550 °C; 5.5 kV). The non-targeted information-dependent acquisition (IDA) mode was applied to screen the content of the samples. Fragmentation spectra of ions within the m/z range 400–1000, and signal intensity above 500,000 cps were collected, at a collision energy of 60 ± 20 eV. The structures of aeruginosamides were additionally characterized using targeted enhanced product ion (EPI) mode.

3.3. NMR Analysis

The 1D ^{1}H NMR and 2D homo- and heteronuclear NMR (COSY, TOCSY, ROESY, HSQC, and HMBC) were acquired with the application of a Varian Unity Inova 500 spectrometer (500 MHz). Spectra were recorded in dimethyl sulfoxide-d_6 (DMSO-d_6). NMR data were processed and analyzed by TopSpin (Bruker, Billerica, MA, USA) and SPARKY software (3.114, Goddard and Kneller, freeware (https://www.cgl.ucsf.edu/home/sparky).

3.4. Cytotoxicity Assays

The cytotoxic activity of the isolated and identified AEG671 as well as the activity of two other samples containing AEGs as the main components was tested. For the purpose the 3-(4,5-dimethylthiazol-2-yl)-2,5-diphenyltetrazolium-bromide (MTT) assays with the application of a human breast adenocarcinoma cell line T47D (Merck KGaA, Darmstadt, Germany) were performed as described by Felczykowska et al. [48] and Szubert et al. [49]. T47D cells were plated at 1×10^4 cells per well of 96-well plate containing RPMI1640 (Carl Roth GmbH) medium supplemented with 10% fetal bovine serum (Merck KGaA) and penicillin-streptomycin solution (50 u and 0.05 mg per 1 mL of medium respectively; Merck KGaA) (24 h at 37 °C, 5% CO_2). The cytotoxic effects of tested samples dissolved in 1% DMSO, at final concentrations 25, 50, 100 and 200 µg ml^{-1} (in culture medium) were examined after 24 h incubation (37 °C, 5% CO_2) using a microplate reader (Spectramax i3, Molecular Devices, LLC. San Jose, CA, USA). Cell viability was calculated as the ratio of the mean absorbance value, for the six replicates containing the samples, to the mean absorbance of the six replicates of the corresponding solvent control, and expressed as a percentage. The results were considered as significant when cell viability decreased below 50%.

4. Conclusions

In this work, *Limnoraphis* sp. CCNP1324 was revealed to be a new producer of aeruginosamides. Some of the peptides were cytotoxic against a breast cancer cell line. The cytotoxic activity of these compounds is probably determined by the unknown amino acid residues in *N*-terminal position. Unfortunately, the data collected with MS/MS were insufficient to resolve their structures. LC-MS/MS analyses of samples are key elements of bioassay-guided fractionation and structure characterization of bioactive metabolites. Due to high sensitivity and selectivity, trace amounts of the compounds in complex matrices can be detected. However, like any technique, it has also some limitations. The unequivocal elucidation of peptide structure with unknown modifications is impossible or bears a high risk of error. Therefore, in our future work, the chromatographic conditions have to be further optimized, to isolate the bioactive peptides in sufficient amounts for structural analysis by NMR.

Supplementary Materials: The following are available online at http://www.mdpi.com/1660-3397/18/9/446/s1, Figures S1–S13. Enhanced product ion mass spectrum of aeruginosamides: AER595, AEG603, AEG657, AER667, AER681a, AER681b, AER683, AER685, AEG705, AEG707, AEG721, AER735, AER749, Figure S14. ^{1}H NMR Spectrum of aeruginosamide AEG671 in DMSO-d_6, Figure S15. COSY Spectrum of aeruginosamide AEG671 in DMSO-d_6, Figure S16. TOCSY Spectrum of aeruginosamide AEG671 in DMSO-d_6, Figure S17. ROESY Spectrum of aeruginosamide AEG671 in DMSO-d_6, Figure S18. HSQC Spectrum of aeruginosamide AEG671 in DMSO-d_6, Figure S19. HMBC Spectrum of aeruginosamide AEG671 in DMSO-d_6.

Author Contributions: Conceptualization, M.C., A.K. and H.M.-M.; methodology, M.C., H.M.-M.; formal analysis, M.C., K.S.; investigation M.C. (HPLC and LC-MS/MS analysis, MTT assays), K.S. (MTT assays), E.W. (NMR analysis), H.M.-M. (LC-MS/MS analysis); writing—original draft preparation, M.C.; writing—review and editing, M.C., K.S., E.W., A.K., H.M.-M.; visualization, M.C.; funding acquisition, A.K., H.M.-M. All authors have read and agreed to the published version of the manuscript.

Funding: This study was financially supported by the National Science Centre in Poland (project number NCN 2016/21/B/NZ9/02304 to HMM), and by the statutory programme of the Institute of Oceanology, PAS (grant No.II.3).

Conflicts of Interest: The authors declare no conflict of interest.

References

1. Burja, A.M.; Banaigs, B.; Abou-Mansour, E.; Burgess, J.G.; Wright, P.C. Marine cyanobacteria—A prolific source of natural products. *Tetrahedron* **2001**, *57*, 9347–9377. [CrossRef]
2. Chlipala, G.E.; Mo, S.; Orjala, J. Chemodiversity in freshwater and terrestrial cyanobacteria—A source for drug discovery. *Curr. Cancer Drug Targets* **2011**, *12*, 1654–1673. [CrossRef] [PubMed]
3. Dittmann, E.; Gugger, M.; Sivonen, K.; Fewer, D.P. Natural product biosynthetic diversity and comparative genomics of the cyanobacteria. *Trends Microbiol.* **2015**, *23*, 642–652. [CrossRef] [PubMed]
4. Shah, S.A.A.; Akhter, N.; Auckloo, B.N.; Khan, I.; Lu, Y.; Wang, K.; Wu, B.; Guo, Y. Structural diversity, biological properties and applications of natural products from cyanobacteria: A review. *Mar. Drugs* **2017**, *15*, 354. [CrossRef]
5. Seddek, N.H.; Fawzy, M.A.; El-Said, W.A.; Ahmed, M.M.R. Evaluation of antimicrobial, antioxidant and cytotoxic activities and characterization of bioactive substances from freshwater blue-green algae. *Glob. NEST J.* **2019**, *21*, 329–337. [CrossRef]
6. Sivonen, K.; Leikoski, N.; Fewer, D.P.; Jokela, J. Cyanobactins—Ribosomal cyclic peptides produced by cyanobacteria. *Appl. Microbiol. Biotechnol.* **2010**, *86*, 1213–1225. [CrossRef]
7. Martins, J.; Vasconcelos, V. Cyanobactins from cyanobacteria: Current genetic and chemical state of knowledge. *Mar. Drugs* **2015**, *13*, 6910–6946. [CrossRef]
8. Donia, M.S.; Ravel, J.; Schmidt, E.W. A global assembly line for cyanobactins. *Nat. Chem. Biol.* **2008**, *4*, 341–343. [CrossRef]
9. Gu, W.; Dong, S.H.; Sarkar, S.; Nair, S.K.; Schmidt, E.W. The biochemistry and structural biology of cyanobactin pathways: Enabling combinatorial biosynthesis. *Methods Enzymol.* **2018**, *604*, 113–163. [CrossRef]
10. Arnison, P.G.; Bibb, M.J.; Bierbaum, G.; Bowers, A.A.; Bugni, T.S.; Bulaj, G.; Camarero, J.A.; Campopiano, D.J.; Challis, G.L.; Clardy, J.; et al. Ribosomally synthesized and post-translationally modified peptide natural products: Overview and recommendations for a universal nomenclature. *Nat. Prod. Rep.* **2013**, *30*, 108–160. [CrossRef]
11. McIntosh, J.A.; Donia, M.S.; Nair, S.K.; Schmidt, E.W. Enzymatic basis of ribosomal peptide prenylation in cyanobacteria. *J. Am. Chem. Soc.* **2011**, *133*, 13698–13705. [CrossRef] [PubMed]
12. Carroll, A.R.; Feng, Y.; Bowden, B.F.; Coll, J.C. Studies of Australian ascidians. 5. Virenamides A–C, new cytotoxic linear peptides from the colonial didemnid ascidian *Diplosoma Virens*. *J. Org. Chem.* **1996**, *61*, 4059–4061. [CrossRef] [PubMed]
13. Wesson, K.J.; Hamann, M. Keenamide A, a bioactive cyclic peptide from the marine mollusc *Pleurobranchus forskalii*. *J. Nat. Prod.* **1996**, *59*, 631–659. [CrossRef]
14. Rudi, A.; Aknin, M.; Gaydou, E.M.; Kashman, Y. Four new cytotoxic cyclic hexa- and heptapeptides from the marine ascidian *Didemnum molle*. *Tetrahedron* **1998**, *54*, 13203–13210. [CrossRef]
15. Ishida, K.; Nakagawa, H.; Murakami, M. Microcyclamide, a cytotoxic cyclic hexapeptide from the cyanobacterium *Microcystis aeruginosa*. *J. Nat. Prod.* **2000**, *63*, 1315–1317. [CrossRef] [PubMed]
16. Ireland, C.M.; Durso, A.R., Jr.; Newman, R.A.; Hacker, M.P. Antineoplastic cyclic peptides from the marine tunicate *Lissoclinum patella*. *J. Org. Chem.* **1982**, *47*, 1807–1811. [CrossRef]
17. Degnan, B.M.; Hawkins, C.J.; Lavin, M.F.; McCaffrey, E.J.; Parry, D.L.; van den Brenk, A.L.; Watterst, D.J. New cyclic peptides with cytotoxic activity from the ascidian *Lissoclinum patella*. *J. Med. Chem.* **1989**, *32*, 1349–1354. [CrossRef] [PubMed]
18. Linington, R.G.; Gonzàles, J.; Ureña, L.-D.; Romero, L.I.; Ortega-Barria, E.; Gerwick, W.H. Venturamides A and B: Antimalarial constituents of the Panamanian marine cyanobacterium *Oscillatoria* sp. *J. Nat. Prod.* **2007**, *70*, 397–401. [CrossRef]
19. Todorova, A.K.; Jüttner, F.; Linden, A.; Plüss, T.; von Philipsborn, W. Nostocyclamide: A new macrocyclic, thiazole-containing allelochemical from *Nostoc* sp. 31 (cyanobacteria). *J. Org. Chem.* **1995**, *60*, 7891–7895. [CrossRef]
20. Jüttner, F.; Todorova, A.K.; Walch, N.; von Philipsborn, W. Nostocyclamide M: A cyanobacterial cyclic peptide with allelopathic activity from *Nostoc* 31. *Phytochemistry* **2001**, *57*, 613–619. [CrossRef]
21. Ireland, C.; Scheuer, P.J. Ulicyclamide and ulithiacyclamide, two new small peptides from a marine Tunicate. *J. Am. Chem. Soc.* **1980**, *102*, 5688–5691. [CrossRef]

22. Long, P.F.; Dunlap, W.C.; Battershill, C.N.; Jaspars, M. Shotgun cloning and heterologous expression of the patellamide gene cluster as a strategy to achieving sustained metabolite production. *Chem. Biol. Chem.* **2005**, *6*, 1760–1765. [CrossRef] [PubMed]
23. Schmidt, E.W.; Nelson, J.T.; Rasko, D.A.; Sudek, S.; Eisen, J.A.; Haygood, M.G.; Ravel, J. Patellamide A and C biosynthesis by a microcin-like pathway in *Prochloron didemni*, the cyanobacterial symbiont of *Lissoclinum patella*. *Proc. Natl. Acad. Sci. USA* **2005**, *102*, 7315–7320. [CrossRef] [PubMed]
24. Leikoski, N.; Fewer, D.P.; Jokela, J.; Wahlsten, M.; Rouhiainen, L.; Sivonen, K. Highly diverse cyanobactins in strains of the genus *Anabaena*. *Appl. Environ. Microbiol.* **2010**, *76*, 701–709. [CrossRef] [PubMed]
25. Donia, M.S.; Schmidt, E.W. Linking chemistry and genetics in the growing cyanobactin natural products family. *Chem. Biol.* **2011**, *18*, 508–519. [CrossRef]
26. McIntosh, J.A.; Lin, Z.; Tianero, M.D.; Schmidt, E.W. Aestuaramides, a natural library of cyanobactin cyclic peptides resulting from isoprene-derived Claisen rearrangements. *ACS Chem. Biol.* **2013**, *8*, 877–883. [CrossRef]
27. Ishida, K.; Matsuda, H.; Murakami, M.; Yamaguchi, K. Kawaguchipeptin B, an antibacterial cyclic undecapeptide from the cyanobacterium *Microcystis aeruginosa*. *J. Nat. Prod.* **1997**, *60*, 724–726. [CrossRef]
28. Lawton, L.A.; Morris, L.A.; Jaspars, M. A bioactive modified peptide, aeruginosamide, isolated from the cyanobacterium *Microcystis aeruginosa*. *J. Org. Chem.* **1999**, *64*, 5329–5332. [CrossRef]
29. Gesner-Apter, S.; Carmeli, S. Three novel metabolites from a bloom of the cyanobacterium *Microcystis* sp. *Tetrahedron* **2008**, *64*, 6628–6634. [CrossRef]
30. Portmann, C.; Blom, J.F.; Kaiser, M.; Brun, R.; Jüttner, F.; Gademann, K. Isolation of aerucyclamides C and D and structure revision of microcyclamide 7806A: Heterocyclic ribosomal peptides from *Microcystis aeruginosa* PCC 7806 and their antiparasite evaluation. *J. Nat. Prod.* **2008**, *71*, 1891–1896. [CrossRef]
31. Crnkovic, C.M.; Braesel, J.; Krunic, A.; Eustáquio, A.S.; Orjala, J. Scytodecamide from the cultured *Scytonema* sp. UIC 10036 expands the chemical and genetic diversity of cyanobactins. *ChemBioChem* **2020**, *21*, 845–852. [CrossRef] [PubMed]
32. Martins, J.; Leikoski, N.; Wahlsten, M.; Azevedo, J.; Antunes, J.; Jokela, J.; Sivonen, K.; Vasconcelos, V.; Fewer, D.P.; Leão, P.N. Sphaerocyclamide, a prenylated cyanobactin from the cyanobacterium *Sphaerospermopsis* sp. LEGE 00249. *Sci. Rep.* **2018**, *8*, 14537. [CrossRef] [PubMed]
33. Leikoski, N.; Fewer, D.P.; Sivonen, K. Widespread occurrence and lateral transfer of the cyanobactin biosynthesis gene cluster in cyanobacteria. *Appl. Environ. Microbiol.* **2009**, *75*, 853–857. [CrossRef] [PubMed]
34. Leikoski, N.; Liu, L.; Jokela, J.; Wahlsten, M.; Gugger, M.; Calteau, A.; Permi, P.; Kerfeld, C.A.; Sivonen, K.; Fewer, D.P. Genome mining expands the chemical diversity of the cyanobactin family to include highly modified linear peptides. *Chem. Biol.* **2013**, *20*, 1033–1043. [CrossRef] [PubMed]
35. Donia, M.S.; Schmidt, E.W. Comprehensive natural products II chemistry and biology. In *Cyanobactins—Ubiquitous Cyanobacterial Ribosomal Peptide Metabolites*; Elsevier: Oxford, UK, 2010; pp. 539–558.
36. Nagatsu, A.; Kajitani, H.; Sakakibara, J. Muscoride A: A new oxazole peptide alkaloid from freshwater cyanobacterium *Nostoc muscorum*. *Tetrahedron Lett.* **1995**, *36*, 4097–4100. [CrossRef]
37. Mattila, A.; Andsten, R.M.; Jumppanen, M.; Assante, M.; Jokela, J.; Wahlsten, M.; Mikula, K.M.; Sigindere, C.; Kwak, D.H.; Gugger, M.; et al. Biosynthesis of the bis-prenylated alkaloids muscoride A and B. *ACS Chem. Biol.* **2019**, *14*, 2683–2690. [CrossRef]
38. Ziemert, N.; Ishida, K.; Liaimer, A.; Hertweck, C.; Dittmann, E. Ribosomal synthesis of tricyclic depsipeptides in bloom-forming cyanobacteria. *Angew. Chem. Int. Ed. Engl.* **2008**, *47*, 7756–7759. [CrossRef]
39. Botta, B.; Vitali, A.; Menendez, P.; Misiti, D.; Monache, G. Prenylated flavonoids: Pharmacology and biotechnology. *Curr. Med. Chem.* **2005**, *12*, 717–739. [CrossRef]
40. Wang, M.; Casey, P.J. Protein prenylation: Unique fats make their mark on biology. *Nat. Rev. Mol. Cell Biol.* **2016**, *17*, 110–122. [CrossRef]
41. Wong, C.P.; Awakawa, T.; Nakashima, Y.; Mori, T.; Zhu, Q.; Liu, X.; Abe, I. Two distinct substrate binding modes for the normal and reverse prenylation of hapalindoles by the prenyltransferase AmbP3. *Angew. Chem. Int. Ed. Engl.* **2018**, *57*, 560–563. [CrossRef]
42. Wätjen, W.; Weber, N.; Lou, Y.J.; Wang, Z.Q.; Chovolou, Y.; Kampkötter, A.; Kahl, R.; Proksch, P. Prenylation enhances cytotoxicity of apigenin and liquiritigenin in rat H4IIE hepatoma and C6 glioma cells. *Food Chem. Toxicol.* **2007**, *45*, 119–124. [CrossRef] [PubMed]

43. López-Ogalla, J.; García-Palomero, E.; Sánchez-Quesada, J.; Rubio, L.; Delgado, E.; García, P.; Medina, M.; Castro, A.; Muñoz, P. Bioactive prenylated phenyl derivatives derived from marine natural products: Novel scaffolds for the design of BACE inhibitors. *Med. Chem. Commun.* **2014**, *5*, 474. [CrossRef]
44. Fu, X.; Do, T.; Schmitz, F.J.; Andrusevich, V.; Engel, M.H. New cyclic peptides from the ascidian *Lissoclinum patella*. *J. Nat. Prod.* **1998**, *61*, 1547–1551. [CrossRef] [PubMed]
45. Wang, Y.-J.; Li, Y.-Y.; Liu, X.-Y.; Lu, X.-L.; Cao, X.; Jiao, B.-H. Marine antibody-drug conjugates: Design strategies and research progress. *Mar. Drugs* **2017**, *15*, 18. [CrossRef] [PubMed]
46. Luesch, H.; Moore, R.E.; Paul, V.J.; Mooberry, S.L.; Corbett, T.H. Isolation of dolastatin 10 from the marine cyanobacterium Symploca species VP642 and total stereochemistry and biological evaluation of its analogue symplostatin 1. *J. Nat. Prod.* **2001**, *64*, 907–910. [CrossRef]
47. Senter, P.D.; Sievers, E.L. The discovery and development of brentuximab vedotin for use in relapsed hodgkin lymphoma and systemic anaplastic large cell lymphoma. *Nat. Biotechnol.* **2012**, *30*, 631–637. [CrossRef] [PubMed]
48. Felczykowska, A.; Pawlik, A.; Mazur-Marzec, H.; Toruńska-Sitarz, A.; Narajczyk, M.; Richert, M.; Węgrzyn, G.; Herman-Antosiewicz, A. Selective inhibition of cancer cells' proliferation by compounds included in extracts from Baltic Sea cyanobacteria. *Toxicon* **2015**, *108*, 1–10. [CrossRef]
49. Szubert, K.; Wiglusz, M.; Mazur-Marzec, H. Bioactive metabolites produced by *Spirulina subsalsa* from the Baltic Sea. *Oceanologia* **2018**, *60*, 245–255. [CrossRef]

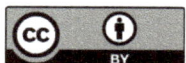

© 2020 by the authors. Licensee MDPI, Basel, Switzerland. This article is an open access article distributed under the terms and conditions of the Creative Commons Attribution (CC BY) license (http://creativecommons.org/licenses/by/4.0/).

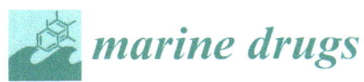

Article

New Thiodiketopiperazine and 3,4-Dihydroisocoumarin Derivatives from the Marine-Derived Fungus *Aspergillus terreus*

Jing-Shuai Wu [1,2], Xiao-Hui Shi [1,2], Guang-Shan Yao [1,2,3], Chang-Lun Shao [1,2], Xiu-Mei Fu [1,2], Xiu-Li Zhang [1,2], Hua-Shi Guan [1,2,*] and Chang-Yun Wang [1,2,*]

1. Key Laboratory of Marine Drugs, The Ministry of Education of China, School of Medicine and Pharmacy, Institute of Evolution & Marine Biodiversity, Ocean University of China, Qingdao 266003, China; wujingshuai0110@sina.cn (J.-S.W.); 13061461893@163.com (X.-H.S.); ygshan@126.com (G.-S.Y.); shaochanglun@163.com (C.-L.S.); fuxiumei92@163.com (X.-M.F.); xiulizhang@ouc.edu.cn (X.-L.Z.)
2. Laboratory for Marine Drugs and Bioproducts, Qingdao National Laboratory for Marine Science and Technology, Qingdao 266237, China
3. Institute of Oceanography, Minjiang University, Fuzhou 350108, China
* Correspondence: hsguan@ouc.edu.cn (H.-S.G.); changyun@ouc.edu.cn (C.-Y.W.); Tel.: +86-53282031667 (H.-S.G.); +86-53282031536 (C.-Y.W.)

Received: 7 February 2020; Accepted: 24 February 2020; Published: 26 February 2020

Abstract: *Aspergillus terreus* has been reported to produce many secondary metabolites that exhibit potential bioactivities, such as antibiotic, hypoglycemic, and lipid-lowering activities. In the present study, two new thiodiketopiperazines, emestrins L (**1**) and M (**2**), together with five known analogues (**3**–**7**), and five known dihydroisocoumarins (**8**–**12**), were obtained from the marine-derived fungus *Aspergillus terreus* RA2905. The structures of the new compounds were elucidated by analysis of the comprehensive spectroscopic data, including high-resolution electrospray ionization mass spectrometry (HRESIMS), one-dimensional (1D) and two-dimensional (2D) nuclear magnetic resonance (NMR), and electronic circular dichroism (ECD) data. This is the first time that the spectroscopic data of compounds **3**, **8**, and **9** have been reported. Compound **3** displayed antibacterial activity against *Pseudomonas aeruginosa* (minimum inhibitory concentration (MIC) = 32 μg/mL) and antifungal activity against *Candida albicans* (MIC = 32 μg/mL). In addition, compound **3** exhibited an inhibitory effect on protein tyrosine phosphatase 1 B (PTP1B), an important hypoglycemic target, with an inhibitory concentration (IC)$_{50}$ value of 12.25 μM.

Keywords: marine-derived fungus; *Aspergillus terreus*; thiodiketopiperazines; dihydroisocoumarins

1. Introduction

Marine fungi, and particularly the genus *Aspergillus*, have proven to be a prolific source of structurally novel and biologically active secondary metabolites that play an eminent role in drug discovery progress [1,2]. A wide array of bioactive compounds, including xanthones, alkaloids, cyclic peptides, and terpenes, have been isolated from marine-derived fungi of *Aspergillus* species [3,4]. Among them, thiodiketopiperazines alkaloids (TDKPs) are an important class of secondary metabolites divided into nearly twenty distinct families, and characterized by the presence of a diketopiperazine core featuring thiomethyl groups and/or transannular sulfide bridges [5]. These compounds have been reported to exhibit a broad range of biological properties, including immunosuppressive [6], cytotoxic [7], antibacterial [8], antiviral [9], and anti-angiogenic activities [10]. Specifically, *Aspergillus terreus* has been reported to produce diverse secondary metabolites that display multiple bioactivities, such as antibiotic, hypoglycemic, and lipid-lowering activities [3,4,11].

During our ongoing research for novel bioactive secondary metabolites from marine-derived *Aspergillus* species, we found a series of bioactive natural products with antifungal, antibacterial, antiviral, antifouling, and cytotoxic activities [12]. In the present study, the chemical investigation of the ethyl acetate (EtOAc) extract of *Aspergillus terreus* RA2905, isolated from the fresh inner tissue of the sea hare *Aplysia pulmonica*, resulted in the identification of two new thiodiketopiperazines, emestrins L (**1**) and M (**2**), as well as five known analogues (**3**–**7**), and five known dihydroisocoumarins (**8**–**12**) (Figure 1). Herein, we report the isolation, structural determination, and bioactivity evaluation of these compounds.

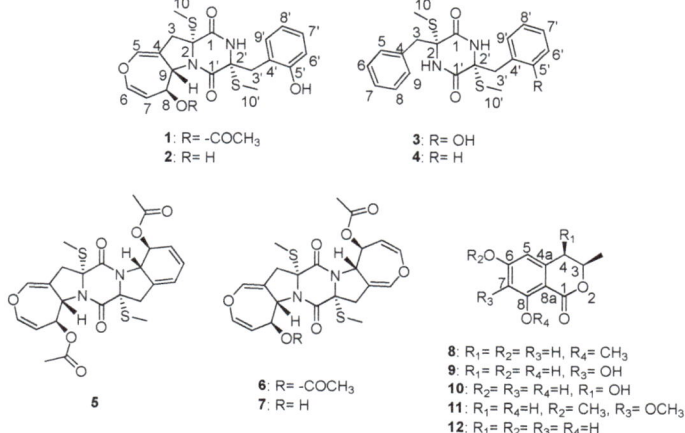

Figure 1. The structures of the compounds.

2. Results

The marine-derived fungus *Aspergillus terreus* RA2905 demonstrated a rapid growth rate on the potato dextrose agar (PDA) plate and produced mature colonies in 3 days. The colonies were characterized by a brown velvety surface (Figure S1). They were cultivated in starch liquid medium at 180 rpm and 28 °C for 7 days. The EtOAc extract (12.5 g) was subjected to column chromatography and semi-preparative high-performance liquid chromatography (HPLC) to yield compounds **1**–**12**, which consisted of two new thiodiketopiperazines, emestrins L (**1**) and M (**2**), five known thiodiketopiperazines, emethacin C (**3**) [13], emethacin B (**4**) [14], bisdethiobis(methylsulfanyl)acetylapoaranotin (**5**) [15], bisdethiobis(methylsulfanyl)acetylaranotin (**6**) [16], and alternarosin A (**7**) [17], and five known dihydroisocoumarins, (3R)-8-methoxy-6-hydroxymellein (**8**) [18], (3R)-6,7,8-trihydroxymellein (**9**) [19], cis-4,6-dihydroxymellein (**10**) [20], (3R)-6,7-dimethoxymellein (**11**) [21], and (3R)-6-hydroxymellein (**12**) [22].

2.1. Structure Elucidation

Emestrin L (**1**) was obtained as a white powder with the molecular formula $C_{22}H_{24}N_2O_6S_2$ established by the HRESIMS spectrum, indicating 12 degrees of unsaturation. The stretch signals at 3600, 3395, 2998, 2913, 1646, 1436, and 1314 cm^{-1} in the infrared (IR) spectrum suggested the presence of aromatic and carbonyl groups in **1**. The ^{1}H NMR spectroscopic data revealed the signal characteristics of the *ortho*-substituted phenyl group (H-6' to H-9') (Table 1), which were supported by the corresponding ^{1}H-^{1}H correlation spectroscopy (COSY) and heteronuclear multiple bond correlation (HMBC) correlations, as shown in Figure 2. A total of 22 carbon atoms, including two thiomethyl carbons (δ_H 2.13, δ_C 14.4; δ_H 2.25, δ_C 13.8), one acetyl methyl (δ_H 1.99, δ_C 21.3), two heteroatom-substituted methane carbons, two methylene carbons, two saturated quaternary carbons (heteroatom-substituted), ten olefinic carbons (seven protonated), and three carbonyl carbons were observed in the ^{13}C NMR spectrum (Table 1). The HMBC correlations from H-10 to C-2, from H-10' to C-2', from H-3 to C-1, and from H-3' to C-1' indicated the presence of a disulfide diketopiperazine skeleton in **1** (Figure 2). The *ortho*-substituted aromatic ring was connected with the diketopiperazine moiety via a methylene bridge of C-3' based on the HMBC correlations from H-3' to C-4'/C-5'/C-9'. The ^{1}H–^{1}H COSY data showed the presence of an isolated spin system corresponding to the C-6–C-7–C-8–C-9 fragment. A 4,5-dihydrooxepine existed in **1** based on the key HMBC correlations from H-5 to C-3/C-6/C-9 and from H-6 to C-5/C-7/C-8, along with the chemical shifts of C-5 (δ_C 137.6), C-6 (δ_C 140.3), and C-9 (δ_C 61.5). The HMBC correlations from H-3 to C-1/C-5/C-9 indicated that the 4,5-dihydrooxepine moiety was located at C-2 of the diketopiperazine core (Figure 2). As the presence of cyclic dipeptide, aromatic ring, 4,5-dihydrooxepine, and the other carbonyl in the molecule occupied 11 degrees of unsaturation, C-9 should be attached to the 2-N atom to form a pyrrolidine ring on the basis of the chemical shifts of C-9 (δ_H 4.79, δ_C 61.5). The carbethoxy was anchored at C-8 on the basis of the HMBC correlation from H-8 to C-11. Collectively, these data permitted the assignment of the planar structure of **1**.

Table 1. ^{1}H Nuclear Magnetic Resonance (NMR) and ^{13}C NMR Data for **1** and **2** [a].

Position	1		2	
	δ_C, Type	δ_H (J in Hz)	δ_C, Type	δ_H (J in Hz)
1	165.0, C		166.6, C	
2	70.1, C		68.9, C	
3	39.9, CH$_2$	2.78, d (15.0)	39.9, CH$_2$	2.74, d (15.0)
		1.98, d (15.0)		1.92, d (15.0)
4	110.4, C		109.5, C	
5	137.6, CH	6.70, t (2.3)	137.2, CH	6.60, t (2.3)
6	140.3, CH	6.44, dd (8.3, 2.3)	138.2, CH	6.28, dd (8.3, 2.3)
7	105.9, CH	4.71, dd (8.3, 2.0)	111.4, CH	4.81, dd (8.3, 2.0)
8	71.5, CH	5.67, dt (7.9, 2.0)	71.8, CH	4.43, dt (7.9, 2.0)
9	61.5, CH	4.79, d (7.9)	64.9, CH	4.54, d (7.9)
10	14.4, CH$_3$	2.13, s	14.4, CH$_3$	2.17, s
11	169.9, C			
12	21.3, CH$_3$	1.99, s		
1'	164.8, C		165.0, C	
2'	68.2, C		68.4, C	
3'	39.1, CH$_2$	3.43, d (13.7)	39.2, CH$_2$	3.45, d (13.7)
		3.19, d (13.7)		3.19, d (13.7)
4'	121.7, C		121.4, C	
5'	156.3, C		156.2, C	
6'	115.8, CH	6.79, dd (8.0, 1.3)	115.7, CH	6.79, dd (8.0, 1.3)
7'	128.8, CH	7.03, td (8.0, 1.7)	128.8, CH	7.04, td (8.0, 1.7)
8'	119.3, CH	6.67, td (7.7, 1.3)	119.2, CH	6.68, dd (7.8, 1.3)
9'	131.7, CH	6.92, dd (7.7, 1.7)	131.8, CH	6.95, dd (7.8, 1.7)
10'	13.8, CH$_3$	2.25, s	14.0, CH$_3$	2.29, s
8-OH				5.44, d (6.0)

[a] 500 MHz for ^{1}H NMR and 125 MHz for ^{13}C NMR in Dimethyl Sulfoxide (DMSO)-d_6.

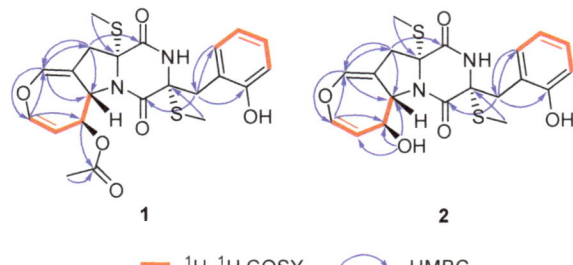

Figure 2. The ^{1}H-^{1}H Correlation Spectroscopy (COSY) and Key Heteronuclear Multiple Bond Correlation (HMBC) Correlations for **1** and **2**.

The coupling constants of $^3J_{\text{H-6–H-7}}$ = 8.3 Hz indicated that the double bond was a Z-configuration. The 7.9 Hz coupling constants between H-8 and H-9 suggested their *anti*-relationship. The nuclear Overhauser effects (NOE) were observed for H-8 and H-10′ when on irradiation of H-10, which demonstrated that they should be on the same face (Figure 3). The absolute configurations of C-2 and C-2′ were assigned as *R* and *R*, respectively, determined by the similar electronic circular dichroism (ECD) data and the same biogenetic pathway as the co-isolated known compound **6** (Figures 4 and 5), for which the absolute configuration was confirmed by X-ray data (Figure S41). Thus, the absolute configurations of **1** were established as 2*R*,2′*R*,8*S*,9*S*.

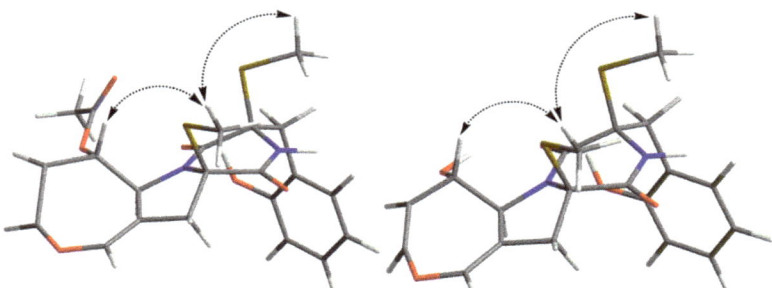

Figure 3. The Nuclear Overhauser Effect (NOE) Correlations for **1** and **2**.

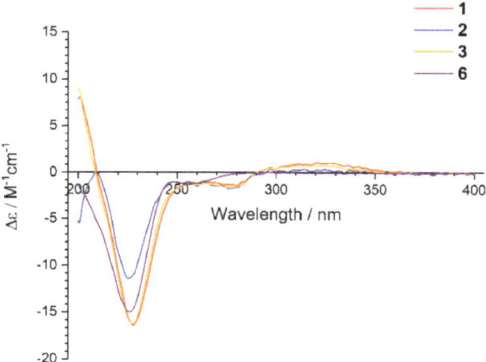

Figure 4. The Electronic Circular Dichroism (ECD) Spectra of **1–3** and **6**.

Emestrin M (**2**) was assigned the molecular formula $C_{20}H_{22}N_2O_5S_2$, with 11 degrees of unsaturation, on the basis of its HRESIMS data, less 42 Da compared with **1**. The ^{1}H and ^{13}C NMR data were very similar to those of **1** (Table 1), which revealed the presence of a thiodiketopiperazine, an *ortho*-substituted phenyl, and a 4,5-dihydrooxepine structure. The main differences were the disappearance of the carbethoxy (δ_H 1.99, δ_C 21.3; δ_C 169.9) in **1**, and the appearance of one hydroxyl (δ_H 5.44). The hydroxyl was anchored at C-8 based on the HMBC correlations from 8-OH to C-7/C-8/C-9. Thus, the planar structure of **2** was established. The similar coupling constants of **2** and **1** between H-6 and H-7, and between H-8 and H-9, respectively, suggested that the relative configurations of the 4,5-dihydrooxepine of **2** were consistent with those of **1** (Figure 3). The absolute configurations of **2** were identical to those of **1** on the basis of the similar ECD data and of the same biogenetic pathway (Figures 4 and 5).

Emethacin C (**3**) was isolated as a white powder. Its molecular formula was defined as $C_{20}H_{22}N_2O_3S_2$ by HRESIMS, with more than 16 Da compared with the known compound emethacin B (**4**). The ^{1}H NMR and ^{13}C NMR spectroscopic data of **3** were closely related to those of **4**, which revealed the presence of a thiodiketopiperazine structure. The distinction was that one aromatic hydrogen in **4** was replaced by one hydroxyl in **3**. The hydroxyl was anchored at C-5' based on the ^{1}H–^{1}H COSY correlations of H-6'/H-7'/H-8'/H-9' and the HMBC correlations from H-3' to C-5'/C-9' (Figure S40). The absolute configurations of **3** were identical to those of **1** and **2** on the basis of the similar ECD data and of the same biogenetic pathway (Figures 4 and 5). It should be noted that the known compound **3** is listed in SciFinder Scholar with the CAS Registry Number 2166398-50-9, but this is the first time that its spectroscopic data have been reported.

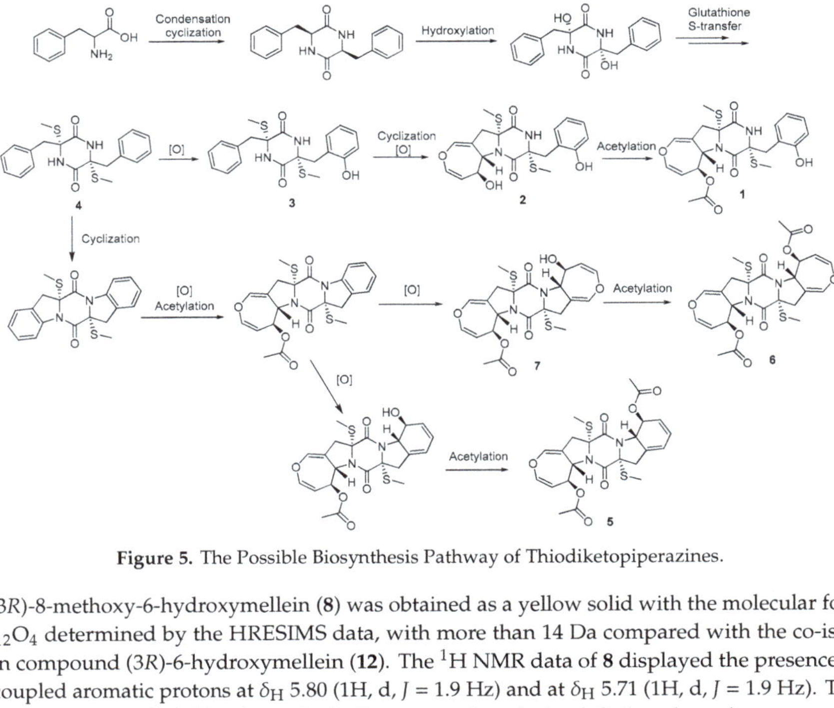

Figure 5. The Possible Biosynthesis Pathway of Thiodiketopiperazines.

(3*R*)-8-methoxy-6-hydroxymellein (**8**) was obtained as a yellow solid with the molecular formula $C_{11}H_{12}O_4$ determined by the HRESIMS data, with more than 14 Da compared with the co-isolated known compound (3*R*)-6-hydroxymellein (**12**). The ^{1}H NMR data of **8** displayed the presence of the *meta*-coupled aromatic protons at δ_H 5.80 (1H, d, *J* = 1.9 Hz) and at δ_H 5.71 (1H, d, *J* = 1.9 Hz). The ^{13}C NMR spectrum revealed 17 carbons, including one carbonyl, six olefinic carbons (two oxygenated), one oxygenated methine carbon, one methylene, and two methyl carbons (one oxygenated). These spectroscopic features were similar to those of (3*R*)-6-hydroxymellein (**12**) except for an additional oxygenated methyl group. The HMBC correlation from H-9 to C-8 was observed for **8** (Figure S42), suggesting that the methoxy group was attached to C-8. The negative Cotton effect at 270 nm in the ECD spectrum of **8** suggested that the absolute configuration of C-3 was *R* (Figure S43) [23]. Compound

8 is listed in SciFinder Scholar with the CAS Registry Number 2247026-31-7, but this is the first time that its spectroscopic data have been reported.

(3R)-6,7,8-trihydroxymellein (9) was established as $C_{10}H_{10}O_5$ on the basis of the HRESIMS data, with more than 16 Da compared with compound 12. The ^{1}H NMR and ^{13}C NMR spectroscopic data of 9 were nearly identical to those of 12, except that one proton at the aromatic ring in 12 was replaced by one hydroxyl in 9. The HMBC correlations from H-5 to C-4/C-7/C-8a indicated that the hydroxyl group was located at C-7 (Figure S42). Similar to 8, the absolute configuration of C-3 in 9 was also determined as R by the negative Cotton effect at 270 nm (Figure S44). Compound 9 is also listed in SciFinder Scholar with the CAS Registry Number 2407423-58-7, but this is the first time that its spectroscopic data have been reported.

2.2. Bioassays

All of the isolated compounds were tested for their antibacterial, antifungal, cytotoxic, and 1,10-diphenyl-2-picryl-hydazyl (DPPH) scavenging activities. Their protein tyrosine phosphatase 1 B (PTP1B) inhibitory activities were also measured—PTP1B is an important hypoglycemic target in diabetes. We found that compounds 2 and 3 displayed antibacterial activities against *Pseudomonas aeruginosa* ATCC 27853 with minimum inhibitory concentration (MIC) values of 64 µg/mL and 32 µg/mL, respectively. Intriguingly, compound 3 also exhibited antifungal activity against *Candida albicans* ATCC10231 with a MIC value of 32 µg/mL. Compounds 3, 5, and 7 showed PTP1B inhibitory activities with inhibitory concentration (IC)$_{50}$ values of 12.25, 25.70 and 24.32 µM, respectively. In addition, compound 9 exhibited a weak DPPH scavenging activity, with an IC$_{50}$ value of 147 µM. All of the isolated compounds showed no cytotoxicity.

3. Materials and Methods

3.1. Instrumentation

Optical rotations were measured with a JASCO P-1020 digital polarimeter (Jasco Corp., Tokyo, Japan). UV spectra were recorded with a HITACHI UH 5300 UV spectrophotometer (Hitachi, Tokyo, Japan). ECD data were acquired on a J-815-150S Circular Dichroism spectrometer (JASCO Electric Co., Ltd., Tokyo, Japan). IR spectra were recorded with a Nicolet-Nexus-470 spectrometer (Thermo Electron Co., Madison, WI, USA) using KBr pellets. NMR spectra were acquired by a JEOL JEM-ECP NMR spectrometer (500 MHz for ^{1}H and 125 MHz for ^{13}C, JEOL, Tokyo, Japan), using tetramethylsilane (TMS) as an internal standard. High-resolution electrospray ionization mass spectrometry (HRESIMS) was measured with a Thermo MAT95XP high resolution mass spectrometer (Thermo Fisher Scientific, Bremen, Germany), and electron ionization mass spectrometry (EIMS) spectra with a Thermo DSQ EImass spectrometer (Thermo Fisher Scientific, Bremen, Germany). Single-crystal X-ray crystallographic analysis was performed on an Agilent Xcalibur Eos Gemini diffractometer (Agilent Technologies, Yarnton, England). Samples were analyzed and prepared using a Hitachi L-2000 HPLC system coupled with a Hitachi L-2455 photodiode array detector, and using a semi-preparative C$_{18}$ column (Kromasil 250 mm × 10 mm, 5 µm). Silica gel (Qing Dao Hai Yang Chemical Group Co., Qing Dao China; 300−400 mesh) and Sephadex LH-20 (Amersham Biosciences, Inc., USA) were used for column chromatography (CC). Precoated silica gel plates (Yan Tai Zi Fu Chemical Group Co., Qing Dao China; G60, F-254) were used for thin-layer chromatography. PTP1B (human recombinant) was purchased from Abcam (ab51277).

3.2. Fungal Material

The fungal strain *Aspergillus terreus* RA2905 was isolated from a piece of fresh tissue from the inner part of the sea hare *Aplysia pulmonica*, collected from the Weizhou coral reefs in the South China Sea in April 2010. The fungus was identified as *Aspergillus terreus* according to its morphological traits and a molecular protocol by amplification and sequencing of the DNA sequences of the internal transcribed spacer (ITS) region of the ribosomal RNA (rRNA) gene by using ITS 1 and ITS 4. Its GenBank (NCBI) access number is MK611650. The phylogenetic tree of the ITS gene was constructed by the Neighbor-Joining method with the aid of MEGA 7 (Figure S1). The strain was deposited in the Key Laboratory of Marine Drugs, Ministry of Education of China, School of Medicine and Pharmacy, Ocean University of China, Qingdao, P. R. China.

3.3. Extraction and Isolation

Sixty 500-mL Erlenmeyer flasks of the fungal strain were cultivated in a starch liquid medium (soluble starch 10 g/L, peptone 1 g/L, artificial sea salt 30 g/L, 200 mL each flask) at 150 rpm and 28 °C for 7 days. The fermentation broth was filtered through a cheesecloth and extracted repeatedly with an equal amount of EtOAc three times, and then it was evaporated in vacuo to obtain an EtOAc extract (12.5 g). The crude extract was isolated on silica gel CC using a step gradient elution with petroleum ether/EtOAc (10:1 to 1:4, v/v) to provide five fractions (Fr.1–Fr.5). Fr.3 was subjected to a silica gel CC eluted with Hexane/CH$_2$Cl$_2$/MeOH (10:1:0 to 0:1:1) to obtain four subfractions (Fr.3.1–Fr.3.4). Fr.3.2 was further separated by the semi-preparative HPLC with MeOH/H$_2$O (60:40) to give compounds **8** (5.5 mg) and **12** (7.1 mg). Fr.3.3 was separated by Sephadex LH-20 CC eluted with CH$_2$Cl$_2$/MeOH (1:1) and the semi-preparative HPLC with MeOH/H$_2$O (45:55) further, to obtain compounds **9–11** (3.2 mg, 3.7 mg, and 2.1 mg, respectively). Fr.4 was separated on a silica gel CC eluted with CH$_2$Cl$_2$/MeOH (100:1 to 1:1) to provide four subfractions (Fr.4.1–Fr.4.4). Fr.4.1 was further subjected to Sephadex LH-20 CC eluted with CH$_2$Cl$_2$/MeOH (1:1) to obtain compounds **6** and **7**. Fr.4.3 was separated by the semi-preparative HPLC with MeOH/H$_2$O (45:55) to give compounds **1–5** (3.3 mg, 3.1 mg, 4.2 mg, 4.5 mg, and 4.3 mg, respectively).

Emestrin L (**1**). White powder; $[\alpha]_D^{20}$-70.4 (*c* 0.42, MeOH); UV (MeOH) λ_{max} (log ε) 229 (3.83), 275 (1.61) nm; IR (KBr) v_{max} 3600, 3395, 2998, 2913, 1646, 1436, 1314 cm^{-1}; ^{1}H and ^{13}C NMR (see Table 1); (−)-HRESIMS *m/z* 475.1007 [M − H]$^-$ (calcd for C$_{22}$H$_{23}$N$_2$O$_6$S$_2$, 475.1003).

Emestrin M (**2**). White powder; $[\alpha]_D^{20}$-85.1 (*c* 0.43, MeOH); UV (MeOH) λ_{max} (log ε) 229 (3.75), 275 (1.75) nm; IR (KBr) v_{max} 3600, 3000, 2912, 2138, 1663, 1438, 1315, 1043 cm^{-1}; ^{1}H NMR (500 MHz, DMSO-d_6) and ^{13}C NMR (125 MHz, DMSO-d_6) (see Table 1); (−)-HRESIMS *m/z* 433.0896 [M − H]$^-$ (calcd for C$_{20}$H$_{21}$N$_2$O$_5$S$_2$, 433.0897).

Emethacin C (**3**). White powder; $[\alpha]_D^{20}$-64.4 (*c* 0.52, MeOH); UV (MeOH) λ_{max} (log ε) 229 (3.89), 275 (2.54) nm; IR (KBr) v_{max} 2952, 2868, 1802, 1715, 1459, 1200, 1139 cm^{-1}; ^{1}H NMR (500 MHz, DMSO-d_6): 8.97 (1H, s, 2-NH), 8.36 (1H, br s, 2'-NH), 7.18 (1H, m, H-7), 7.10 (4H, m, H-5, H-6, H-8, H-9), 6.89 (1H, td, *J* = 7.8, 1.7 Hz, H-7'), 6.67 (1H, td, *J* = 7.8, 1.2 Hz, H-8'), 6.26 (1H, dd, *J* = 7.8, 1.7 Hz, H-9'), 6.22 (1H, dd, *J* =7.8, 1.2 Hz, H-6'), 3.47 (1H, d, *J* = 13.6 Hz, H-3a), 3.05 (1H, d, *J* = 15.4 Hz, H-3'a), 3.01 (1H, d, *J* = 15.4 Hz, H-3'b), 2.96 (1H, d, *J* = 13.6 Hz, H-3b), 2.25 (3H, s, H-10), 2.17 (3H, s, H-10'); ^{13}C NMR (125 MHz, DMSO-d_6): 166.3 (C, C-1'), 165.6 (C, C-1), 155.6 (C, C-5'), 135.4 (C, C-4), 130.8 (CH × 2, C-5, C-9), 129.9 (CH, C-9'), 128.3(CH×2, C-6, C-8), 127.7 (CH, C-7'), 127.2 (CH, C-7), 122.3 (C, C-4'), 119.4 (CH, C-6'), 115.2 (CH, C-8'), 65.5 (C, C-2), 65.2 (C, C-2'), 43.5 (CH$_2$, C-3), 37.0 (CH$_2$, C-3'), 14.0 (CH$_3$, C-10), 13.9 (CH$_3$, C-10'); (−)-HRESIMS *m/z* 401.1003 [M − H]$^-$ (calcd for C$_{20}$H$_{21}$N$_2$O$_3$S$_2$, 401.0999).

(3R)-8-methoxy-6-hydroxymellein (**8**). Yellow solid; $[\alpha]_D^{20}$-47.8 (*c* 1.00, MeOH); UV (MeOH) λ_{max} (log ε) 238 (2.11), 251 (0.95), 319 (0.41) nm; IR (KBr) v_{max} 3749, 3674, 2360, 1736, 1581, 1418 cm^{-1}; ^{1}H NMR (500 MHz, DMSO-d_6): 5.80 (1H, d, *J* = 1.9 Hz, H-5), 5.71 (1H, d, *J* = 1.9 Hz, H-7), 4.25 (1H, m, H-3), 3.59 (3H, s, H-9), 2.57 (1H, dd, *J* = 15.8, 3.3 Hz, H-4a), 2.55 (1H, m, overlapped, H-4b), 1.26 (3H, d, *J* = 6.2 Hz, H-10); ^{13}C NMR (125 MHz, DMSO-d_6): 172.3 (C, C-1), 163.4 (C-6), 162.1 (C, C-8), 142.5 (C, C-4a), 109.4 (CH, C-5), 100.1 (C, C-8a), 97.1 (CH, C-7), 72.0 (CH, C-3), 54.7 (CH$_3$, C-9), 36.2 (CH$_2$, C-4), 20.6 (CH$_3$, C-10); (+)-HRESIMS *m/z* 209.0809 [M + H]$^+$ (calcd for C$_{11}$H$_{13}$O$_4$, 209.0808).

(3R)-6,7,8-trihydroxymellein (**9**). Yellow solid; $[\alpha]_D^{20}$-50.1 (*c* 0.37, MeOH); UV (MeOH) λ_{max} (log ε) 238 (2.03), 251 (1.05), 317 (0.23) nm; IR (KBr) v_{max} 3749, 3674, 2360, 1736, 1651, 1384 cm^{-1}; ^{1}H NMR

(500 MHz, DMSO-d_6): 6.26 (1H, s, H-5), 4.64 (1H, m, H-3), 2.82 (1H, dd, J = 16.2, 3.3 Hz, H-4a), 2.71 (1H, dd, J = 16.2, 1.3 Hz, H-4b), 1.37 (3H, d, J = 6.2 Hz, H-9); ^{13}C NMR (125 MHz, DMSO-d_6): 170.0 (C, C-1), 153.2 (C-6), 151.1 (C, C-8), 131.3 (C, C-7), 131.0 (C, C-4a), 106.5 (CH, C-5), 100.0 (C, C-8a), 75.9 (CH, C-3), 33.2 (CH$_2$, C-4), 20.4 (CH$_3$, C-9); (−)-HRESIMS m/z 209.0458 [M − H]$^−$ (calcd for C$_{10}$H$_9$O$_5$, 209.0455).

Crystal data for **6**: C$_{18}$H$_{18}$N$_2$O$_7$S$_2$, Mr = 534.11, monoclinic, a = 6.8830(3) Å, b = 12.4383(5) Å, c = 14.6020(6) Å, α = 90.00°, β = 94.415(4)°, γ = 90.00°, V = 1246.41(9) Å^3, space group P2$_1$, Z = 2, Dx = 1.135 mg/m^3, μ (Cu Kα) = 0.670 mm^{-1}, and F (000) = 425. Crystal dimensions: 0.12 × 0.11 × 0.11 mm^3. Independent reflections: 7369/4117 (R_{int} = 0.0422). The final R1 value was 0.0481, $wR2$ = 0.1180 ($I > 2\sigma(I)$). Flack parameter = −0.012(13). Crystallographic data for **6** are deposited at the Cambridge Crystallographic Data Centre as supplementary publication number CCDC 1911625.

3.4. Antibacterial Assays

The antibacterial activity was evaluated following the standards recommended by the Clinical and Laboratory Standards Institute [24]. Six pathogenic bacterial strains, *Staphylococcus epidermidis* ATCC 12228, *Staphylococcus aureus* ATCC 25923, *Pseudomonas aeruginosa* ATCC 27853, *Bacillus cereus* ATCC 14579, *Escherichia coli* ATCC 25922, and *Sarcina lutea* ATCC 9341, were used, and vancomycin was used as a positive control.

3.5. Antifungal Assays

The antifungal bioassays were conducted following the standards recommended by the Clinical and Laboratory Standards Institute [24]. Three pathogenic fungal strains, *Candida albicans* ATCC 24433, *Candida tropicalis* ATCC 20962, and *Candida parapsilosis* ATCC 22019, were used. Amphotericin B was used as a positive control.

3.6. PTP1B Inhibition Assays

The PTP1B Inhibition assay was performed in 96-well plates [25]. The compound (10 μL) was added to the 99-μL reaction buffer solution, which consisted of 10 mM Tris (pH 7.4), 50 mM NaCl, 2 mM dithiothreitol (DTT), 1 mM MnCl$_2$, and 10 mM para-nitrophenyl phosphate (pNPP). The reaction mix was pre-warmed using a block heater at 37 °C. The recombinant PTP1B solution (1 mg/mL, 1 μL) was mixed in each well. An NaOH solution (10 μL, 0.1 M) was added to stop the reaction. The absorbance was recorded at 405 nm using a microplate. Sodium vanadate was used as a positive control.

3.7. DPPH Scavenging Activities

The DPPH scavenging assays were performed using the method described by Aquino et al. [26]. The reaction mixture consisted of freshly prepared 100 μM DPPH in methanol, mixed with different concentrations of the compounds. The reaction mixture was incubated for 20 min at room temperature in the dark, and the optical density was recorded at 517 nm.

3.8. Cytotoxicity Assays

The cytotoxic activities were evaluated with the sulforhodamine B (SRB) assay [27], using five human tumor cell lines: A549, HCT116, MCF-7, Hela, and Hep G2. Adriamycin was used as a positive control.

Supplementary Materials: The following are available online at http://www.mdpi.com/1660-3397/18/3/132/s1, Figure S1. *Aspergillus terreus* RA2905 and its phylogenetic tree of ITS gene, Figures S2–S39: the NMR, ESIMS and HRESIMS spectra, Figure S40: Key HMBC correlations of compound **3**, Figure S41: crystal diagram of compound **6**, Figure S42: key HMBC correlations of compounds **8** and **9**, Figure S43: the CD spectrum of compound **8**, Figure S44: the CD spectrum of compound **9**.

Author Contributions: Conceptualization, C.-Y.W. and H.-S.G.; Methodology, J.-S.W.; Data analysis, J.-S.W., X.-H.S., C.-L.S., and X.-L.Z.; Bioassays, J.-S.W., X.-H.S., and G.-S.Y.; Writing—Original draft preparation, J.-S.W.

and X.-H.S.; Writing—Review and editing, J.-S.W., X.-M.F., and C.-Y.W. All authors have read and agreed to the published version of the manuscript.

Funding: This research was funded by the Marine S&T Fund of Shandong Province for Pilot National Laboratory for Marine Science and Technology (Qingdao, China) (No. 2018SDKJ0406-5), the National Science and Technology Major Project for Significant New Drugs Development, China (No. 2018ZX09735-004), the Shandong Provincial Natural Science Foundation (Major Basic Research Projects) (No. ZR2019ZD18), the Program of Open Studio for Druggability Research of Marine Natural Products, the Pilot National Laboratory for Marine Science and Technology (Qingdao, China) directed by Kai-Xian Chen and Yue-Wei Guo, and the Taishan Scholars Program, China.

Conflicts of Interest: The authors declare no conflict of interest.

References

1. Carroll, A.R.; Copp, B.R.; Davis, R.A.; Keyzers, R.A.; Prinsep, M.R. Marine natural products. *Nat. Prod. Rep.* **2019**, *36*, 122. [CrossRef]
2. Jin, L.; Quan, C.; Hou, X.; Fan, S. Potential pharmacological resources: Natural bioactive compounds from marine-derived fungi. *Mar. Drugs* **2016**, *14*, 76. [CrossRef]
3. Wang, K.W.; Ding, P. New bioactive metabolites from the marine-derived fungi *Aspergillus*. *Mini-Rev. Med. Chem.* **2018**, *18*, 1072–1094. [CrossRef]
4. Lee, Y.M.; Kim, M.J.; Li, H.; Zhang, P.; Bao, B.; Lee, K.J.; Jung, J.H. Marine-derived *Aspergillus* species as a source of bioactive secondary metabolites. *Mar. Biotechnol.* **2013**, *15*, 499–519. [CrossRef]
5. Welch, T.R.; Williams, R.M. Epidithiodioxopiperazines. occurrence, synthesis and biogenesis. *Nat. Prod. Rep.* **2014**, *31*, 1376–1404. [CrossRef]
6. Fujimoto, H.; Sumino, M.; Okuyama, E.; Ishibashi, M. Immunomodulatory constituents from an ascomycete, *Chaetomium Seminudum*. *J. Nat. Prod.* **2004**, *67*, 98–102. [CrossRef]
7. Sun, Y.; Takada, K.; Takemoto, Y.; Yoshida, M.; Nogi, Y.; Okada, S.; Matsunaga, S. Gliotoxin analogues from a marine-derived fungus, *Penicillium* sp., and their cytotoxic and histone methyltransferase inhibitory activities. *J. Nat. Prod.* **2011**, *75*, 111–114. [CrossRef]
8. Zheng, C.J.; Kim, C.J.; Bae, K.S.; Kim, Y.H.; Kim, W.G. Bionectins A–C, epidithiodioxopiperazines with anti-MRSA activity, from *Bionectra byssicola* F120. *J. Nat. Prod.* **2006**, *69*, 1816–1819. [CrossRef]
9. Curtis, P.J.; Greatbanks, D.; Hesp, B.; Cameron, A.F.; Freer, A.A. Sirodesmins A, B, C, and G, antiviral epipolythiopiperazine-2,5-diones of fungal origin: X-Ray analysis of sirodesmin A diacetate. *J. Chem. Soc. Perkin Trans.* **1977**, *1*, 180–189. [CrossRef]
10. Lee, H.J.; Lee, J.H.; Hwang, B.Y.; Kim, H.S.; Lee, J.J. Anti-angiogenic activities of gliotoxin and its methylthio-derivative, fungal metabolites. *Arch. Pharmacal Res.* **2001**, *24*, 397. [CrossRef]
11. Mayer, A.; Rodríguez, A.D.; Taglialatela-Scafatim, O.; Fusetani, N. Marine pharmacology in 2012–2013: Marine compounds with antibacterial, antidiabetic, antifungal, anti-inflammatory, antiprotozoal, antituberculosis, and antiviral activities; affecting the immune and nervous systems, and other miscellaneous mechanisms of action. *Mar. Drugs* **2017**, *15*, 273.
12. Liu, L.; Zheng, Y.Y.; Shao, C.L.; Wang, C.Y. Metabolites from marine invertebrates and their symbiotic microorganisms: Molecular diversity discovery, mining, and application. *Mar. Life Sci. Tech.* **2019**, *1*, 60–94. [CrossRef]
13. Niu, S.W.; Liu, D.; Shao, Z.; Proksch, P.; Lin, W.H. Eutypellazines N–S, new thiodiketopiperazines from a deep sea sediment derived fungus *Eutypella* sp. with anti-VRE activities. *Tetrahedron Lett.* **2017**, *58*, 3695–3699. [CrossRef]
14. Kawahara, N. Sulfur-containg dioxopiperazine derivatives from *Emericella heterothallica*. *Heterocycles* **1989**, *29*, 397–402.
15. Neuss, N.; Nagarajan, R.; Molloy, B.B.; Huckstep, L.L. Aranotin and related metabolites. II. Isolation, characterization, and structures of two new metabolites. *Tetrahedron Lett.* **1968**, *9*, 4467–4471. [CrossRef]
16. Kamata, S.; Sakai, H.; Hirota, A. Isolation of acetylaranotin, bisdethiodi (methylthio)-acetylaranotin and terrein as plant growth inhibitors from a strain of *Aspergillus terreus*. *Agric. Biol. Chem.* **1983**, *47*, 2637–2638. [CrossRef]
17. Nagarajan, R.; Huckstep, L.L.; Lively, D.H.; DeLng, D.C.; Marsh, M.M.; Neuss, N. Aranotin and related metabolites from *Arachniotus aureus*. I. Determination of structure. *J. Am. Chem. Soc.* **1968**, *90*, 2980–2982. [CrossRef]

18. Dethoup, T.; Manoch, L.; Kijjoa, A.; Pinto, M.; Gales, L.; Damas, A.M.; Silva, A.M.S.; Eaton, G.; Herz, W. Merodrimanes and other constituents from *Talaromyces thailandiasis*. *J. Nat. Prod.* **2007**, *70*, 1200–1202. [CrossRef]
19. Zaehle, C.; Gressler, M.; Shelest, E.; Geib, E.; Hertweck, C.; Brock, M. Terrein biosynthesis in *Aspergillus terreus* and its impact on phytotoxicity. *Chem. Biol.* **2014**, *21*, 719–731. [CrossRef]
20. Takenaka, Y.; Morimoto, N.; Hamada, N.; Tanahashi, T. Phenolic compounds from the cultured mycobionts of *Graphis proserpens*. *Phytochemistry* **2011**, *72*, 1431–1435. [CrossRef]
21. Choudhary, M.I.; Musharraf, S.G.; Mukhmoor, T.; Shaheen, F.; Ali, S.; Rahman, A. Isolation of bioactive compounds from *Aspergillus terreus*. *Z. Naturforsch. B J. Chem. Sci.* **2004**, *59*, 324–328. [CrossRef]
22. Islam, M.S.; Ishigami, K.; Watanabe, H. Synthesis of (−)-mellein, (+)-ramulosin, and related natural products. *Tetrahedron* **2006**, *63*, 1074–1079. [CrossRef]
23. Krohn, K.; Bahramsari, R.; Flörke, U.; Ludewig, K.; Kliche-Spory, C.; Michel, A.; Aust, H.J.; Draeger, S.; Schulz, B.; Antus, S. Dihydroisocoumarins from fungi: Isolation, structure elucidation, circular dichroism and biological activity. *Phytochemisty* **1997**, *45*, 313–320. [CrossRef]
24. Clinical and Laboratory Standards Institute. *Performance Standards for Antimicrobial Susceptibility Testing*; Twenty-Second Informational Supplement. M100-S22; Clinical and Laboratory Standards Institute (CLSI): Wayne, PA, USA, 2012.
25. Tian, J.L.; Liao, X.J.; Wang, Y.H.; Si, X.; Shu, C.; Gong, E.-S.; Xie, X.; Ran, X.L.; Li, B. Identification of cyanidin-3-arabinoside extracted from blueberry as selective PTP1B inhibitor. *J. Agric. Food Chem.* **2019**, *67*, 13624–13634. [CrossRef]
26. Aquino, R.; Morelli, S.; Lauro, M.R.; Abdo, S.; Saija, A.; Tomaino, A. Phenolic constituents and antioxidant activity of an extract of *Anthurium versicolor* leaves. *J. Nat. Prod.* **2001**, *64*, 1019–1023. [CrossRef]
27. Skehan, P.; Storeng, R.; Scudiero, D.; Monks, A.; McMahon, J.; Vistica, D.; Warren, J.T.; Bokesch, H.; Kenney, S.; Boyd, M.R. New colorimetric cytotoxicity assay for anticancer-drug screening. *J. Natl. Cancer Inst.* **1990**, *82*, 1107–1112. [CrossRef]

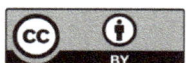

© 2020 by the authors. Licensee MDPI, Basel, Switzerland. This article is an open access article distributed under the terms and conditions of the Creative Commons Attribution (CC BY) license (http://creativecommons.org/licenses/by/4.0/).

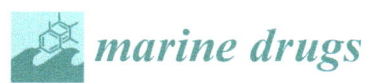

Article

Cytotoxic Thiodiketopiperazine Derivatives from the Deep Sea-Derived Fungus *Epicoccum nigrum* SD-388

Lu-Ping Chi [1,2,3], Xiao-Ming Li [1,2], Li Li [1,2,3], Xin Li [1,2,*] and Bin-Gui Wang [1,2,4,*]

1. Key Laboratory of Experimental Marine Biology, Institute of Oceanology, Chinese Academy of Sciences, Nanhai Road 7, Qingdao 266071, China; chiluping@qdio.ac.cn (L.-P.C.); lixmqdio@126.com (X.-M.L.); 15738367975@163.com (L.L.)
2. Laboratory of Marine Biology and Biotechnology, Qingdao National Laboratory for Marine Science and Technology, Wenhai Road 1, Qingdao 266237, China
3. University of Chinese Academy of Sciences, Yuquan Road 19A, Beijing 100049, China
4. Center for Ocean Mega-Science, Chinese Academy of Sciences, Nanhai Road 7, Qingdao 266071, China
* Correspondence: lixin@qdio.ac.cn (X.L.); wangbg@ms.qdio.ac.cn (B.-G.W.); Tel.: +86-532-8289-8890 (X.L.); +86-532-8289-8553 (B.-G.W.)

Received: 8 February 2020; Accepted: 11 March 2020; Published: 13 March 2020

Abstract: Four new thiodiketopiperazine alkaloids, namely, 5′-hydroxy-6′-ene-epicoccin G (**1**), 7-methoxy-7′-hydroxyepicoccin G (**2**), 8′-acetoxyepicoccin D (**3**), and 7′-demethoxyrostratin C (**4**), as well as a pair of new enantiomeric diketopiperazines, (±)-5-hydroxydiphenylalazine A (**5**), along with five known analogues (**6–10**), were isolated and identified from the culture extract of *Epicoccum nigrum* SD-388, a fungus obtained from deep-sea sediments (−4500 m). Their structures were established on the basis of detailed interpretation of the NMR spectroscopic and mass spectrometric data. X-ray crystallographic analysis confirmed the structures and established the absolute configurations of compounds **1–3**, while the absolute configurations for compounds **4** and **5** were determined by ECD calculations. Compounds **4** and **10** showed potent activity against Huh7.5 liver tumor cells, which were comparable to that of the positive control, sorafenib, and the disulfide bridge at C-2/C-2′ is likely essential for the activity.

Keywords: *Epicoccum nigrum*; deep-sea-derived fungus; thiodiketopiperazines; diketopiperazine enantiomers; cytotocxic activity

---

1. Introduction

Natural products have historically been a rich source of new drugs or drug candidates. Strikingly, deep-sea-derived microorganisms survive under extreme environments, leading to special biological diversity and prolific metabolisms differing from those of terrestrial microorganisms. Recently, deep-sea-sourced microbial natural products have been reported with high hit-rates from bioactivity screening, particularly in the antitumor area [1,2].

Epicoccum nigrum is a chemically distinct fungal species with potential to produce structurally unique secondary metabolites including thiodiketopiperazines (TDKPs) [3,4], polyketides [5], and polysaccharides [6]. Some of these metabolites exhibited intriguing biological properties, such as antimicrobial [3], cytotoxic [4], and antioxidant activities [5,6].

The TDKP derivatives are a family of diketopiperazines which have been isolated from several fungal sources, such as *Epicoccum nigrum* [3], *Exserohilum rostratum* [7], *Penicillium brocae* [8], and *Penicillium adametzioides* [9].

In continuation of our research aimed at discovery of bioactive metabolites from marine-derived microorganisms [10–12], a fungal strain of *Epicoccum nigrum* SD-388 was isolated from a deep-sea sediment sample collected at a depth of 4500 m. Chemical investigation of the fungus resulted in the isolation of spiroepicoccin A, an unusual spiro-TDKP derivative, whose stereochemistry could not be elucidated by conventional NMR methods and was solved based on residual chemical shift anisotropies [12]. This result encouraged us to perform a further study of the fungus and has led to the isolation of four new TDKPs including 5'-hydroxy-6'-ene-epicoccin G (**1**), 7-methoxy-7'-hydroxyepicoccin G (**2**), 8'-acetoxyepicoccin D (**3**), and 7'-demethoxyrostratin C (**4**), as well as a pair of new enantiomeric diketopiperazines (DKPs), (±)-5-hydroxydiphenylalazine A ((±)-**5**), together with five known analogues including diphenylalazine A (**6**) [4], emeheterone (**7**) [13], epicoccins E (**8**) and G (**9**) [4], and rostratin C (**10**) [7] (Figure 1). Details of the isolation and purification, structural elucidation, and cytotoxic potency against Huh7.5 liver tumor cells of compounds **1–10** are described herein.

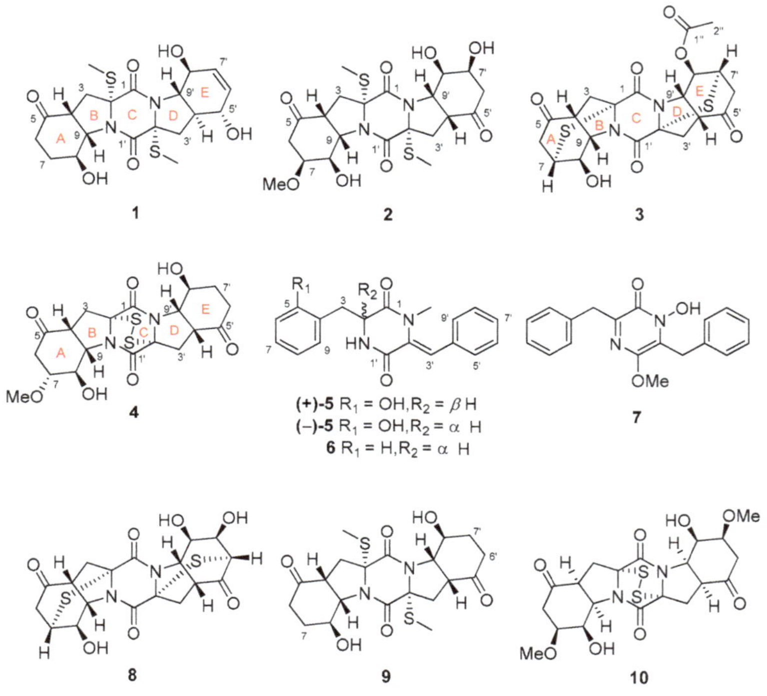

Figure 1. Structures of the isolated compounds **1–10**.

2. Results and Discussion

2.1. Structure Elucidation of the New Compounds

The fungal strain *E. nigrum* SD-388 was cultured on the rice solid medium, which was further exhaustively extracted with EtOAc to afford an extract. Fractionation of the extracts by a combination of column chromatography (CC) over silica gel, Lobar LiChroprepRP-18, SephadexLH-20, as well as semi-preparative HPLC, yielded compounds **1–10**.

Compound **1**, initially obtained as colorless gum, gave a pseudomolecular ion peak at *m/z* 455.1293 [M + H]$^+$ by HR-ESI-MS, consistent with a molecular formula of $C_{20}H_{26}N_2O_6S_2$, indicating 9 degrees of unsaturation. The ^{1}H-, ^{13}C-NMR, and DEPT spectroscopic data (Tables 1 and 2) revealed the presence of two methyls, four sp^3 hybridized methylenes, nine methines (with five oxygenated/nitrogenated and two olefinic), five nonprotonated carbons (with one ketone and two amide carbonyls), as well as three exchangeable protons. Detailed analysis of the NMR data disclosed that the structure of **1** was similar to that of epicoccin G (**9**), a well described TDKP derivative identified from a *Cordyceps*-colonizing fungus *Epicoccum nigrum* XZC04-CS-302 in 2009 [4]. However, signals for two CH$_2$ groups at δ_H/δ_C 2.20 and 2.59/33.8 (C-6') and at δ_H/δ_C 1.88 and 2.12/25.8 (C-7') in compound **9**, were replaced by two olefinic CH groups at δ_H/δ_C 5.68/133.3 (C-6') and δ_H/δ_C 5.53/129.9 (C-7') in the NMR spectra of **1**. Furthermore, the signal for the ketone group (C-5') of **9** (δ_C 207.7) was replaced by an oxygenated methine (δ_H/δ_C 4.11/71.3) in **1**. The COSY correlations for the spin system from H-3' through H-9' via H-4'~H-8' and the HMBC correlations from H-5' to C-7' and C-9', from H-6' to C-4' and C-5', and from H-7' to C-9', confirmed the proposed structure of **1** (Figure 2).

Table 1. ^{1}H NMR spectroscopic data for compounds **1–5** [a].

No.	1	2	3	4	5
2					4.17, t (6.4)
3	α 2.80, d (13.4)	α 2.75, d (13.5)	α 3.13, d (17.7)	α 2.68, m	a 3.02, dd (13.3, 6.4)
	β 2.28, m	β 2.35, dd (13.5, 8.5)	β 2.89, m	β 2.99, dd (14.8, 7.9)	b 2.95, dd (13.3, 6.4)
4	2.98, t (8.0)	2.92, t (8.5)	3.06, t (8.3)	3.18, t (7.9)	
6	α 2.22, m	α 2.54, dd (17.1, 4.7)	α 2.85, m	α 2.71, m	6.79, d (7.3)
	β 2.61, m	β 2.65, m	β 2.92, m	β 2.61, m	
7	α 2.19, m	3.82, ddd (10.1, 4.7, 2.0)	3.73, m	3.29, ddd (10.9, 4.7, 1.5)	6.96, m
	β 1.92, m				
8	4.36, m	4.56, m	4.01, dt (4.6, 2.4)	5.03, t (4.7)	6.67, td (7.3, 1.2)
9	4.33, m	4.33, m	4.67, dd (8.3, 2.4)	4.41, dd (7.9, 4.7)	6.98, m
3'	α 2.42, dd (12.5, 4.9)	α 2.73, d (13.4)	α 2.93, m	α 2.74, m	6.83, s
	β 2.26, m	β 2.34, dd (13.4, 8.5)	β 3.29, d (19.4)	β 2.93, dd (14.8, 8.0)	
4'	2.09, m	2.91, t (8.5)	3.17, d (8.1)	3.23, t (8.0)	
5'	4.11, m				7.27, d (7.3)
6'	5.68, d (9.8)	α 2.40, dd (16.8, 4.4)	α 2.89, m	α 2.66, m	7.40, t (7.3)
		β 2.61, m	β 2.97, m	β 2.27, dt (16.7, 4.1)	
7'	5.53, d (9.8)	4.12, ddd (10.2, 4.4, 2.0)	3.92, m	α 1.62, td (12.5, 5.0)	7.32, t (7.3)
				β 1.89, m	
8'	4.08, m	4.29, s	5.04, dd (4.3, 2.0)	4.81, m	7.40, t (7.3)
9'	3.41, dd (12.0, 8.1)	4.34, m	4.83, dd (8.1, 2.0)	4.36, m	7.27, d (7.3)
1-NMe					2.69, s
1'-NH					[b]
2-SMe	1.95, s	1.93, s			
2'-SMe	2.08, s	1.92, s			
2''			2.04, s		
5-OH					8.50, br s
8-OH	5.36, d (3.2)	5.44, br s	6.25, d (2.4)	5.64, d (4.7)	
5'-OH	5.92, s				
7'-OH		5.19, br s			
8'-OH	5.28, d (5.8)	5.44, br s		5.49, d (4.0)	
7-OMe		3.25, s		3.21, s	

[a] Data collected at 500 MHz in DMSO-d_6. [b] Data not detected.

The relative configuration of **1** was deduced from analysis of the NOESY spectrum. NOE correlations from H-9 to H-3β and H-4, and from the proton of 8-OH to H-4, H-6β, and H-7β, indicated the cofacial orientation of these groups (Figure 3). Besides, NOEs from H-3α to 2-SMe placed them on another face, opposite to that of H-4, H-9, and 8-OH. Moreover, NOE cross-peaks from H-8' to H-3'α and H-4', and from H-3'α to 2'-SMe, confirmed them on the same spatial orientation, while NOE correlations from H-5' to H-9' and H-3'β placed these groups on the opposite face. On the basis of the above observation, the relative configurations for rings A/B and D/E were determined respectively. However, the relationship between these two units could not be correlated based on the NOESY experiment, because no diagnostic NOE cross-peak could be detected between rings A/B and D/E.

Table 2. ^{13}C NMR spectroscopic data for compounds **1–5** [a].

No.	1	2	3	4	5
1	168.7, C	165.5, C	158.3, C	162.2, C	167.2, C
2	71.4, C	71.6, C	71.1, C	76.2, C	55.6, CH
3	34.3, CH$_2$	34.4, CH$_2$	41.4, CH$_2$	32.6, CH$_2$	34.8, CH$_2$
4	44.0, CH	43.8, CH	45.0, CH	46.4, CH	122.0, C
5	207.5, C	206.6, C	207.1, C	207.8, C	156.1, C
6	33.8, CH$_2$	40.4, CH$_2$	43.2, CH$_2$	40.7, CH$_2$	115.1, CH
7	25.9, CH$_2$	75.8, CH	41.3, CH	75.5, CH	127.8, CH
8	63.6, CH	61.5, CH [b]	65.2, CH	61.9, CH	118.4, CH
9	64.8, CH	63.2, CH	60.3, CH	63.2, CH	131.2, CH
1′	165.5, C	165.4, C	158.9, C	162.2, C	162.4, C
2′	72.9, C	71.6, C	71.7, C	76.4, C	132.2, C
3′	35.1, CH$_2$	34.1, CH$_2$	41.5, CH$_2$	32.2, CH$_2$	117.7, CH
4′	43.4, CH	43.5, CH	45.3, CH	46.7, CH	133.8, C
5′	71.3, CH	207.4, C	206.3, C	208.6, C	129.4, CH
6′	133.3, CH	43.3, CH$_2$	43.5, CH$_2$	33.9, CH$_2$	128.1, CH
7′	129.9, CH	65.7, CH	38.8, CH	25.4, CH$_2$	127.9, CH
8′	68.9, CH	68.1, CH [b]	67.4, CH	60.8, CH	128.1, CH
9′	67.8, CH	62.7, CH	57.5, CH	65.8, CH	129.4, CH
1″			168.8, C		
2″			20.6, CH$_3$		
1-NMe					34.5, CH$_3$
2-SMe	14.4, CH$_3$	14.2, CH$_3$			
2′-SMe	14.2, CH$_3$	13.9, CH$_3$			
7-OMe		55.8, CH$_3$		56.0, CH$_3$	

[a] Data collected at 125 MHz in DMSO-d_6. [b] Assigned by HSQC experiment.

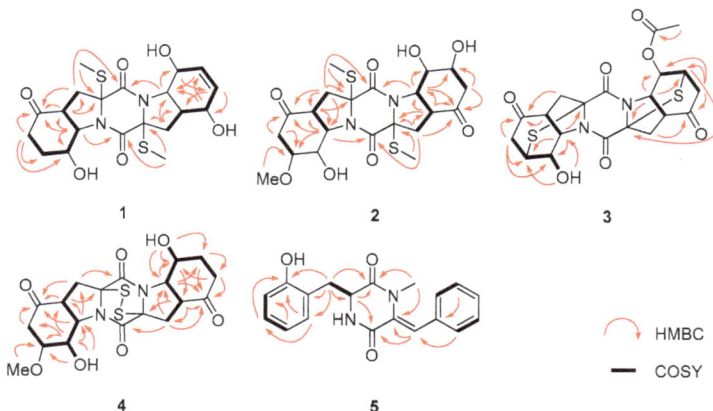

Figure 2. Key ^{1}H-^{1}H COSY (bold lines) and HMBC (red arrows) correlations of compounds **1–5**.

To fully assign the configuration of compound **1**, efforts toward a single crystal X-ray study were performed. By slow evaporation of the solvent (MeOH–H$_2$O, 100:1) under refrigeration, quality crystals of **1** were obtained, making it feasible for an X-ray crystallographic experiment which confirmed not only the planar structure, but also the relative configuration of compound **1** (Figure 4). The defined Flack parameter 0.01(3) determined the absolute configuration of **1** as 2*R*, 4*R*, 8*S*, 9*S*, 2′*R*, 4′*S*, 5′*S*, 8′*S*, and 9′*S*, and the trivial name 5′-hydroxy-6′-ene-epicoccin G was assigned to compound **1**.

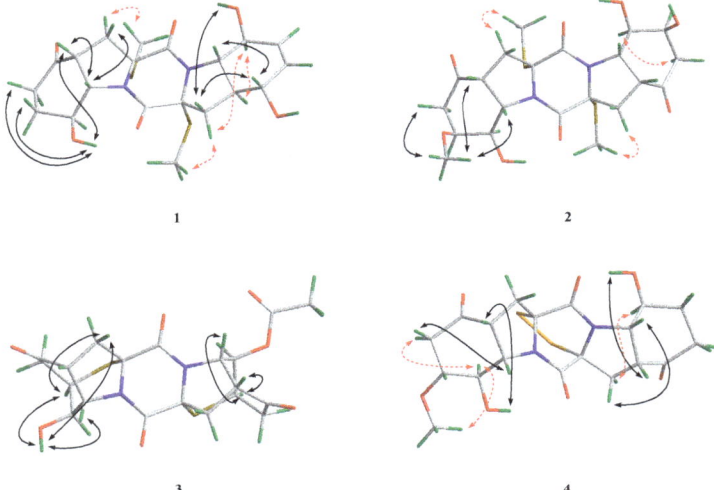

Figure 3. Key NOE correlations of compounds **1–4** (black solid lines: β-orientation; red dashed lines: α-orientation).

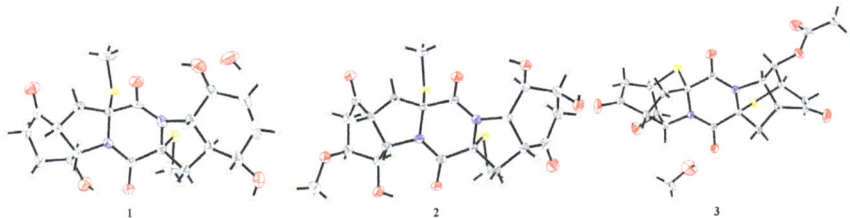

Figure 4. X-ray crystallographic structures of compounds **1–3**.

The elemental composition of **2** was established to be $C_{21}H_{28}N_2O_8S_2$ by analysis of HR-ESI-MS and NMR data, indicating nine degrees of unsaturation. The ^{1}H- and ^{13}C-NMR data of **2** were similar to those of epicoccin G (**9**), a symmetrical TDKP derivative characterized from *E. nigrum* XZC04-CS-302 [4], except that the signals of two methylene groups at δ_H/δ_C 1.88 and 2.12/25.8 (CH_2-7 and CH_2-7′) in **9** were replaced by two oxygenated methine groups at δ_H/δ_C 3.82/75.8 (CH-7) and δ_H/δ_C 4.12/65.7 (CH-7′) in **2**, respectively. Moreover, signals for a methoxy group at δ_H/δ_C 3.25/55.8 (7-OMe) were also observed (Tables 1 and 2). The methoxy group was assigned at C-7 based on the observed HMBC correlation from 7-OMe to C-7. Supported by key COSY correlations from H-6 to H-7, and from H-6′ to H-7′, as well as by HMBC correlations from H-6 and H-9 to C-7 and from H-6′ and H-9′ to C-7′ (Figure 2), the planar structure of compound **2** was determined.

The relative configuration of **2** was assigned by analysis of *J*-coupling constants and NOESY data. A coupling constant of 8.5 Hz between H-4 and H-9 as well as between H-4′ and H-9′ suggested their *cis* relationships, as reported in the previous literature [7]. NOE correlations from the proton of 7-OMe to H-4 and H-9 indicated the cofacial orientation of these groups. However, the relative configurations of **2** could not be fully assigned due to the lack of some key NOE correlations.

A single crystal of **2** was cultivated, after attempts by dissolving the samples in MeOH–H_2O (100:1) followed by slow evaporation under refrigeration for two weeks. Once the Cu/Kα X-ray crystallographic experiment was conducted (Figure 4), the structure and absolute configuration of

2 were assigned as 2R, 4R, 7S, 8R, 9S, 2'R, 4'R, 7'S, 8'R, and 9'S, with a Flack parameter of 0.02(4). Compound **2** was named 7-methoxy-7'-hydroxyepicoccin G.

The accurate mass data measured by HR-ESI-MS of compound **3** assigned its molecular formula, $C_{20}H_{20}N_2O_7S_2$ (12 degrees of unsaturation), and was supported by the NMR data. The ^{1}H- and ^{13}C-NMR data of **3** (Tables 1 and 2) showed close similarity to those of epicoccin D, a TDKP derivative isolated from the fungal strain *E. nigrum* (2203) in 2007 [3]. However, resonances for an ester carbonyl carbon (δ_C 168.8, C-1'') and a methyl group (δ_H/δ_C 2.04/20.6, CH$_3$-2'') were observed in the NMR spectra of **3**. Deshielded shift at δ_H 5.04 for H-8' in **3** was detected, compared to that of δ_H 4.00 in epicoccin D. The above observation suggested that compound **3** was a C-8' acetylated derivative of epicoccin D. The relative configuration of **3** was assigned on the basis of the NOESY experiment and J-coupling constants. For ring A of **3**, NOE correlations from the proton of OH-8 to H-7 and H-9 revealed the same orientation of these groups (Figure 3). In addition, the *cis* relationship between H-4 and H-9 was established by the coupling constant (J = 8.3 Hz) which is in agreement with that of rostratin B (J = 7.2 Hz) [7]. However, the relative configurations of ring E could not be solved as it lacked some key NOE correlations. To unequivocally determine the relative and absolute configurations, single crystals for **3** were cultivated upon slow evaporation of the solvent (MeOH) and a Cu/Kα X-ray diffraction analysis was conducted (Figure 4). The final refinement of the X-ray data resulted in a 0.02(3) Flack parameter, allowing for the assignment of the absolute configuration as 2R, 4R, 7R, 8R, 9S, 2'R, 4'R, 7'R, 8'R, and 9'S.

Compound **4** was initially isolated as a colorless powder. Its molecular formula was postulated as $C_{19}H_{22}N_2O_7S_2$ through HR-ESI-MS analysis, indicating 10 degrees of unsaturation. The 1D NMR data of **4** were similar to those of rostratin C (**10**), a DKP derivative isolated from the marine-derived fungal strain *Exserohilum rostratum* CNK-630 [7], with the exception of the disappeared signals for the oxygenated methine (C-7') and the methoxy group attached to C-7'. In contrast, signals for a methylene group at δ_H 1.62/1.89 and δ_C 25.4 (CH$_2$-7') were observed in the NMR spectra of **4** (Tables 1 and 2), indicating that **4** is a 7'-demethoxy derivative of **10**. The 2D NMR correlations supported this inference by the COSY correlations from H-7' to H-6' and H-8', and HMBC correlations from H-7' to C-5' and from H-9' to C-7' (Figure 2).

The relative configuration for rings A and E of **4** were determined by analysis of NOESY data. NOE correlations, with respect to ring A from H-8 to H-3α and 7-OMe, placed them on the same face. Meanwhile, NOEs from the proton of 8-OH to H-4, and from H-3β to H-9, disclosed the cofacial orientation of these groups. As for ring E, the coupling constant (J = 8.0 Hz) observed between H-4' and H-9' revealed their *cis* relationship [7]. In addition, NOEs from the proton of 8'-OH to H-4', and from H-3'β to H-9', revealed them on the cofacial orientation. Whereas NOE from H-3'α to H-8' revealed that these groups were on the other face (Figure 3).

The assignment of the absolute configurations at C-2/C-2' were established by analysis of ECD cotton effects (CEs) following the rules reported by the previous reference [14]. The ECD spectrum of **4** showed a positive CE near 265 nm, which was characteristic for the 2R/2'R configurations in TDKPs. The whole absolute configuration of **4** was further studied using the time-dependent density functional (TDDFT)-ECD calculation in Gaussian 09. The ECD spectra of four possible stereoisomers of **4**, including (2R, 4R, 7R, 8R, 9S, 2'R, 4'R, 8'S, 9'S)-**4**, (2R, 4R, 7R, 8R, 9S, 2'R, 4'S, 8'R, 9'R)-**4**, (2R, 4S, 7S, 8S, 9R, 2'R, 4'R, 8'S, 9'S)-**4**, and (2R, 4S, 7S, 8S, 9R, 2'R, 4'S, 8'R, 9'R)-**4**, were calculated. The experimental ECD spectrum for **4** showed agreement with that calculated for (2R, 4R, 7R, 8R, 9S, 2'R, 4'R, 8'S, 9'S)-**4** (Figure 5a), allowing the elucidation of whole chiral centers as 2R, 4R, 7R, 8R, 9S, 2'R, 4'R, 8'S, and 9'S.

Compound **5**, obtained as a yellow oil, was assigned the molecular formula $C_{19}H_{18}N_2O_3$ by HR-ESI-MS, and required 12 degrees of unsaturation. Analysis of the ^{1}H- and ^{13}C-NMR data (Tables 1 and 2) revealed that compound **5** had same basic structure as that of the previously reported diphenylalazine A (**6**), which was identified from the fungus *E. nigrum* XZC04-CS-302 [4]. However, the aromatic methine at C-5 in **6** (δ_H/δ_C 7.18/129.82) was replaced by a nonprotonated and hydroxylated carbon (δ_C 156.1) in **5**. HMBC correlations from H-3, H-7, and H-9 to C-5, supported this deduction. The planar structure of **5** was thus established as 5-hydroxydiphenylalazine A. However, the specific optical rotation value of $[\alpha]_{25}^{D} = 0$ (c 0.10, MeOH) revealed the racemic nature of compound **5**, which was also confirmed by the fact that no cotton effects were observed in the ECD spectrum (Figure S36). Separation of **5** by HPLC using the Daicel Chiral-pak IC column yielded (+)-**5** and (−)-**5** (Figure S37), which were individually determined absolute configurations by experimental and calculated ECD spectra (Figure 5b), and assigned (+)-**5** as 2R and (−)-**5** as 2S.

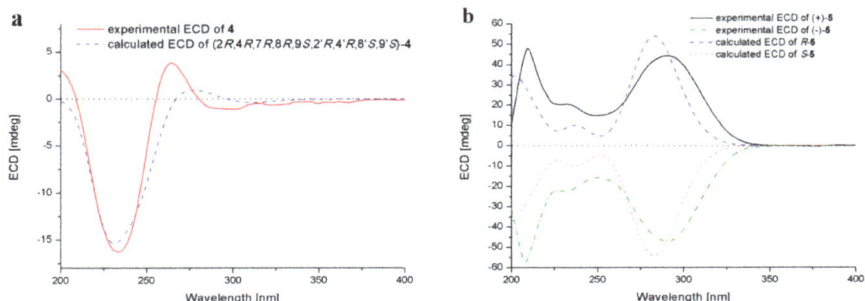

Figure 5. Experimental and calculated ECD spectra of compounds **4** (**a**) and **5** (**b**).

In addition to compounds **1–5**, five known analogues (**6–10**) were also isolated. By detailed spectroscopic analysis as well as comparison with reported data, the structures of compounds **6–10** were identified as diphenylalazines A (**6**) [4], emeheterone (**7**) [13], epicoccins E (**8**) and G (**9**) [4], and rostratin C (**10**) [7].

2.2. Biological Activities of the Isolated Compounds

All of the isolated compounds were assayed for their activities against Huh7.5 liver tumor cells. Among them, only compounds **4** and **10** displayed significant cytotoxic effects against Huh7.5 with cell viability less than 30% at the concentration of 20 µM. As shown in Figure 6, the growth-inhibiting effects of **4** and **10** were concentration-dependent, with IC$_{50}$ values of 9.52 and 4.88 µM, respectively, which were comparable to that of the positive control, sorafenib (IC$_{50}$ 8.2 µM). Compounds **4** and **10** were also measured for their cytotoxicity against human normal liver LO2 cell line. The results showed that compound **4** exhibited the inhibitory effects against normal liver cells, similar to that of cancer cells (Figure 6). However, compound **10** was less sensitive to normal liver cells than liver cancer cells, only at a narrow concentration range of 4~10 µM. The results suggested that the disulfide bridge at C-2/C-2' is likely essential for the activity.

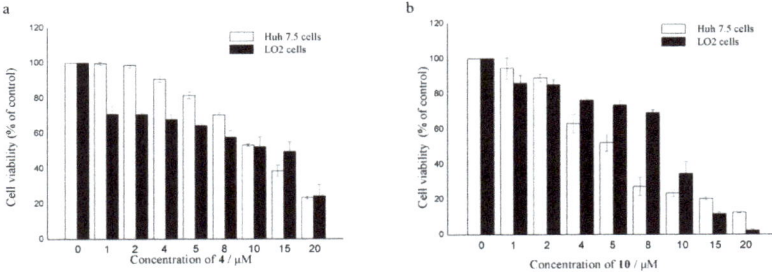

Figure 6. Cell viability of Huh7.5 liver cancer cells and LO2 normal liver cells treated with compounds **4** (**a**) and **10** (**b**).

3. Experimental Section

3.1. General Experimental Procedures

Melting points were acquired through an SGW X-4 micro-melting-point apparatus (Shanghai Shenguang Instrument Co. Ltd, Shanghai, China). Optical rotations were measured using an Optical Activity AA-55 polarimeter (Optical Activity Ltd., Cambridgeshire, UK). UV spectra were determined by a PuXi TU-1810 UV-visible spectrophotometer (Shanghai Lengguang Technology Co. Ltd., Shanghai, China), and ECD spectra were obtained with a JASCO J-715 spectropolarimeter (JASCO, Tokyo, Japan). NMR spectra were recorded on a Bruker Avance 500 spectrometer (Bruker Biospin Group, Karlsruhe, Germany), using solvent chemical shifts (DMSO-d_6: δ_H/δ_C 2.50/39.52) as reference. HR-ESI-MS were measured on an API QSTAR Pulsar 1 mass spectrometer (Applied Biosystems, Foster, Waltham, MA, USA). Analytical and semi-preparative reversed-phase HPLC separations were performed by a Dionex HPLC system, equipped with P680 pump (Dionex, Sunnyvale, CA, USA), ASI-100 automated sample injector, and UVD340U multiple wavelength detector controlled by Chromeleon software (version 6.80). Commercially available Lobar LiChroprep RP-18 (40–63 μm, Merck, Darmstadt, Germany), Si gel (200–300 mesh, Qingdao Haiyang Chemical Co., Qingdao, China), and Sephadex LH-20 (Pharmacia, Pittsburgh, PA, USA) were used for column chromatography. Thin-layer chromatography (TLC) was carried out using precoated Si gel GF$_{254}$ plates (Merck, Darmstadt, Germany). All solvents used were distilled prior to use.

3.2. Fungal Material

The fungal strain *Epicoccum nigrum* SD-388 was isolated from the deep-sea sediment collected in the West Pacific (depth 4500 m) on March 2015. The fungus was identified using a molecular biological protocol by DNA amplification and sequencing of the ITS (internal transcript spacer) region. The sequence data for the fungus have been deposited in GenBank with the accession no. MN089646. Through the BLAST searching, the fungus was identified as *Epicoccum nigrum* according to the ITS region sequence, which is the same (100%) as that of *E. nigrum* (accession no. KU254609). The strain is preserved at the Key Laboratory of Experimental Marine Biology, Institute of Oceanology, Chinese Academy of Sciences (IOCAS).

3.3. Fermentation

For chemical investigations, the fresh mycelia of the fungus were grown on PDA medium at 28 °C for one week and were then inoculated into 1 L Erlenmeyer flasks. The fungus was fermented statically at room temperature for 35 days in rice solid medium containing rice (70 g/flask), peptone (0.3%), yeast extract (0.5%), corn steep liquor (0.2%), monosodium glutamate (0.1%), $Fe_2(SO_4)_3$ (0.002%), $MgSO_4·7H_2O$ (0.07%), $ZnSO_4$ (0.0001%), KH_2PO_4 (0.025%), and naturally sourced and filtered seawater (obtained from the Huiquan Gulf of the Yellow Sea near the campus of IOCAS, 100 mL/flask).

3.4. Extraction and Isolation

The fermented rice substrate was mechanically fragmented after incubation, and then extracted with petroleum ether (PE) to remove the low-polarity chemical constituents. The remaining culture was extracted thoroughly with EtOAc, which was filtered and evaporated under reduced pressure to give EtOAc extract (75.5 g).

The EtOAc extract was fractionated by Si gel VLC (vacuum liquid chromatography), using solvents of increasing polarity (PE-EtOAc, 20:1 to 1:1, and then CH_2Cl_2-MeOH, 20:1 to 1:1) to yield nine fractions (Frs. 1–9). Fr. 5 (6.6 g) was further separated by CC (Column Chromatography) over Lobar LiChroprep RP-18 with a MeOH-H_2O gradient (from 1:9 to 10:0) to yield 10 subfractions (Frs. 5.1–5.10). Fr. 5.4 (453.8 mg) was subjected to CC on Si gel eluting with a CH_2Cl_2-MeOH gradient (from 500:1 to 200:1) to yield compounds **6** (187.6 mg) and **7** (15.5 mg). Fr. 6 (29.2 g) was repeatedly subjected to Si gel VLC and then fractionated by solvents of increasing polarity from CH_2Cl_2 to acetone to yield four subfractions (Frs. 6.1–6.4) based on HPLC and TLC analysis. Purification of Fr. 6.1 (6.2 g) by CC over Lobar LiChroprep RP-18 with a MeOH-H$_2$O gradient (from 1:9 to 10:0) yielded 10 subfractions (Frs. 6.1.1–6.1.10). Fr. 6.1.1 (14.3 mg) was recrystallized from mixed solvents (MeOH-H$_2$O, 10:1) to give **3** (6.7 mg). Fr. 6.1.2 (53.7 mg) was purified by prep-TLC and CC on Sephadex LH-20 (MeOH) to obtain **10** (34.1 mg). Fr. 6.1.3 (44.8 mg) was also recrystallized from MeOH to give **9** (21.9 mg). Fr. 6.1.4 (79.2 mg) was applied to semi-preparative HPLC (Elite ODS-BP column, 10 μm; 20 × 250 mm; 70% MeOH-H$_2$O, 16 mL/min) to afford **4** (18.3 mg, t_R 29.6 min). Fr. 6.1. 5 (207.3 mg) was subjected to repeated CC on silica gel (CH$_2$Cl$_2$-MeOH, 140:1) and purified by prep-TLC and CC on Sephadex LH-20 (MeOH) to give **5** (9.4 mg). Fr. 6.2 (6.0 g) was split by CC over Lobar LiChroprep RP-18, silica gel, and Sephadex LH-20 to yield **2** (12.5 mg). Fr. 6.3 (6.5 g) was subjected to CC over Lobar LiChroprep RP-18, eluted with a MeOH-H$_2$O gradient (from 1:9 to 10:0) to yield 10 subfractions (Frs. 6.3.1–6.3.10). Fr. 6.3.1 (32.1 mg) was recrystallized from mixed solvents (MeOH-H$_2$O, 10:1) to afford **8** (13.7 mg). Fr. 6.3.3 (108.9 mg) was purified by semi-preparative HPLC (Elite ODS-BP column, 10 μm; 20 × 250 mm; 72% MeOH-H$_2$O, 16 mL/min) to afford **1** (46.8 mg, t_R 31.2 min).

5′-Hydroxy-6′-ene-epicoccin G (**1**): Colorless cube crystal (MeOH-H$_2$O); mp 161–163 °C; $[\alpha]_{25}^{D}$ −95.7 (c 0.23, MeOH); UV (MeOH) λ_{max} (log ε) 204 (3.99) nm; ECD (4.18 mM, MeOH) λ_{max} (Δε) 200 (−1.96), 233 (+2.46), 260 (−3.07) nm; ^{1}H and ^{13}C NMR data, Tables 1 and 2; ESIMS m/z 455 [M + H]$^+$; HRESIMS m/z 455.1293 [M + H]$^+$ (calcd for C$_{20}$H$_{27}$O$_6$N$_2$S$_2$, 455.1305).

7-Methoxy-7′-hydroxyepicoccin G (**2**): Colorless cube crystal (MeOH); mp 173–175 °C; $[\alpha]_{25}^{D}$ −138.9 (c 0.18, MeOH); UV (MeOH) λ_{max} (log ε) 204 (4.16) nm; ECD (4.80 mM, MeOH) λ_{max} (Δε) 200 (−3.35), 231 (+3.91), 259 (−2.53)nm; ^{1}H and ^{13}C NMR data, Tables 1 and 2; ESIMS m/z 501 [M + H]$^+$; HRESIMS m/z 501.1360 [M + H]$^+$ (calcd for C$_{21}$H$_{29}$O$_8$N$_2$S$_2$, 501.1360).

8′-Acetoxyepicoccin D (**3**): Colorless needle crystal (MeOH); mp 233–235 °C; $[\alpha]_{25}^{D}$ +225.6 (c 0.02, MeOH); UV (MeOH) λ_{max} (log ε) 204 (3.75) nm; ECD (2.15 mM, MeOH) λ_{max} (Δε) 218 (+1.24), 252 (+0.31), 290 (−0.10) nm; ^{1}H and ^{13}C NMR data, Tables 1 and 2; ESIMS m/z 482 [M + NH$_4$]$^+$, m/z 487 [M + Na]$^+$; HRESIMS m/z 482.1045 [M + NH$_4$]$^+$ (calcd for C$_{20}$H$_{24}$O$_7$N$_3$S$_2$, 482.1050), 487.0601 [M + Na]$^+$ (calcd for C$_{20}$H$_{20}$O$_7$N$_2$NaS$_2$, 487.0604).

7′-Demethoxyrostratin C (**4**): Colorless amorphous powder; $[\alpha]_{25}^{D}$ −215.4 (c 0.13, MeOH); UV (MeOH) λ_{max} (log ε) 201 (4.06) nm; ECD (2.20 mM, MeOH) λ_{max} (Δε) 200 (+0.43), 234 (−2.24), 265 (+0.53) nm; ^{1}H and ^{13}C NMR data, Tables 1 and 2; ESIMS m/z 455 [M + H]$^+$; HRESIMS m/z 455.0930 [M + H]$^+$ (calcd for C$_{19}$H$_{23}$O$_7$N$_2$S$_2$, 455.0941).

(±)-5-Hydroxydiphenylalazine A (**5**): Yellow oil; UV (MeOH) λ_{max} (log ε) 200 (4.49) nm, 216 (4.19) nm, 283 (4.14) nm; ^{1}H and ^{13}C NMR data, Tables 1 and 2; ESIMS m/z 323 [M + H]$^+$; HRESIMS m/z 323.1383 [M + H]$^+$ (calcd for C$_{19}$H$_{19}$O$_3$N$_2$, 323.1390).

(+)-**5**: $[\alpha]_{25}^{D}$ +350 (c 0.18, MeOH); ECD (5.59 mM, MeOH) λ_{max} (Δε) 209 (+2.59), 233 (+1.11), 291 (+2.41) nm.

(−)-**5**: $[\alpha]_{25}^{D}$ −345 (c 0.18, MeOH); ECD (5.59 mM, MeOH) λ_{max} (Δε) 206 (−3.11), 242 (−1.21), 288 (−2.55) nm.

3.5. X-Ray Crystallographic Analysis

Crystallographic data have been deposited in the Cambridge Crystallographic Data Centre [15]. Crystallographic data were collected on an Agilent Xcalibur Eos Gemini CCD plate diffractometer equipped with a graphite-monochromatic Cu-Kα radiation (λ = 1.54178) Å at 293 (2) K. The data were corrected for absorption by using the program SADABS [16]. The structures were solved by direct methods with the SHELXTL software package [17]. All non-hydrogen atoms were refined anisotropically. The H atoms connected to C atoms were calculated theoretically, and those to O atoms were assigned by difference Fourier maps [18]. The absolute structure was determined by refinement of the Flack parameter [19], based on anomalous scattering. The structures were optimized by full-matrix least-squares techniques.

Crystal data of compound **1**: $C_{20}H_{26}N_2O_6S_2 \cdot H_2O$, F.W. = 472.56, orthorhombic space group $P2(1)2(1)2(1)$, unit cell dimensions a = 8.5746 (5) Å, b = 10.9602 (8) Å, c = 24.3158 (16) Å, V = 2285.2 (3) Å^3, $\alpha = \beta = \gamma = 90°$, Z = 4, d_{calcd} = 1.374 mg/m^3, crystal dimensions 0.40 × 0.21× 0.13 mm, μ = 2.491 mm^{-1}, $F(000)$ = 1000. The 5006 measurements yielded 3321 independent reflections after equivalent data were averaged. The final refinement gave R_1 = 0.0525 and wR_2 = 0.1263 [$I > 2\sigma(I)$]. The absolute structure parameter was 0.01(3).

Crystal data of compound **2**: $C_{21}H_{28}N_2O_8S_2$, F.W. = 500.57, monoclinic space group $P2(1)$, unit cell dimensions a = 6.8423 (4) Å, b = 20.5136 (10) Å, c = 8.2231 (5) Å, V = 1130.48 (11) Å^3, $\alpha = \gamma = 90°$, β = 101.635 (2)°, Z = 2, d_{calcd} = 1.471 mg/m^3, crystal dimensions 0.20 × 0.17× 0.10 mm, μ = 2.587 mm^{-1}, $F(000)$ = 528. The 6832 measurements yielded 2789 independent reflections after equivalent data were averaged. The final refinement gave R_1 = 0.0514 and wR_2 = 0.1199 [$I > 2\sigma(I)$]. The absolute structure parameter was 0.02(4).

Crystal data of compound **3**: $C_{20}H_{20}N_2O_7S_2 \cdot CH_3OH$, F.W. = 496.54, orthorhombic space group $P2(1)2(1)2(1)$, unit cell dimensions a = 10.1030 (6) Å, b = 10.8478 (5) Å, c = 19.6848 (10) Å, V = 2157.4 (2) Å^3, $\alpha = \beta = \gamma = 90°$, Z = 4, d_{calcd} = 1.529 mg/m^3, crystal dimensions 0.25 × 0.17× 0.13 mm, μ = 2.711 mm^{-1}, $F(000)$ = 1040. The 4782 measurements yielded 3033 independent reflections after equivalent data were averaged. The final refinement gave R_1 = 0.0510 and wR_2 = 0.1001 [$I > 2\sigma(I)$]. The absolute structure parameter was 0.02(3).

3.6. Computational Section

Conformational searches were carried out via molecular mechanics with the MM+ method in HyperChem 8.0 software (Gainesville, FL, USA). Afterwards, the geometries were optimized at the gas-phase B3LYP/6-31G level in Gaussian09 software to afford the energy-minimized conformers. Then, the optimized conformers were subjected to the calculations of ECD spectra using the TD-DFT at BH&HLYP/TZVP level for **4** and PBE0/TZVP level for **5**. Simultaneously, solvent effects of the MeOH solution were evaluated at the same DFT level using the SCRF/PCM method [20].

3.7. Cytotoxic Assays

3.7.1. Cell Culture

Liver cancer Huh7.5 cell line used was obtained from the American Type Culture Collection (ATCC). Human normal liver LO2 cell line used was purchased from China Center for Type Culture Collection (CCTCC). Huh7.5 cells and LO2 cells were cultured at 37 °C in RPMI-1640 medium and DMEM medium, respectively, supplemented with 10% fetal bovine serum (FBS, PAN Biotech, Aidenbach, Germany), 100 U/mL penicillin, and 100 mg/mL streptomycin. All experiments were carried out with the same batch of cell line between passages 2 and 5 [21].

3.7.2. Cell Proliferation Assay

The cytotoxic activities of compounds **1–10** against Huh7.5 liver tumor cells and human normal liver LO2 cell line were determined by the 3-(4,5-dimethylthiazolyl-2)-2,5-diphenyltetrazolium bromide (MTT) assay. Briefly, 6 × 10^3 of logarithmically growing Huh7.5 cells and human normal liver LO2 cell line were plated in the 96-well plate at 37 °C for 24 h. Then, cells were treated with DMSO (as the vehicle control) and increasing concentrations of test compounds (with the final concentration of 1, 2, 4, 5, 8, 10, 15, 20 μM) for 48 h, respectively. MTT solution (5 mg/mL, 20 μL per well) was added and incubated for another 4 h. After supernate from the wells were removed, DMSO was added to each well to dissolve purple crystals of formazan with gentle shaking for 10 min, and optical density at 490 nm was read by a multi-detection microplate reader (Infinite M1000 Pro, Tecan, Switzerland). Sorafenib was used as positive control. All the compounds and positive control were dissolved and diluted in DMSO. All tests were performed in triplicate. The values of relative cell viability were calculated as percentages of absorbance from the treated samples to absorbance from the vehicle control [21].

4. Conclusions

In conclusion, ten diketopiperazine alkaloids including four new derivatives, 5′-hydroxy-6′-ene-epicoccin G (**1**), 7-methoxy-7′-hydroxyepicoccin G (**2**), 8′-acetoxyepicoccin D (**3**), and 7′-demethoxyrostratin C (**4**), and a pair of new enantiomeric diketopiperazines (±)-5-hydroxydiphenylalazine A ((±)-**5**), along with five known analogues (**6–10**) were characterized from the deep sea-derived fungus *E. nigrum* SD-388. The discovery of these compounds might provide further insight into the biosynthesis of the diketopiperazine family and provide new targets for synthetic or biosynthetic studies. Compounds **4** and **10** exhibited potent cytotoxic activities against Huh7.5 liver cancer cells and may provide useful candidates for further study as antitumor agents.

Supplementary Materials: Selected 1D and 2D NMR, HRESIMS, and ECD spectra of compounds **1–5** are available online at: http://www.mdpi.com/1660-3397/18/3/160/s1.

Author Contributions: L.-P.C. performed the experiments for the isolation, structure elucidation, and prepared the manuscript; X.-M.L. performed the 1D and 2D NMR experiments; L.L. participated in the isolation of the fungus *Epicoccum nigrum*. X.L. contributed to ECD calculations and revised the manuscript; B.-G.W. All authors have read and agreed to the published version of the manuscript.

Funding: This research work was financially supported by the Strategic Priority Research Program of the Chinese Academy of Sciences (XDA22050401) and the Aoshan Scientific and Technological Innovation Project of Qingdao National Laboratory for Marine Science and Technology (2016ASKJ14). X.L. appreciates the China Postdoctoral Science Foundation (2017M612360) for project funding. B.-G.W. acknowledges the support of the Research Vessel KEXUE of the National Major Science and Technology Infrastructure from the Chinese Academy of Sciences (KEXUE2018G28) and the Taishan Scholar Project from Shandong Province.

Acknowledgments: The authors appreciate Chao-min Sun and Ge Liu at the Institute of Oceanology, Chinese Academy of Sciences, for their support in cytotoxic assays, and the High Performance Computing Environment Qingdao Branch of the Chinese Academy of Science (CAS)–High Performance Computing Center of Institute of Oceanology of CAS for CPU time.

Conflicts of Interest: The authors declare no conflicts of interest.

References

1. Niu, S.; Xia, M.; Chen, M.; Liu, X.; Li, Z.; Xie, Y.; Shao, Z.; Zhang, G. Cytotoxic polyketides isolated from the deep-sea-derived fungus *Penicillium chrysogenum* MCCC 3A00292. *Mar. Drugs* **2019**, *17*, 686. [CrossRef] [PubMed]
2. Liu, Z.; Fan, Z.; Sun, Z.; Liu, H.; Zhang, W. Dechdigliotoxins A–C, three novel disulfide-bridged gliotoxin dimers from deep-sea sediment derived fungus *Dichotomomyces cejpii*. *Mar. Drugs* **2019**, *17*, 596. [CrossRef] [PubMed]
3. Zhang, Y.; Liu, S.; Che, Y.; Liu, X. Epicoccins A–D, epipolythiodioxopiperazines from a *Cordyceps*-colonizing isolate of *Epicoccum nigrum*. *J. Nat. Prod.* **2007**, *70*, 1522–1525. [CrossRef] [PubMed]
4. Guo, H.; Sun, B.; Gao, H.; Chen, X.; Liu, S.; Yao, X.; Liu, X.; Che, Y. Diketopiperazines from the *Cordyceps*-colonizing fungus *Epicoccum nigrum*. *J. Nat. Prod.* **2009**, *72*, 2115–2119. [CrossRef] [PubMed]
5. Yan, Z.; Wen, S.; Ding, M.; Guo, H.; Huang, C.; Zhu, X.; Huang, J.; She, Z.; Long, Y. The purification, characterization, and biological activity of new polyketides from mangrove-derived endophytic fungus *Epicoccum nigrum* SCNU-F0002. *Mar. Drugs* **2019**, *17*, 414. [CrossRef] [PubMed]
6. Sun, H.H.; Mao, W.J.; Jiao, J.Y.; Xu, J.C.; Li, H.Y.; Chen, Y.; Xu, J.; Zhao, C.Q.; Hou, Y.J.; Yang, Y.P. Structural characterization of extracellular polysaccharides produced by the marine fungus *Epicoccum nigrum* JJY-40 and their antioxidant activities. *Mar. Biotechnol.* **2011**, *13*, 1048–1055. [CrossRef] [PubMed]

7. Tan, R.X.; Jensen, P.R.; Williams, P.G.; Fenical, W. Isolation and structure assignments of rostratins A–D, cytotoxic disulfides produced by the marine-derived fungus *Exserohilum rostratum*. *J. Nat. Prod.* **2004**, *67*, 1374–1382. [CrossRef] [PubMed]
8. Meng, L.H.; Li, X.M.; Lv, C.T.; Huang, C.G.; Wang, B.G. Brocazines A–F, cytotoxic bisthiodiketopiperazine derivatives from *Penicillium brocae* MA-231, an endophytic fungus derived from the marine mangrove plant *Avicennia marina*. *J. Nat. Prod.* **2014**, *77*, 1921–1927. [CrossRef] [PubMed]
9. Liu, Y.; Li, X.M.; Meng, L.H.; Jiang, W.L.; Xu, G.M.; Huang, C.G.; Wang, B.G. Bisthiodiketopiperazines and acorane sesquiterpenes produced by the marine-derived fungus *Penicillium adametzioides* AS-53 on different culture media. *J. Nat. Prod.* **2015**, *78*, 1294–1299. [CrossRef] [PubMed]
10. Cao, J.; Li, X.M.; Meng, L.H.; Konuklugil, B.; Li, X.; Li, H.L.; Wang, B.G. Isolation and characterization of three pairs of indolediketopiperazine enantiomers containing infrequent N-methoxy substitution from the marine algal-derived endophytic fungus *Acrostalagmus luteoalbus* TK-43. *Bioorg. Chem.* **2019**, *90*, 103030. [CrossRef] [PubMed]
11. Li, X.D.; Li, X.M.; Li, X.; Xu, G.M.; Liu, Y.; Wang, B.G. Aspewentins D–H, 20-nor-isopimarane derivatives from the deep sea sediment-derived fungus *Aspergillus wentii* SD-310. *J. Nat. Prod.* **2016**, *79*, 1347–1353. [CrossRef] [PubMed]
12. Li, X.; Chi, L.P.; Navarro-Vázquez, A.; Hwang, S.; Schmieder, P.; Li, X.M.; Li, X.; Yang, S.Q.; Lei, X.; Wang, B.G.; et al. Stereochemical elucidation of natural products from residual chemical shift anisotropies in a liquid crystalline phase. *J. Am. Chem. Soc.* **2019**. [CrossRef] [PubMed]
13. Kawahara, N.; Nozawa, K.; Nakajima, S.; Kawai, K.I. Emeheterone, a pyrazinone derivative from *Emericella heterothallica*. *Phytochemistry* **1988**, *27*, 3022–3024. [CrossRef]
14. Wang, J.M.; Jiang, N.; Ma, J.; Yu, S.S.; Tan, R.X.; Dai, J.G.; Si, Y.K.; Ding, G.Z.; Ma, S.G.; Qu, L.; et al. Study on absolute configurations of α/α' chiral carbons of thiodiketopiperazines by experimental and calculated circular dichroism spectra. *Tetrahedron* **2013**, *69*, 1195–1201. [CrossRef]
15. Crystallographic data of compounds 1–3 have been deposited in the Cambridge Crystallographic Data Centre as CCDC 1935572, CCDC 1935573 and CCDC 1935571, respectively. Available online: https://www.ccdc.cam.ac.uk/structures/? (accessed on 13 March 2020).
16. Sheldrick, G.M. *SADABS, Software for empirical absorption correction*; University of Gottingen: Gottingen, Germany, 1996.
17. Sheldrick, G.M. *SHELXTL, Structure determination software programs*; Bruker Analytical X-ray System Inc.: Madison, WI, USA, 1997.
18. Sheldrick, G.M. *SHELXL-97 and SHELXS-97, Program for X-ray Crystal Structure Solution and Refinement*; University of Gottingen: Gottingen, Germany, 1997.
19. Flack, H.D. On enantiomorph-polarity estimation. *Acta Cryst.* **1983**, *39*, 876–881. [CrossRef]
20. Gaussian09, RevisionC.01. Available online: http://gaussian.com/g09citation/ (accessed on 13 March 2020).
21. Liu, G.; Kuang, S.; Cao, R.; Wang, J.; Peng, Q.; Sun, C. Sorafenib kills liver cancer cells by disrupting SCD1-mediated synthesis of monounsaturated fatty acids via the ATP-AMPK-mTOR-SREBP1 signaling pathway. *FASEB J.* **2019**, *33*, 10089–10103. [CrossRef] [PubMed]

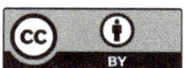

© 2020 by the authors. Licensee MDPI, Basel, Switzerland. This article is an open access article distributed under the terms and conditions of the Creative Commons Attribution (CC BY) license (http://creativecommons.org/licenses/by/4.0/).

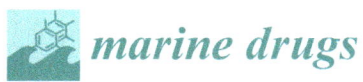

Communication

Lysophosphatidylcholines and Chlorophyll-Derived Molecules from the Diatom *Cylindrotheca closterium* with Anti-Inflammatory Activity

Chiara Lauritano [1,*], Kirsti Helland [2], Gennaro Riccio [1], Jeanette H. Andersen [2], Adrianna Ianora [1] and Espen H. Hansen [2]

1. Department of Marine Biotechnology, Stazione Zoologica Anton Dohrn, CAP80121 Naples, Italy; gennaro.riccio@szn.it (G.R.); adrianna.ianora@szn.it (A.I.)
2. Marbio, UiT—The Arctic University of Norway, Breivika N-9037 Tromsø, Norway; kirsti.helland@uit.no (K.H.); jeanette.h.andersen@uit.no (J.H.A.); espen.hansen@uit.no (E.H.H.)
* Correspondence: chiara.lauritano@szn.it; Tel.: +39-081-5833-221

Received: 17 January 2020; Accepted: 13 March 2020; Published: 17 March 2020

Abstract: Microalgae have been shown to be excellent producers of lipids, pigments, carbohydrates, and a plethora of secondary metabolites with possible applications in the pharmacological, nutraceutical, and cosmeceutical sectors. Recently, various microalgal raw extracts have been found to have anti-inflammatory properties. In this study, we performed the fractionation of raw extracts of the diatom *Cylindrotheca closterium*, previously shown to have anti-inflammatory properties, obtaining five fractions. Fractions C and D were found to significantly inhibit tumor necrosis factor alpha (TNF-α) release in LPS-stimulated human monocyte THP-1 cells. A dereplication analysis of these two fractions allowed the identification of their main components. Our data suggest that lysophosphatidylcholines and a breakdown product of chlorophyll, pheophorbide a, were probably responsible for the observed anti-inflammatory activity. Pheophorbide a is known to have anti-inflammatory properties. We tested and confirmed the anti-inflammatory activity of 1-palmitoyl-sn-glycero-3-phosphocholine, the most abundant lysophosphatidylcholine found in fraction C. This study demonstrated the importance of proper dereplication of bioactive extracts and fractions before isolation of compounds is commenced.

Keywords: diatoms; marine biotechnology; anti-inflammatory; drug discovery; *Cylindrotheca closterium*

---

1. Introduction

Inflammation is a complex set of interactions among soluble factors and cells (e.g., chemokines, cytokines, adhesion molecules, recruitment, and activation of leukocytes) that can arise in any tissue helping to protect the host from systemic infection and to restore tissue homeostasis after injury, infection, and irritation [1–3]. Therefore, it represents a crucial defense mechanism that is important for maintenance of health [1,2]. However, if targeted destruction and assisted repair are not properly controlled by its mediators, the so-called "non-resolving inflammation", they can lead to persistent tissue damage and the insurgence of various pathologies [2]. Inflammation has important pathogenic roles in several pathologies, such as asthma, atherosclerosis, atopic dermatitis, Crohn's disease, multiple sclerosis, cystic fibrosis, psoriasis, neurodegenerative diseases, as well as cancer [1,4]. It is a protective response that involves immune cells, blood vessels, and different molecular mediators (e.g., TNF-α, IL1, nitric oxide, and prostaglandins) and anti-inflammatory assays that are used in the literature, generally include the study of one or more of these characteristics and mediators.

Oceans account for 71% of the earth's surface and represent a huge, relatively untapped, reservoir of new compounds for drug discovery [5]. One such source is the Phytoplankton, photosynthetic eukaryotes at the base of marine and freshwater food webs that are essential in the transfer of organic material to top consumers such as fish [6]. These micro-organisms have shorter generation times as compared with macro-organisms and can easily be cultivated in closed photobioreactors or in open ponds providing access to larger amounts of biomass necessary for an eco-sustainable and eco-friendly approach to drug discovery [7]. Diatoms, with over 100,000 species, constitute one of the major components of marine phytoplankton, comprise up to 40% of annual productivity at sea [8] and represent 25% of global carbon-fixation [9]. Different studies have shown that diatoms are excellent sources and producers of pigments, lipids, and bioactive compounds [7,10]. Anti-inflammatory properties have previously been found for various diatoms, such as *Porosira glacialis*, *Attheya longicornis* [11], *Cylindrotheca closterium*, *Odontella mobiliensis*, *Pseudonitzschia pseudodelicatissima* [12], and *Phaeodactylum tricornutum* [13]. The activity was assessed on lipopolysaccharide (LPS)-stimulated human THP-1 macrophages, except for *P. tricornutum* which was tested on murine RAW 264.7 macrophages. However, there is very little information available on the actual compounds responsible for the observed anti-inflammatory activity.

Anti-inflammatory properties have also been found for flagellates. Extracts of *Tetraselmis suecica* [14], *Chlorella ovalis*, *Nannochloropsis oculata*, and *Amphidinium carterae* [13], and a sterol-rich fraction of *Nannochloropsis oculata* [15] were active in LPS-stimulated RAW 264.7 macrophages. Oxylipin-containing lyophilized biomass from *Chlamydomonas debaryana* have been shown to have anti-inflammatory properties in an induced colitis rat model [16–18] and *Dunaliella bardawil* was found to protect against acetic acid-induced small bowel inflammation in rats [16,17]. Regarding studies on LPS-stimulated human THP-1 monocytic leukemia cells, lipid extracts of *Pavlova lutheri* [19] and monogalactosyldiacylglycerols (MGDGs) and digalactosyldiacylglycerols (DGDGs) mixtures, and the isolated DGDGs 11 and 12 from *Isochrysis galbana* [20] were reported as active. Regarding the compounds responsible for anti-inflammatory properties from flagellates, lycopene was purified from *Chlorella marina* and the activity was confirmed in a rat model of arthritis [21], and phytosterols from *Dunaliella tertiolecta* were tested in a sheep model of inflammation [22]. In addition, carotenoids, the most abundant lipid-soluble phytochemicals, have shown anti-inflammatory properties [23].

In this study, we investigated the capacity of extracts of *C. closterium* to inhibit the release of one of the main effectors of inflammation, TNF-α [3], in LPS-stimulated human THP-1 monocytic leukemia cells. Bioactivity-guided fractionation was performed, and chemical contents of the active fraction are described for the first time. This study is perfectly aligned with recent trends in analyzing possible microalgal properties for cancer prevention and improving general human health and well-being [24,25].

2. Results and Discussion

2.1. Testing for Anti-Inflammatory Activity in Algal Fractions

Previous studies have shown that raw extracts of the diatom *C. closterium* had anti-inflammatory properties [12]. In the present study, a raw extract of *C. closterium* was pre-fractionated to obtain five fractions (Fractions A to E). These were amino acids and saccharides rich fraction (named Fraction A), nucleosides rich fraction (named fraction B), glycol- and phospholipid rich fraction (named fraction C), free fatty acids and sterols rich fraction (named fraction D), and triglycerides rich fraction (named fraction E), as reported in the solid phase extraction (SPE) protocol to fractionate organic extracts of Cutignano et al. [26]. Bioactivity testing of these fractions identified fraction C as the most active, able to inhibit TNF-α release at 100 μg/mL and 50 μg/mL concentrations (Figure 1). In particular, at 100 μg/mL, fraction C showed 60% inhibition of TNF-α release ($p < 0.01$), and 40% inhibition at 50 μg/mL ($p < 0.001$). Fraction D showed almost 40% TNF-α inhibition at 100 μg/mL ($p < 0.01$) and 30% at 50 μg/mL ($p < 0.001$). The other fractions did not show any significant TNF-α inhibition activity ($p > 0.05$). Both fractions C and D were selected for dereplication and further characterization.

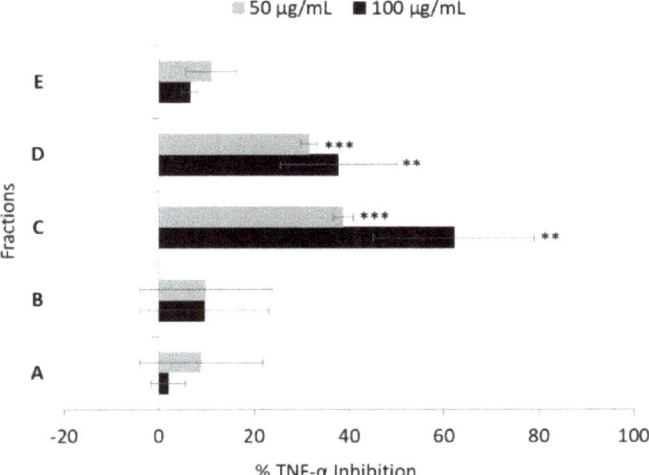

Figure 1. Anti-inflammatory assay. Inhibition of TNF-α secretion from LPS-stimulated THP-1 cells treated with fractions A, B, C, D, and E of *Cylindrotheca closterium* extracts ($n = 3$, ** for $p < 0.01$ and *** for $p < 0.001$, Student's *t*-test).

2.2. Anti-Proliferative Activity Assay

In order to test if the active anti-inflammatory fractions of *C. closterium* also had antiproliferative activities, the 3-(4,5-dimethyl-2-thizolyl)-2,5-diphenyl-2H-tetrazolium bromide (MTT) assay was performed. In particular, A549, A2058, and HepG2 cells were incubated in the presence or in the absence of three different concentrations (1, 10, and 100 µg/mL) of both fractions C and D. After 72 h of incubation at 37 °C, cell survival was measured with the MTT assay. As shown in Figure 2, fractions C and D did not show any significant inhibition of cell proliferation ($p > 0.05$). These results suggest that these two fractions have no antiproliferative or cytotoxicity activity but specific anti-inflammatory activity.

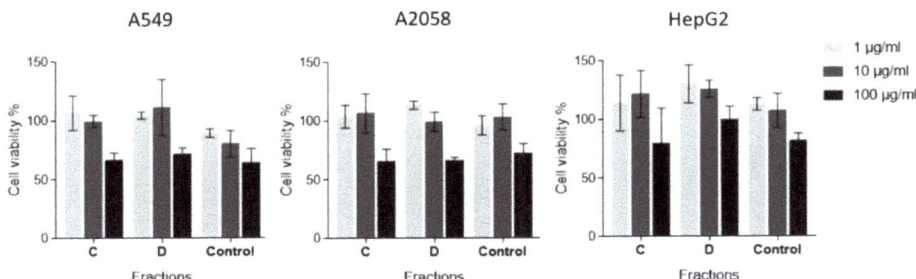

Figure 2. Antiproliferative assay. The histograms show the antiproliferative effects of fractions C and D of *C. closterium* extracts, on A549, A2058, and HepG2 cell lines. Control sample, containing only DMSO, was also tested (named as control). Results are expressed as percent survival after 72 h exposure ($n = 3$).

2.3. Dereplication

Since isolation of new compounds is very time consuming and costly [27,28], it is important to perform an early dereplication to identify already known components. In order to identify the bioactive compounds in the active fractions C and D, they were analyzed by UHPLC-HR-MS/MS and compared to the inactive fractions A and B (Figure 3). In fraction C, we found a series of compounds that all had a common fragment at *m/z* 184.0740 corresponding to a molecular formula of $C_5H_{15}NO_4P$ (see Figure S1, Supplementary Information). This is a common fragment observed when the head group of phosphocholines is cleaved off in tandem mass spectrometry. Phosphocholines are a class of phospholipids where the phosphocholine head group can be esterified to one or two fatty acids. Phosphocholines with two fatty acids are common membrane-forming phospholipids known as phosphatidylcholines (PC). When one fatty acid is removed from a PC, either enzymatically or by spontaneous hydrolysis, lysophosphatidylcholines (LysoPCs) are formed. After calculating the elemental compositions of the related molecules in fraction C and searching the ChemSpider database for known compounds, they were all identified as LysoPCs with different fatty acids attached. From the UHPLC-HR-MS/MS data we were able to determine the length of the fatty acids and the degree of unsaturation, but we were not able to directly determine the position of any double bonds and if the fatty acid was attached to carbon one or two on the glycerol backbone. In order to confirm our identification of LysoPCs, we injected a commercial standard of a C16:0 LysoPC (1-palmiotyl-sn-glycero-3-phosphocholine). The standard had the same retention time, mass, collisional cross section, and fragmentation pattern as one of the most intense compounds in fraction C (see Figure S2 and S3, Supplementary Information). The dominating LysoPCs in fraction C were 16:0, 16:1, 18:1, and 18:2 (approximately equal amounts) and minor LysoPCs were 14:0 and 18:3 (each approximately 20% of the most intense LysoPCs). A summary of the most intense LysoPCs and their retention times is given in Table S1 (Supplementary Information). There is current interest in LysoPCs because some of these are proposed for treatment of systemic inflammatory disorders [29–35]. However, their biological roles are not completely understood and some studies even found a putative pro-inflammatory activity [29]. Plasma LysoPC levels are diminished in human patients with sepsis [31,36], and in rodent models of sepsis and ischemia, LysoPC treatments in ex vivo and in vivo studies suggesting a potential role to relieve serious inflammatory conditions [29]. LysoPCs have also been shown to prevent neuronal death both in an in vivo model of transient global ischemia and in an in vitro model of excitotoxicity using primary cultures of cerebellar granule cells exposed to high extracellular concentrations of glutamate (20 to 40 micromol/L).

In fraction D, trace amounts of the same LysoPCs were present. However, the most intense peak in fraction D had a *m/z* value of 593.2752 with a corresponding elemental composition of $C_{35}H_{37}N_4O_5$ ($[M + H]^+$). When searching in the ChemSpider database, the elemental composition, as well as the fragmentation pattern, indicated that the compound was pheophorbide a, a breakdown product of chlorophyll (see Figure S4, Supplementary Information). Another peak in fraction D was identified as a related breakdown product of chlorophyll, hydroxypheophorbide a ($C_{35}H_{36}N_4O_6$, *m/z* 609.2708 $[M + H]^+$), see Figure S5 (Supplementary Information). Both pheophorbide a and its derivatives are known to have anti-inflammatory and anticancer properties [37–43], but, to our knowledge, this is the first case in a marine microalgae where the bioactivity was attributed to pheophorbide a. Pheophorbide a has already been extracted from a range of different marine organisms. Examples are the seaweed *Grateloupia ellittica* [40], the brown alga *Saccharina japonica* [39], marine diatoms [44,45], and the freshwater glaucophyte *Cyanophora paradoxa* [37]. Hydroxypheophorbide a has been previously isolated from the terrestrial plants *Clerodendrum calamitosum*, *Neptunia oleracea*, the freshwater unicellular green alga *Chlorella* sp., and from the marine tunicate *Trididemnum solidum*, but never from a marine diatom species. It is mainly known to have anticancer but not anti-inflammatory activity ([38,41], Patents No. 185220/82 and US4709022A). Hence we suggest that the possible anti-inflammatory activity observed in our experiments was due to the presence of LysoPCs and the known anti-inflammatory pheophorbide a. In fact, pheophorbide a is known to induce a dose-dependent inhibition against lipopolysaccharide (LPS)-induced nitric oxide (NO) production at nontoxic concentrations in RAW 264.7 murine macrophage cells and to suppress the expression of nitric oxide synthase (iNOS) [39].

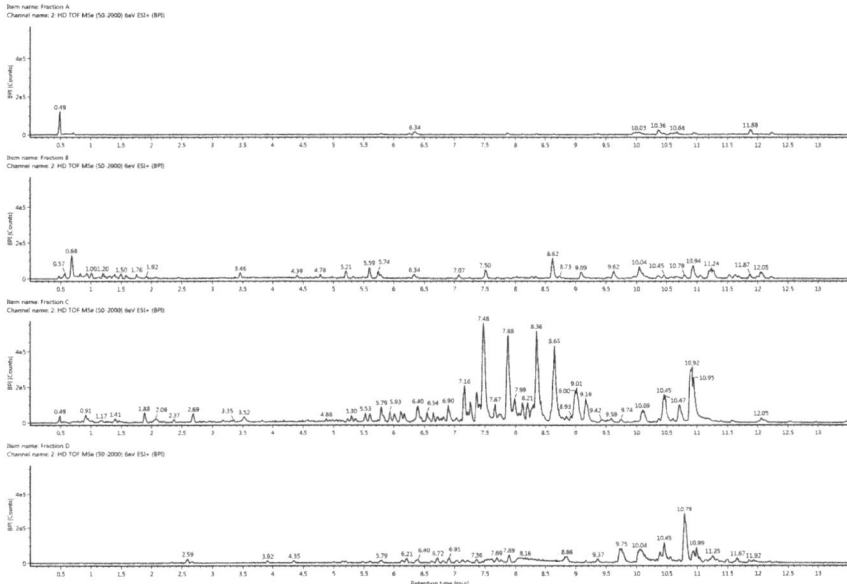

Figure 3. Base peak intensity chromatograms of fraction A, B, C, and D from the UHPLC-HR-MS/MS analysis using positive electrospray.

2.4. Anti-Inflammatory Activity of 1-Palmitoyl-sn-glycero-3-phosphocholine

Considering that the most active fraction mainly contained various phosphocholines, we tested one of these, 1-palmitoyl-sn-glycero-3-phosphocholine (which was the most abundant compound in fraction C) in our AIF-assay. The effect of 1-palmitoyl-sn-glycero-3-phosphocholine on secretion of TNF-α showed a dose-response relationship and was active at 25 µg/mL ($p < 0.05$) and 50 µg/mL ($p < 0.01$), as shown in Figure 4.

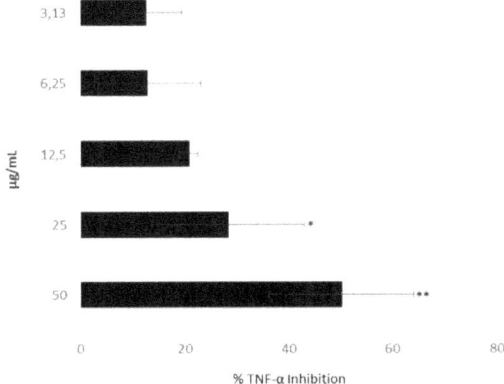

Figure 4. Anti-inflammatory assay. Inhibition of TNF-α secretion from LPS-stimulated THP-1 cells treated with 3.13, 6.25, 12.5, 25, and 50 µg/mL of 1-Palmitoyl-sn-glycero-3-phosphocholine ($n = 3$; * for $p < 0.05$ and ** for $p < 0.01$, Student's *t*-test).

3. Conclusions

Considering that inflammation plays a crucial role in the pathogenicity of several diseases, marine drug discovery is often directed to finding new natural products with anti-inflammatory properties [46,47]. Our results indicate that lysophosphatidylcholines (lysoPCs) and a breakdown product of chlorophyll, pheophorbide a, were probably responsible for the observed anti-inflammatory activity of the diatom *C. closterium*, giving new insights into microalgal compound bioactivities and their possible applications. This is the first time that a marine diatom is reported to produce these anti-inflammatory compounds. Pheophorbide a is known to inhibit the production of NO via inhibition of iNOS protein expression, thereby suggesting its potential use in the treatment of various inflammatory diseases (37), but there is no further information on its anti-inflammatory mechanism of action. Hence our study shows, for the first time, that it can inhibit TNF-α release in THP1 cells.

LysoPCs are products of phospholipase A2 enzyme activity, and similar to the enzyme, have a direct role in pro-inflammatory [48] and anti-inflammatory responses, in a variety of organ systems. Our results indicate that one of these LysoPCs, 1-palmitoyl-sn-glycero-3-phosphocholine (which was the most abundant compound in fraction C), had a strong anti-inflammatory activity which has not been demonstrated before. Microalgae, and in particular diatoms, therefore, can be considered potentially important producers of compounds to prevent and treat different human pathologies. In recent years they have been shown to have anti-inflammatory, antimicrobial, anticancer, antidiabetic, antiepileptic and even antituberculosis properties [10–12,49–55]. A better understanding of the potential health benefits from these marine organisms, the compounds they produce, and the environmental conditions affecting their production should allow for the sustainable development of these valuable marine resources in the future.

4. Materials and Methods

4.1. Cell Culturing and Harvesting

The diatom *Cylindrotheca closterium* (FE2), which has previously been shown to have anti-inflammatory activity [12], was cultured in Guillard's f/2 medium [56] in ten-liter polycarbonate carboys (4 replicates). Cultures were constantly bubbled with air filtered through 0.2 µm membrane filters and kept in a climate chamber at 19 °C and a 12:12 h light:dark cycle (100 µmol photons m^{-2} s^{-1}). Initial cell concentration was about 5000 cells/mL per bottle; culture growth was monitored daily by fixing 1 ml of culture with one drop of Lugol (final concentration of about 2%) and counting cells in a Bürker counting chamber under an Axioskop 2 microscope (20×) (Carl Zeiss GmbH, Jena, Germany). At the end of the stationary phase, cultures were centrifuged for 15 min at 4 °C at 3900 g using a cooled centrifuge with a swing-out rotor (DR 15P, Braun Biotechnology International, Allentown, PA, USA). The supernatant was discarded, and pellets freeze-dried and kept at −80 °C until chemical extraction.

4.2. Extraction and Fractionation

For extraction and fractionation, the protocol by Cutignano et al. [26] was used, but with some modifications. Briefly, a methanolic extract was firstly prepared by adding 5 mL methanol (MeOH) for each g of pellet (algae were cultured in three different occasions in triplicate batches), sonicating the samples for 30 s, centrifuging them at 4000 rpm for 5 min at room temperature and drying the supernatant with a rotovapor.

For the fractionation, columns were activated (column type: 6 mL/500 mg resin) with 6 mL methanol and 17 mL of distilled water. The resin used was a spherical poly(styrene-divinylbenzene) resin for SPE (Chromabond®HR-X, Düren, Germany). One mL of distilled water was added for each 20 mg of methanolic extract. Samples were sonicated to obtain a good suspension and added to the columns. The column was eluted as follows: (1) wash step with 2 mL of distilled water, throwing away 1.5 mL to eliminate salts, (2) addition of 18 mL of distilled water to obtain fraction A, (3) addition of 24 mL of methanol (CH$_3$OH)/water (50:50) to obtain fraction B, (4) addition of 18 mL Acetonitrile

(CH$_3$CN)/water (70:30) to obtain fraction C, (5) addition of 18 mL acetonitrile (100%) to obtain fraction D, (6) and finally addition of 18 mL of dichloromethane/methanol (CH$_2$Cl$_2$/CH$_3$OH; 90:10) to obtain fraction E.

4.3. Anti-Inflammatory Assay

The anti-inflammatory assay was performed as in Lauritano et al. [12]. Briefly, ~10^6 human monocyte THP-1 cells/mL (ATCC®TIB-202™) supplemented with 50 ng/mL phorbol 12- myristate 13-acetate (PMA, Sigma-Aldrich) were seeded in 96-well plates and incubated at 37 °C, 5% CO$_2$ for 48 h in RPMI-1640 medium (Biochrom). After 72 h, 80 µL fresh RPMI medium and 10 µL/well of test sample were added. In particular, fractions A, B, C, D, and E were tested at 100 and 50 µg/mL, while 1-palmitoyl-sn-glycero-3-phosphocholine (Sigma L5254) was tested at 3.13, 6.25, 12.5, 25, and 50 µg/mL. The tests were performed at least in triplicate. After incubation for 1 h, all samples were incubated with 1 ng/mL lipopolysaccharide (LPS) for 6 h at 37 °C and plates were then frozen at −80 °C. Enzyme-linked immunosorbent assay (ELISA) was used to test TNF-α inhibition. ELISA was performed as in Lauritano et al. [12]. Results were read at 405 nm.

4.4. In Vitro Anti-Proliferative Assay

Human cells were bought at ATCC (https://www.lgcstandards-atcc.org/). Human hepatocellular liver carcinoma cells (HepG2; ATCC®HB-8065™) were cultured in EMEM medium, human melanoma cells (A2058; ATCC®CRL-11147™) were cultured in DMEM, adenocarcinomic human alveolar basal epithelial cells (A549; ATCC®CL-185™) were cultured in F-12K medium. The media were supplemented with 10% fetal bovine serum, 50 U/ml penicillin, and 50 µg/ml streptomycin.

To evaluate the in vitro antiproliferative effects of the fractions, HepG2, A2058, and A549 cell lines were seeded in 96-well microtiter plates at a density of 1×10^4 cells/well and incubated at 37 °C to allow for cell adhesion in the plates. After 16 h, the medium was replaced with fresh medium containing increasing concentrations of the fractions (1, 10, and 100 µg/mL) for 72 h. Each concentration was tested at least in triplicate. After 72 h, cell viability was assessed using the MTT test (3-(4,5-dimethyl-2-thizolyl)-2,5-diphenyl-2H-tetrazolium bromide; A2231,0001, AppliChem Panreac Tischkalender, Darmstadt, GmbH). Briefly, the medium was replaced with medium containing MTT at 0.5 mg/ml and the plates were incubated for 3 h at 37 °C. After incubation, cells were treated with isopropyl alcohol (used as MTT solvent) for 30 minutes at room temperature. Absorbance was measured at OD = 570 nm using a microplate reader (Multiskan™ FC Microplate Photometer, Thermo Fisher Scientific, Waltham, MA, USA). Cell survival was expressed as a percentage of viable cells in the presence of the tested samples, with respect to untreated control cultures.

4.5. Statistical Analysis

Student's t-test was performed using GraphPad Prism statistic software, V4.00 (GraphPad Software, San Diego, CA, USA). Data were considered significant when p values were <0.05 (* for $p < 0.05$, ** for $p < 0.01$, and *** for $p < 0.001$).

4.6. Dereplication of Fractions

One mg of each fraction A to E were resuspended in 100 µL 80% aqueous methanol, centrifuged at 13,000 rpm for 5 min, and the supernatants were transferred to UHPLC injection vials. UHPLC-HR-MS/MS analysis of the fractions was performed using a Waters Acquity I-class UPLC system interfaced with a PDA Detector and a VION IMS-qTOF (Milford, MA, USA) using electrospray ionization (ESI) in positive mode. The VION IMS- qTOF was operated with a capillary voltage of 0.80 kV, desolvation gas flow (N$_2$) of 800 L/h, desolvation temperature of 450 °C, cone gas flow (N$_2$) of 50 L/h and an ion source temperature of 120 °C. Data were acquired between *m/z* 50 and 2000 with a scan time of 0.2 s. Fragment data were acquired by ramping the energy of the collision cell from 15 to 45 V, and high and low energy data were acquired in the same run. Leucine-enkephalin was used for internal calibration and the system was tuned to a resolution of 45,000 (FWHM). The system was controlled, and data were processed using UNIFI 1.9.4 (Waters). Chromatographic separation was achieved by injecting 3 µL of the dissolved fractions on a BEH C18 1.7 µm (2.1 × 100 mm) column (Waters) operated at 40 °C. The fractions were eluted with a gradient of 10% to 100% acetonitrile in water over 10 min (both containing 0.1% formic acid), followed by maintaining 100% acetonitrile until 13.5 min.

Supplementary Materials: The following are available online at http://www.mdpi.com/1660-3397/18/3/166/s1, Figure S1: Top: Base peak intensity chromatogram from the UHPLC-HR-MS/MS analysis of fraction C using positive electrospray. Bottom: Ion chromatogram of m/z 184. 0740 from fraction C indicating the presence of phosphocholines, Figure S2: Top: Ion chromatogram of m/z 496.3396 from fraction C showing the presence of LysoPC. Bottom: Base peak intensity chromatogram from the UHPLC-HR-MS/MS analysis of fraction C using positive electrospray, Figure S3: Top: Low energy mass spectrum of 1-Palmiotyl-sn-glycero-3-phosphocholine from fraction C. Bottom: High energy mass spectrum of 1-Palmiotyl-sn-glycero-3-phosphocholine showing fragments and mass deviations corresponding with the commercial standard, Figure S4: Top: Low energy mass spectrum of pheophorbide A from fraction D. Bottom: High energy mass spectrum of pheophorbide A showing fragments and mass deviations corresponding with the theoretical fragmentation of the database hit, Figure S5: Top: Low energy mass spectrum of hydroxypheophorbide A from fraction D. Bottom: High energy mass spectrum of hydroxypheophorbide A showing fragments and mass deviations corresponding with the theoretical fragmentation of the database hit, Table S1: The most abundant lysophosphatidylcholines in fraction C. The type indicates number of carbons and double bonds in the fatty acid moiety of the respective LysoPCs, and the retention times are given in minutes.

Author Contributions: C.L. and E.H.H. conceived and designed the experiments; C.L., K.H., G.R., and E.H.H. performed the experiments; C.L., K.H., G.R., and E.H.H. analyzed the data. All authors (C.L., K.H., G.R., J.H.A., A.I. and E.H.H.) co-wrote the paper. All authors have read and agreed to the published version of the manuscript.

Funding: This research was funded by the "Antitumor Drugs and Vaccines from the Sea (ADViSE)" project (PG/2018/0494374).

Acknowledgments: We thank Massimo Perna and Mariano Amoroso for their technical support.

Conflicts of Interest: The authors declare no conflict of interest.

References

1. Nathan, C. Points of control in inflammation. *Nature* **2002**, *420*, 846–852. [CrossRef] [PubMed]
2. Nathan, C.; Ding, A. Nonresolving inflammation. *Cell* **2010**, *140*, 871–882. [CrossRef] [PubMed]
3. Newton, K.; Dixit, V.M. Signaling in innate immunity and inflammation. *Cold Spring Harb. Perspect. Biol.* **2012**, *4*, a006049. [CrossRef] [PubMed]
4. Korniluk, A.; Koper, O.; Kemona, H.; Dymicka-Piekarska, V. From inflammation to cancer. *Ir. J. Med. Sci.* **2017**, *186*, 57–62. [CrossRef]
5. Jaspars, M.; De Pascale, D.; Andersen, J.H.; Reyes, F.; Crawford, A.D.; Ianora, A. The marine biodiscovery pipeline and ocean medicines of tomorrow. *J. Mar. Biol. Assoc. U. K.* **2016**, *96*, 151–158. [CrossRef]
6. Carotenuto, Y.; Esposito, F.; Pisano, F.; Lauritano, C.; Perna, M.; Miralto, A.; Ianora, A. Multi-generation cultivation of the copepod *Calanus helgolandicus* in a re-circulating system. *J. Exp. Mar. Biol. Ecol.* **2012**, *418–419*, 46–58. [CrossRef]
7. Romano, G.; Costantini, M.; Sansone, C.; Lauritano, C.; Ruocco, N.; Ianora, A. Marine microorganisms as a promising and sustainable source of bioactive molecules. *Mar. Environ. Res.* **2017**, *128*, 58–69. [CrossRef]
8. Falkowski, P.G. The role of phytoplankton photosynthesis in global biogeochemical cycles. *Photosyn. Res.* **1994**, *39*, 235–258. [CrossRef]
9. Nelson, D.M.; Tréguer, P.; Brzezinski, M.A.; Leynaert, A.; Quéguiner, B. Production and dissolution of biogenic silica in the ocean: Revised global estimates, comparison with regional data and relationship to biogenic sedimentation. *Glob. Biogeochem. Cycles* **1995**, *9*, 359–372. [CrossRef]
10. Martínez Andrade, K.; Lauritano, C.; Romano, G.; Ianora, A. Marine microalgae with anti-cancer properties. *Mar. Drugs* **2018**, *16*, 165. [CrossRef]
11. Ingebrigtsen, R.A.; Hansen, E.; Andersen, J.H.; Eilertsen, H.C. Light and temperature effects on bioactivity in diatoms. *J. Appl. Phycol.* **2016**, *28*, 939–950. [CrossRef]

12. Lauritano, C.; Andersen, J.H.; Hansen, E.; Albrigtsen, M.; Escalera, L.; Esposito, F.; Helland, K.; Hanssen, K.Ø.; Romano, G.; Ianora, A. Bioactivity screening of microalgae for antioxidant, anti-inflammatory, anticancer, anti-diabetes, and antibacterial activities. *Front. Mar. Sci.* **2016**, *3*, 68. [CrossRef]
13. Samarakoon, K.W.; Ko, J.-Y.; Shah, M.R.; Lee, J.-H.; Kang, M.-C.; O-Nam, K.; Lee, J.-B.; Jeon, Y.-J. In vitro studies of anti-inflammatory and anticancer activities of organic solvent extracts from cultured marine microalgae. *Algae* **2013**, *28*, 111–119. [CrossRef]
14. Jo, W.S.; Choi, Y.J.; Kim, H.J.; Nam, B.H.; Hong, S.H.; Lee, G.A.; Lee, S.W.; Seo, S.Y.; Jeong, M.H. Anti-inflammatory effect of microalgal extracts from *Tetraselmis suecica*. *Food Sci. Biotechnol.* **2010**, *19*, 1519–1528. [CrossRef]
15. Sanjeewa, K.K.A.; Fernando, I.P.S.; Samarakoon, K.W.; Lakmal, H.H.C.; Kim, E.-A.; Kwon, O.-N.; Dilshara, M.G.; Lee, J.-B.; Jeon, Y.-J. Anti-inflammatory and anti-cancer activities of sterol rich fraction of cultured marine microalga *Nannochloropsis oculata*. *Algae* **2016**, *31*, 277–287. [CrossRef]
16. Lavy, A.; Naveh, Y.; Coleman, R.; Mokady, S.; Werman, M.J. Dietary *Dunaliella bardawil*, a beta-carotene-rich alga, protects against acetic acid-induced small bowel inflammation in rats. *Inflamm. Bowel Dis.* **2003**, *9*, 372–379. [CrossRef] [PubMed]
17. Lee, J.-C.; Hou, M.-F.; Huang, H.-W.; Chang, F.-R.; Yeh, C.-C.; Tang, J.-Y.; Chang, H.-W. Marine algal natural products with anti-oxidative, anti-inflammatory, and anti-cancer properties. *Cancer Cell Int.* **2013**, *13*, 55. [CrossRef]
18. Ávila-Román, J.; Talero, E.; Rodríguez-Luna, A.; García-Mauriño, S.; Motilva, V. Anti-inflammatory effects of an oxylipin-containing lyophilised biomass from a microalga in a murine recurrent colitis model. *Br. J. Nutr.* **2016**, *116*, 2044–2052. [CrossRef]
19. Robertson, R.C.; Guihéneuf, F.; Bahar, B.; Schmid, M.; Stengel, D.B.; Fitzgerald, G.F.; Ross, R.P.; Stanton, C. The anti-inflammatory effect of algae-derived lipid extracts on lipopolysaccharide (LPS)-stimulated human THP-1 macrophages. *Mar. Drugs* **2015**, *13*, 5402–5424. [CrossRef]
20. de los Reyes, C.; Ortega, M.J.; Rodríguez-Luna, A.; Talero, E.; Motilva, V.; Zubía, E. Molecular characterization and anti-inflammatory activity of galactosylglycerides and galactosylceramides from the microalga *Isochrysis galbana*. *J. Agric. Food Chem.* **2016**, *64*, 8783–8794. [CrossRef]
21. Renju, G.L.; Muraleedhara Kurup, G.; Saritha Kumari, C.H. Anti-inflammatory activity of lycopene isolated from *Chlorella marina* on type II collagen induced arthritis in Sprague Dawley rats. *Immunopharmacol. Immunotoxicol.* **2013**, *35*, 282–291. [CrossRef] [PubMed]
22. Caroprese, M.; Albenzio, M.; Ciliberti, M.G.; Francavilla, M.; Sevi, A. A mixture of phytosterols from *Dunaliella tertiolecta* affects proliferation of peripheral blood mononuclear cells and cytokine production in sheep. *Vet. Immunol. Immunopathol.* **2012**, *150*, 27–35. [CrossRef] [PubMed]
23. Kaulmann, A.; Bohn, T. Carotenoids, inflammation, and oxidative stress–implications of cellular signaling pathways and relation to chronic disease prevention. *Nutr. Res.* **2014**, *34*, 907–929. [CrossRef] [PubMed]
24. Nicoletti, M. Microalgae nutraceuticals. *Foods* **2016**, *5*, 54. [CrossRef]
25. García, J.L.; de Vicente, M.; Galán, B. Microalgae, old sustainable food and fashion nutraceuticals. *Microb. Biotechnol.* **2017**, *10*, 1017–1024. [CrossRef]
26. Cutignano, A.; Nuzzo, G.; Ianora, A.; Luongo, E.; Romano, G.; Gallo, C.; Sansone, C.; Aprea, S.; Mancini, F.; D'Oro, U.; et al. Development and application of a novel SPE-method for bioassay-guided fractionation of marine extracts. *Mar. Drugs* **2015**, *13*, 5736–5749. [CrossRef]
27. Cordell, G.A.; Shin, Y.G. Finding the needle in the haystack. The dereplication of natural product extracts. *Pure Appl. Chem.* **1999**, *71*, 1089–1094. [CrossRef]
28. Hubert, J.; Nuzillard, J.-M.; Renault, J.-H. Dereplication strategies in natural product research: How many tools and methodologies behind the same concept? *Phytochem. Rev.* **2017**, *16*, 55–95. [CrossRef]
29. Cunningham, T.J.; Yao, L.; Lucena, A. Product inhibition of secreted phospholipase A2 may explain lysophosphatidylcholines' unexpected therapeutic properties. *J. Inflamm.* **2008**, *5*, 17. [CrossRef]
30. Mehta, D. Lysophosphatidylcholine: An enigmatic lysolipid. *Am. J. Physiol.-Lung Cell. Mol. Physiol.* **2005**, *289*, L174–L175. [CrossRef]
31. Drobnik, W.; Liebisch, G.; Audebert, F.-X.; Frohlich, D.; Gluck, T.; Vogel, P.; Rothe, G.; Schmitz, G. Plasma ceramide and lysophosphatidylcholine inversely correlate with mortality in sepsis patients. *J. Lipid Res.* **2003**, *44*, 754–761. [CrossRef] [PubMed]

32. Chen, G.; Li, J.; Qiang, X.; Czura, C.J.; Ochani, M.; Ochani, K.; Ulloa, L.; Yang, H.; Tracey, K.J.; Wang, P.; et al. Suppression of HMGB1 release by stearoyl lysophosphatidylcholine: An additional mechanism for its therapeutic effects in experimental sepsis. *J. Lipid Res.* **2005**, *46*, 623–627. [CrossRef] [PubMed]
33. Blondeau, N.; Lauritzen, I.; Widmann, C.; Lazdunski, M.; Heurteaux, C. A potent protective role of lysophospholipids against global cerebral ischemia and glutamate excitotoxicity in neuronal cultures. *J. Cereb. Blood Flow Metab.* **2002**, *22*, 821–834. [CrossRef] [PubMed]
34. Yan, J.-J.; Jung, J.-S.; Lee, J.-E.; Lee, J.; Huh, S.-O.; Kim, H.-S.; Jung, K.C.; Cho, J.-Y.; Nam, J.-S.; Suh, H.-W.; et al. Therapeutic effects of lysophosphatidylcholine in experimental sepsis. *Nat. Med.* **2004**, *10*, 161–167. [CrossRef]
35. Murch, O.; Collin, M.; Sepodes, B.; Foster, S.J.; Mota-Filipe, H.; Thiemermann, C. Lysophosphatidylcholine reduces the organ injury and dysfunction in rodent models of gram-negative and gram-positive shock. *Br. J. Pharmacol.* **2006**, *148*, 769–777. [CrossRef]
36. Lissauer, E.; Johnson, B.G.; Shi, S.; Gentle, T.; Scalea, M. 128: Decreased lysophosphatidylcholine levels are associated with sepsis compared to uninfected inflammation prior to onset of sepsis. *J. Surg. Res.* **2007**, *137*, 206. [CrossRef]
37. Baudelet, P.-H.; Gagez, A.-L.; Bérard, J.-B.; Juin, C.; Bridiau, N.; Kaas, R.; Thiéry, V.; Cadoret, J.-P.; Picot, L. Antiproliferative activity of *Cyanophora paradoxa* pigments in melanoma, breast and lung cancer cells. *Mar. Drugs* **2013**, *11*, 4390–4406. [CrossRef]
38. Choi, S.-E.; Sohn, S.; Cho, J.-W.; Shin, E.-A.; Song, P.-S.; Kang, Y. 9-Hydroxypheophorbide alpha-induced apoptotic death of MCF-7 breast cancer cells is mediated by c-Jun N-terminal kinase activation. *J. Photochem. Photobiol. B Biol.* **2004**, *73*, 101–107. [CrossRef]
39. Islam, M.N.; Ishita, I.J.; Jin, S.E.; Choi, R.J.; Lee, C.M.; Kim, Y.S.; Jung, H.A.; Choi, J.S. Anti-inflammatory activity of edible brown alga *Saccharina japonica* and its constituents pheophorbide a and pheophytin a in LPS-stimulated RAW 264.7 macrophage cells. *Food Chem. Toxicol.* **2013**, *55*, 541–548. [CrossRef]
40. Cho, M.; Park, G.-M.; Kim, S.-N.; Amna, T.; Lee, S.; Shin, W.-S. Glioblastoma-specific anticancer activity of pheophorbide a from the edible red seaweed *Grateloupia elliptica*. *J. Microbiol. Biotechnol.* **2014**, *24*, 346–353. [CrossRef]
41. Nakamura, Y.; Murakami, A.; Koshimizu, K.; Ohigashi, H. Inhibitory effect of pheophorbide a, a chlorophyll-related compound, on skin tumor promotion in ICR mouse. *Cancer Lett.* **1996**, *108*, 247–255. [CrossRef]
42. Chan, J.Y.-W.; Tang, P.M.-K.; Hon, P.-M.; Au, S.W.-N.; Tsui, S.K.-W.; Waye, M.M.-Y.; Kong, S.-K.; Mak, T.C.-W.; Fung, K.-P. Pheophorbide a, a major antitumor component purified from *Scutellaria barbata*, induces apoptosis in human hepatocellular carcinoma cells. *Planta Med.* **2006**, *72*, 28–33. [CrossRef] [PubMed]
43. Hibasami, H.; Kyohkon, M.; Ohwaki, S.; Katsuzaki, H.; Imai, K.; Nakagawa, M.; Ishi, Y.; Komiya, T. Pheophorbide a, a moiety of chlorophyll a, induces apoptosis in human lymphoid leukemia molt 4B cells. *Int. J. Mol. Med.* **2000**, *6*, 277–279. [CrossRef] [PubMed]
44. Veuger, B.; Oevelen, D. Long-term pigment dynamics and diatom survival in dark sediment. *Limnol. Oceanogr.* **2011**, *56*, 1065–1074. [CrossRef]
45. Kuczynska, P.; Jemiola-Rzeminska, M.; Strzalka, K. Photosynthetic pigments in diatoms. *Mar. Drugs* **2015**, *13*, 5847–5881. [CrossRef] [PubMed]
46. Hurst, D.; Børresen, T.; Almesjö, L.; Raedemaecker, F.; Bergseth, S. *Marine Biotechnology Strategic Research and Innovation Roadmap-Insights to the Future Direction of European Marine Biotechnology*; Marine Biotechnology ERA-NET: Oostende, Belgium, 2016; ISBN 978-94-92043-27-6.
47. Reen, F.J.; Gutiérrez-Barranquero, J.A.; Dobson, A.D.W.; Adams, C.; O'Gara, F. Emerging concepts promising new horizons for marine biodiscovery and synthetic biology. *Mar. Drugs* **2015**, *13*, 2924–2954. [CrossRef]
48. Law, S.-H.; Chan, M.-L.; Marathe, G.K.; Parveen, F.; Chen, C.-H.; Ke, L.-Y. An updated review of lysophosphatidylcholine metabolism in human diseases. *Int. J. Mol. Sci.* **2019**, *20*, 1149. [CrossRef]
49. Lauritano, C.; Martín, J.; de la Cruz, M.; Reyes, F.; Romano, G.; Ianora, A. First identification of marine diatoms with anti-tuberculosis activity. *Sci. Rep.* **2018**, *8*, 2284. [CrossRef]
50. Brillatz, T.; Lauritano, C.; Jacmin, M.; Khamma, S.; Marcourt, L.; Righi, D.; Romano, G.; Esposito, F.; Ianora, A.; Queiroz, E.F.; et al. Zebrafish-based identification of the antiseizure nucleoside inosine from the marine diatom *Skeletonema marinoi*. *PLoS ONE* **2018**, *13*, e0196195. [CrossRef]

51. Giordano, D.; Costantini, M.; Coppola, D.; Lauritano, C.; Núñez Pons, L.; Ruocco, N.; di Prisco, G.; Ianora, A.; Verde, C. Biotechnological applications of bioactive peptides from marine sources. In *Advances in Microbial Physiology*; Elsevier: Amsterdam, The Netherlands, 2018; Volume 73, pp. 171–220. ISBN 978-0-12-815190-7.
52. Riccio, G.; Lauritano, C. Microalgae with immunomodulatory activities. *Mar. Drugs* **2020**, *18*, 2. [CrossRef]
53. Lauritano, C.; Ianora, A. Marine organisms with anti-diabetes properties. *Mar. Drugs* **2016**, *14*, 220. [CrossRef] [PubMed]
54. Sasso, S.; Pohnert, G.; Lohr, M.; Mittag, M.; Hertweck, C. Microalgae in the postgenomic era: A blooming reservoir for new natural products. *FEMS Microbiol. Rev.* **2012**, *36*, 761–785. [CrossRef] [PubMed]
55. Plaza, M.; Herrero, M.; Cifuentes, A.; Ibáñez, E. Innovative natural functional ingredients from microalgae. *J. Agric. Food Chem.* **2009**, *57*, 7159–7170. [CrossRef] [PubMed]
56. Guillard, R.R.L. Culture of phytoplankton for feeding marine invertebrates. In *Culture of Marine Invertebrate Animals: Proceedings—1st Conference on Culture of Marine Invertebrate Animals Greenport*; Smith, W.L., Chanley, M.H., Eds.; Springer: Boston, MA, USA, 1975; pp. 29–60. ISBN 978-1-4615-8714-9.

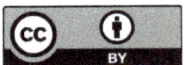

© 2020 by the authors. Licensee MDPI, Basel, Switzerland. This article is an open access article distributed under the terms and conditions of the Creative Commons Attribution (CC BY) license (http://creativecommons.org/licenses/by/4.0/).

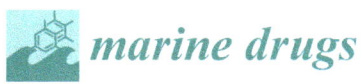

Article

Bioactive Molecules from Mangrove *Streptomyces qinglanensis* 172205

Dongbo Xu [1], Erli Tian [1], Fandong Kong [2] and Kui Hong [1,*]

[1] Key Laboratory of Combinatorial Biosynthesis and Drug Discovery, Ministry of Education, School of Pharmaceutical Sciences, Wuhan University, Wuhan 430071, China; xudongbo1990@gmail.com (D.X.); erlitian@whu.edu.cn (E.T.)
[2] Institute of Tropical Bioscience and Biotechnology, Chinese Academy of Tropical Agricultura Sciences, Haikou 571101, China; kongfandong@itbb.org.cn
* Correspondence: kuihong31@whu.edu.cn; Tel.: +86-27-6875-2442

Received: 17 April 2020; Accepted: 12 May 2020; Published: 13 May 2020

Abstract: Five new compounds 15R-17,18-dehydroxantholipin (**1**), (3E,5E,7E)-3-methyldeca-3,5,7-triene-2,9-dione (**2**) and qinlactone A–C (**3–5**) were identified from mangrove *Streptomyces qinglanensis* 172205 with "genetic dereplication," which deleted the highly expressed secondary metabolite-enterocin biosynthetic gene cluster. The chemical structures were established by spectroscopic methods, and the absolute configurations were determined by electronic circular dichroism (ECD). Compound **1** exhibited strong anti-microbial and antiproliferative bioactivities, while compounds **2–4** showed weak antiproliferative activities.

Keywords: mangrove *Streptomyces*; genetic dereplication; anti-microbial; antiproliferative

1. Introduction

Microbial natural products are an important source of drug lead. Mangrove streptomycetes were reported as a potential source of plenty of antiproliferative or anti-microbial chemicals with novel structures [1]. The bioinformatics of easily available genome information from microorganisms breaks the bottleneck of traditional natural product discovery to a certain extent, and secondary metabolites isolation guided by genome sequence has increasingly become a research frontier [2]. Genome mining and silent gene cluster activation unveil the potential of diverse secondary metabolites in bacteria [3–5]. The OSMAC (One Strain Many Compounds) approach has been proven to be a simple and powerful tool to mine new natural products [6,7]. Due to complexity profiles of secondary metabolites including intermediates, a strategy named "genetic dereplication" was also developed to simplify the profiles by eliminating the major known secondary metabolites' biosynthetic pathway, so that more easily detecting other novel compounds and/or reversing the precursor pools for other low expressed pathways in the microorganisms [8].

Previous studies reported that enterocin and its metabolites are the main and high-yield products in *Streptomyces qinglanensis* 172205 [9]. After the whole genome sequence was obtained, we analyzed the gene clusters of secondary metabolites, and found that more than 50% of them are coding for unknown compounds. However, enterocin was always detected in all of the media used during the OSMAC study. Hence, in this study, to mine the unknown compounds in strain 172205, we carried out the genetic dereplication strategy by which we deleted the enterocin biosynthetic gene cluster in genome and then detected the diversity of secondary metabolites profiles by OSMAC method. A mutant strain 172205Δenc was generated by the whole enterocin biosynthetic gene cluster deletion using double-crossover homologous recombination and tested by HPLC fingerprint profiles for diverse products of crude extracts from 10 kinds of liquid fermentation media. The results showed that strain 172205Δenc could produce the most diverse peaks on HPLC under fermentation in D.O.

(dextrin-oatmeal) medium. Subsequently, a large-scale fermentation with D.O. medium was performed. After isolation and purification of the compounds from the crude extract, five new compounds including 15R-17,18-dehydroxantholipin (**1**), (3E,5E,7E)-3-methyldeca-3,5,7-triene-2,9-dione (**2**) and qinlactone A–C (**3–5**) were identified. Their structures were elucidated by one-dimensional (1D)/two-dimensional (2D) nuclear magnetic resonance spectroscopy (NMR) data, as well as electronic circular dichroism (ECD) calculation. In anti-microbial bioassay tests, compound **1** showed strong anti-*Staphylococcus aureus* and anti-*Candida albicans* activities with MIC (minimum inhibitory concentration) values of 0.78 μg/mL and 3.13 μg/mL, respectively. For antiproliferative bioactivity, compound **1** exhibited strong cytotoxicities against human breast cancer cell line MCF-7 and human cervical cancer cell line HeLa with IC_{50} values of 5.78 μM and 6.25 μM, respectively, while compound **2–4** showed weaker antiproliferative activities with IC_{50} values ranging from 129 to 207 μM. Therefore, the "genetic dereplication" strategy is useful to find compounds that synthesized by low expression gene clusters and would be of interest to colleagues in natural product discovery.

2. Results

Strain 172205Δ*enc* was obtained by the enterocin biosynthetic gene cluster deletion (Figure 1a) and confirmed by PCR (polymerase chain reaction) amplification (Supplementary Figure S1 and Table S1). The HPLC profile of crude extract in D.O. medium (Figure 1b) showed that enterocin biosynthesis were totally blocked in mutant strain 172205Δ*enc*, including its intermediate metabolite-cinnamic acid.

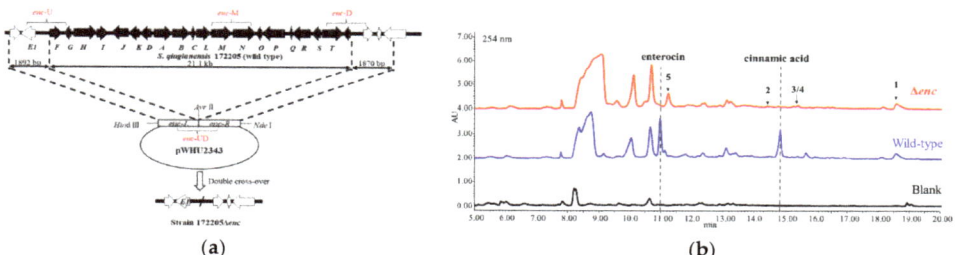

Figure 1. (**a**) The organization of enterocin biosynthetic gene cluster before and after deletion. Amplification fragments by verifying primers were labeled by fronts in red; (**b**) HPLC detection of crude extracts of strain 172205 wild type and Δ*enc* in D.O. medium.

Almost 80 grams crude extract was obtained from extraction of 60 L fermentation broth of mutant 172205Δ*enc* and subjected to column chromatography and semi-preparative HPLC purification to afford compounds **1–5**. The chemical structures were showed in Figure 2.

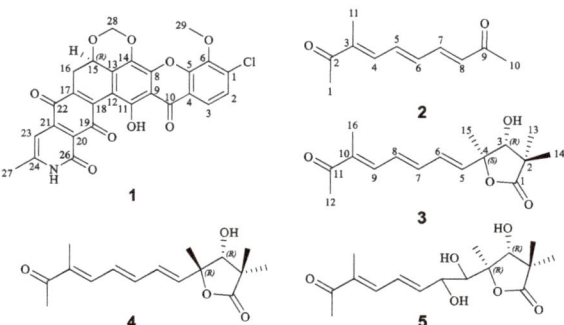

Figure 2. Chemical structures of compound **1–5**.

15R-17,18-dehydroxantholipin (**1**) was obtained as a dark red powder with the molecular formula of $C_{27}H_{16}ClNO_9$ (HRESIMS-high resolution electrospray ionisation mass spectrometry m/z 534.0587, calcd 534.0586 for [M + H]$^+$), implying 20 degrees of unsaturation. Detailed comparison of 1D NMR (Table 1) between compound **1** and the reported xantholipin [10,11] showed that **1** had the same NMR data with xantholipin, except for the two sp^2 quaternary carbons C-17 (δ_C 136.0) and C-18 (δ_C 141.5), implying a double bond. The mass spectrum suggested the loss of a H$_2$O group to form a double bond between C-17 and C-18. The correlations in HMBC (heteronuclear multiple bond coherence) from H-16a to C-13, C-15, C-17 and C-18 also located the placement at C-17 and C-18. Thus, the planar structure of **1** was determined. The key HMBC and COSY (homonuclear correlation spectroscopy) correlations are shown in Figure 3. Furthermore, the quantum chemical ECD calculation method was also used to determine the absolute configuration. The calculated ECD spectrum of **1** was compared with the experimental one, which revealed an excellent agreement between them (Figure 4). Therefore, the absolute configuration of **1** was assigned to 15R. Thus, the structure of **1** was determined.

Table 1. ^{1}H and ^{13}C NMR data for Compound **1–2**.

Position	1			2		
	δ_H (J in Hz)	δ_C, Type	HMBC	δ_H (J in Hz)	δ_C, Type	HMBC
1		133.6, C		2.38 s	26.0, CH$_3$	C-2, 4
2	7.63 d (8.8)	125.9, CH	C-1, 4, 6		202.0, C	
3	7.95 d (8.4)	120.8, CH	C-1, 5, 10		140.7, C	
4		120.6, C		7.28 d (11.4)	139.6, CH	C-2, 6, 11
5		149.7, C		7.16 dd (11.5, 14.6)	137.9, CH	C-3, 7
6		144.6, C		6.84 dd (11.2, 14.6)	138.8, CH	C-4, 7, 8
7				7.41 dd (11.1, 15.6)	144.5, CH	C-5, 6, 9
8		143.4, C		6.31 d (15.7)	133.7, CH	C-6, 9, 10
9		108.2 *, C			201.3, C	
10		181.4, C		2.32 s	27.4, CH$_3$	C-7, 8, 9
11		158.9, C		1.94 d (1.0)	12.0, CH$_3$	C-2, 3
12		109.5 *, C				
13		131.4, C				
14		131.3, C				
15	5.15 dd (6.4, 14.0)	71.1, CH				
16	a, 2.37 m b, 2.54 overlapped	25.3, CH$_2$	C-13, 15, 17, 18			
17		136.0 **, C				
18		141.5 **, C				
19		178.6, C				
20		117.3, C				
21		145.1, C				
22		182.8, C				
23	6.55 s	99.6, CH	C-20, 22, 24, 27			
24		154.5, C				
25-NH	12.67 s		C-20, 23, 26, 27			
26		151.9, C				
27	2.36 s	19.5, CH$_3$	C-23, 24			
28	a, 5.71 d (5.9) b, 5.48 d (5.8)	91.3, CH$_2$	C-14, 15 C-15			
29	4.08 s	61.6, CH$_3$	C-6			
11-OH	12.67 s		C-9			

*, ** Assignments are made in comparison with literature data for similar reported compounds. **1** (800 and 200 MHz, DMSO-d_6, δ in ppm); **2** (500 and 125 MHz, CD$_3$OD-d_4, δ in ppm).

(3E,5E,7E)-3-methyldeca-3,5,7-triene-2,9-dione (**2**) was obtained as a yellow powder. The molecular formula of **2** was determined as $C_{11}H_{14}O_2$ (HRESIMS m/z 179.1064, calcd 179.1067 for [M + H]$^+$), indicating 5 degrees of unsaturation. The 1D and HSQC (heteronuclear single quantum coherence) NMR data (Table 1) of **2** revealed the presence of three aliphatic methyls, two carbonyls (ketone) (δ_C 202.0 and 201.3), five olefinic methines (C-4 to C-8) and six olefinic carbons. The ^{1}H-^{1}H COSY correlations (Figure 3) from H-4 to H-8 revealed the conjugated system indicated by bold lines in Figure 3. HMBC correlations from H-5 to C-3 and C-7, H-6 to C-4 and C-7, H-7 to C-5 and C-6 and H-8 to C-6 and C-7 suggested that **2** contained three conjugated double bonds. HMBC correlations from H-11 to C-2 and C-3, and H-4 to C-2 and C-11 located one methyl (H-11) at C-3. HMBC correlations from H-1 to C-2 and C-4, and H-11 to C-2 and C-3 supported one methyl (C-1) located at C-2 and the connection between C-2 and C-3. Moreover, HMBC correlation from H-10 to C-8 and C-9, H-8 to C-9, and H-7 to C-9 assigned another methyl ketone location at C-8. $J_{H-5/H-6}$ = 14.6 Hz and $J_{H-7/H-8}$ = 15.6 Hz revealed two (E)-alkene between C-5-C-8. The ROESY (rotating frame overhauser effect spectroscopy) correlation of H-4 and H-1 supported the (E)-alkene between C-3 and C-4. Thus, the (3E,5E,7E)-triene was identified and chemical structure of **2** was established.

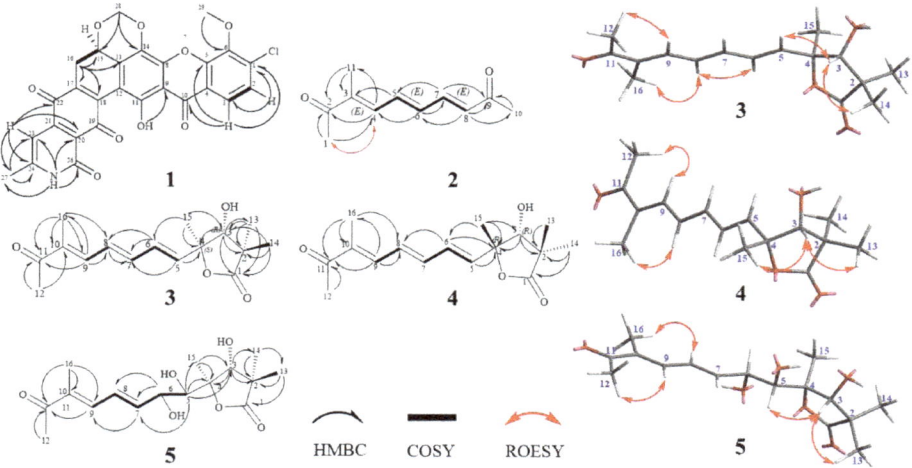

Figure 3. Key heteronuclear multiple bond coherence (HMBC), homonuclear correlation spectroscopy (COSY) and rotating frame overhauser effect spectroscopy (ROESY) correlations of compound **1–5**.

Qinlactone A (**3**) was obtained as a colorless oil. Its HRESIMS data indicated its molecular formula is $C_{16}H_{22}O_4$ (m/z 279.1587, calcd 279.1591 for [M + H]$^+$) with 6 degrees of unsaturation. The 1D (Table 2) and HSQC NMR data of **3** revealed the presence of five aliphatic methyl groups, one carbonyl (ketone, δ_C 202.2) and one carbonyl (ester, δ_C 183.3) and five olefinic methines (C-5 to C-9). The ^1H-^1H correlations of H-5/H-6/H-7 and H-8/H-9 confirmed the same three conjugated double bonds as **2**. The HMBC correlations (Figure 3) from H-12 to C-11 (δ_C 202.2) and C-10, H-9 to C-11 and H-16 to C-8/C-9/C-10/C-11 confirmed the location of one methyl ketone and a methyl (C-16) at C-10. ROESY correlations of H-12/H-9, H-8/H-16 and H-9/H-7 confirmed all the (E)-alkenes from C-5 to C-10. Additionally, HMBC correlations from H-13 to C-1/C-2/C-3/C-14 and H-14 to C-1/C-2/C-3/C-13 suggested two aliphatic methyl groups located at quaternary carbon C-2, and indicated the connection from C1 to C3. HMBC correlations from H-15 to C-3/C-4 located the last methyl (δ_C 22.1) at C-4. Two carbons connected to oxygen atoms (δ_C 81.5 and 88.0) suggested the OH group at C-3 and ester oxygen connected with C-4. Thus, based on the unsaturation and ester group (δ_C 183.8, C-1), a γ-lactone structure was revealed. The HMBC correlations from H-3 to C-1/C-2/C-4/C-5/C-13/C-14 also confirmed γ-lactone in **3**. Meanwhile, the HMBC correlations of H-5 to C-4 and H-6 to C-4 revealed the connection of lactone and conjugated olefin part. Thus, the planar structure of **3** was established. The relative configuration of **3** was established by ROESY experiment. The ROESY correlation of H-3 and H-14/H-5 suggested the relative configuration of 3R*, 4S* (Figure 3). The absolute configuration was confirmed by a good agreement between the calculated ECD spectrum of **3** and experimental one (Figure 4). Therefore, the absolute configuration **3** was assigned to 3R, 4S. Compound **3** was named qinlactone A.

Table 2. ^{1}H and ^{13}C NMR data for Compound 3–5 (500 and 125 MHz, CD$_3$OD-d_4, δ in ppm).

Position	3			4			5		
	$δ_H$ (J in Hz)	$δ_C$, Type	HMBC	$δ_H$ (J in Hz)	$δ_C$, Type	HMBC	$δ_H$ (J in Hz)	$δ_C$, Type	HMBC
1		183.3, C			182.6, C			183.4, C	
2		45.9, C			44.9, C			45.0, C	
3	3.96 s	81.5, CH	C-1, 2, 4, 5, 13, 14	3.98 s	83.8, CH	C-2, 4, 5, 13, 14	4.53 s	75.1, CH	C-2, 4, 5, 14, 15
4		88.0, C			86.2, C			90.4, C	
5	6.14 d (15.4)	142.1, CH	C-3, 4, 7, 15	6.27 d (15.6)	139.0, CH	C-4, 6, 7, 15	3.63 d (2.3)	77.9, CH	C-3, 4, 7, 15
6	6.46 dd (9.9, 15.4)	129.8, CH	C-4, 7, 8	6.46 dd (9.8, 15.6)	130.2, CH	C-4, 5, 8	4.44 d (5.8)	72.8, CH	C-7, 8
7	6.71 overlapped	140.7, CH	C-6	6.71 overlapped	141.0, CH	C-8, 9	6.35 dd (5.6, 15.3)	144.4, CH	C-6, 9
8	6.71 overlapped	130.6, CH	C-6, 7	6.71 overlapped	130.4, CH		6.78 dd (11.2, 15.1)	127.9, CH	C-6, 9, 10
9	7.23 dd (1.0, 10.3)	141.3, CH	C-6, 8, 11, 16	7.23 dd (1.0, 10.0)	141.5, CH	C-7, 8, 11, 16	7.22 d (11.1)	141.1, CH	C-7, 8, 11, 16
10		137.7, C			137.5, C			137.3, C	
11		202.2, C			202.3, C			202.5, C	
12	2.34 s	25.8, CH$_3$	C-9, 10, 11	2.33 s	25.8, CH$_3$	C-9, 10, 11	2.34 s	25.8, CH$_3$	C-9, 10, 11
13	1.19 s	20.5, CH$_3$	C-1, 2, 3, 14	1.21 s	25.3, CH$_3$	C-1, 2, 3, 14	1.24 s	25.6, CH$_3$	C-1, 2, 3, 14
14	1.22 s	26.3, CH$_3$	C-1, 2, 3, 13	1.04 s	19.9, CH$_3$	C-1, 2, 3, 13	1.20 s	21.2, CH$_3$	C-1, 2, 13
15	1.46 s	22.1, CH$_3$	C-3, 4, 5, 6	1.52 s	27.4, CH$_3$	C-3, 4, 5, 6	1.43 s	19.3, CH$_3$	C-3, 4, 5,
16	1.87 d (1.0)	11.7, CH$_3$	C-8, 9, 10, 11	1.87 d (0.8)	11.7, CH$_3$	C-8, 9, 10, 11	1.87 s	11.6, CH$_3$	C-9, 10, 11

Qinlactone B (**4**) was obtained as a colorless oil and assigned the same molecular formula as **3** by HRESIMS (*m/z* 279.1587, [M + H]$^+$). The 1D and 2D NMR data (Table 2) of **4** corresponded closely to those of **3**, which suggested **4** had the same planar structure with **3** as epimer instead of enantiomer. The ROESY correlations of H-3 and H-15/H-13 suggested the relative configuration of 3*R**, 4*R** (Figure 3). The absolute configuration was determined as 3*R*, 4*R* by the similar Cotton effects between the calculated ECD spectrum and experimental one of **4** (Figure 4). Thus, the structure of **4** was determined (Figure 2), named qinlactone B.

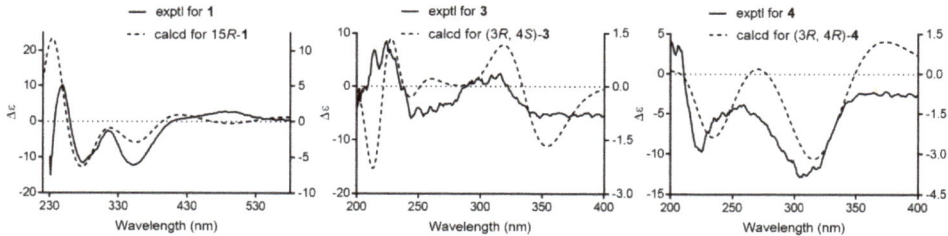

Figure 4. Experimental and calculated electronic circular dichroism (ECD) spectra for compound **1**, **3** and **4**.

Qinlactone C (**5**) was obtained as a light-yellow oil with the molecular formula $C_{16}H_{24}O_6$, determined by HRESIMS *m/z* 313.1650 (calcd 313.1646 for [M + H]$^+$), implying 5 degrees of unsaturation. Compared with **3**, 1D NMR data (Table 2) of **5** revealed the absence of two olefinic methines, but the presence of two methines connected with oxygen atoms ($\delta_{C/H}$ 72.8/4.44 and 77.9/3.63). Based on the formula and unsaturation analysis, **5** contained a vicinal diol at C-5 and C-6, which was also confirmed by ^{1}H-^{1}H COSY correlations from H-5 to H-9 and HMBC correlations from H-5 to C-3 and C-4 (Figure 3). Therefore, the planar structure of **5** was identified. ROESY correlations of H-3 and H-13/H-5 suggested the relative configuration of 3*R**, 4*R** in the lactone ring (Figure 3). However, due to the existing vicinal diol structure, the relative and absolute configuration of **5** could not be determined based on the present data. Thus, compound **5** was named qinlactone C.

In the anti-microbial bioassay test, only compound **1** exhibited strong bioactivity against *Staphylococcus aureus* and *Candida albicans*, with MIC values of 0.78 µg/mL and 3.13 µg/mL, respectively. Meanwhile, in antiproliferative bio-test, **1** showed strong inhibitory effects on MCF-7 and HeLa cell lines with IC$_{50}$ values of 5.78 µM and 6.25 µM, respectively (Table 3). Compound **2**–**4** showed weak activities against MCF-7 and HeLa cell lines with IC$_{50}$ values ranging from 129 to 207 µM (Table 4).

Table 3. MIC (µg/mL) against pathogenic microbes of compounds **1**–**5**. *E. coli*: *Escherichia coli*; *S. aureus*: *Staphylococcus aureus*; *C. albicans*: *Candida albicans*.

Compound.	E. coli	S. aureus	C. albicans
1	>100	0.78	3.13
kanamycin	6.25	6.25	/
nystatin	/	/	3.13

Table 4. Cytotoxicities against MCF-7 and HeLa cells of compound **1**–**5** (µM).

Compound	MCF-7 (IC$_{50}$ ± SD, 48 h)	HeLa (IC$_{50}$ ± SD, 48 h)
1	5.78 ± 0.26	6.25 ± 0.29
2	206.91 ± 9.69	183.03 ± 11.11
3	>179.86	168.13 ± 13.15
4	136.87 ± 10.67	129.14 ± 3.98
Paclitaxel	<0.46	<0.46

3. Discussion

In this study, we identified five new compounds with bioactivities from mangrove *Streptomyces qinglanensis* 172205 with "genetic dereplication." Compound **1** showed strong anti-*Staphylococcus aureus* and anti-*Candida albicans* activities with MIC values of 0.78 μg/mL and 3.13 μg/mL, respectively, and exhibited strong cytotoxicities against MCF-7 and HeLa cell lines with IC_{50} values of 5.78 μM and 6.25 μM, respectively. However, compound **2–4** exhibited only weak antiproliferative activities with IC_{50} values ranging from 129 to 207 μM.

Attempting to activate gene clusters of possible unknown secondary metabolites in strain 172205, we deleted the whole biosynthetic gene cluster of the main product enterocin. Through HPLC detection, we found that this strategy in strain 172205 did not clearly activate any new metabolites in several media. However, we still focused on some low-yield products, which produced in the wild type strain as well (Figure 1). However, the mutant strain without the main product enterocin facilitated detection and isolation of the low-yield products, from which we finally identified five new compounds. Thus, "genetic dereplication" did help simplifying the process of isolation and mining the low-yield products. This strategy would be more effective for identifying multiple types of metabolites in one strain, if combined with other genome mining tools or methods.

15*R*-17,18-dehydroxantholipin is an analog of reported xantholipin [10], which exhibited similar strong antiproliferative and anti-microbial activities. In fact, we firstly identified a gene cluster by antiSMASH analysis in the genome of strain 172205 (Supplementary Figure S41 and Table S2), which had a high similarity with the reported xantholipin gene cluster [12]. Then, we tried at least 10 media to detect the similar UV absorption of xantholipin by HPLC and characterized mass for halogen compounds by HRESIMS, and finally detected analogs in products from D.O. medium, which is the same recipe with the reported medium to produce xantholipin. Compound with the targeted UV absorption was identified as 15*R*-17,18-dehydroxantholipin. Lacking the oxidoreductase gene *xanZ2* which was proposed for the double band reduction at C-17 and C-18 [12], resulted in the production of 15*R*-17,18-dehydroxantholipin in strain 172205. Hence, genome-guided compound discovery combined with OSMAC is an effective method for isolation and identification of some well-known and valuable compounds or potential new analogs. Moreover, multiple strategies of genome mining will be helpful to mine the potential of natural products in one strain.

4. Materials and Methods

4.1. General Experimental Procedures

Ultraviolet (UV) spectra were recorded on a Shimadzu UV-2401 PC UV-Visible spectrophotometer. ECD spectra were recorded on an Applied PhotoPhysics Chirascan. IR spectra were recorded on Bruker Tensor27 spectrometer. Optical rotations were measured with JASCO P-1020. 1D and 2D NMR spectra were recorded in DMSO-d_6 and CD$_3$OD-d_4 on Bruker DRX-500. Chemical shifts (δ) were expressed in ppm with reference to the solvent signals. High resolution mass spectra were recorded on a Thermo Instruments MS system (LTQ Orbitrap) equipped with a Thermo Instruments HPLC system with a Thermo Hypersil GOLD column (150 × 4.6 mm) with electrospray ionization in the positive-ion mode. Analytical HPLC was performed on a Waters 2998 with a photodiode array detector (PDA) detector with a Phenomenex Gemini (C18 250 × 4.6 mm) column. Semi-preparative HPLC was carried out on an Agilent 1260 Infinity with a diode array detector (DAD) with an Agilent Zorbax SBC18 (250 × 9.4 mm) column. Sephadex LH-20 (Shanghai kayon Biological Technology) was used for column chromatography.

4.2. Microorganism Material and Culture

Streptomyces qinglanensis 172205 was isolated from a mangrove soil sample and identified as a novel species [13]. This strain was cultured on ISP2 agar plates at 28 °C. *Escherichia coli* Top 10 was used for cloning and E. coli ET12567/pUZ8002 was used for intergeneric conjugation, which cultured on LB agar plates at 37 °C.

4.3. Gene Cluster Deletion

Strain 177205 was reported to produce the main product enterocin and its biosynthesis gene cluster was located in genome [9]. Hence, strain 172205Δenc was constructed by the whole enterocin biosynthetic gene cluster deletion with double-crossover homologous recombination. To construct the plasmid for gene cluster deletion, two DNA fragments, an 1870 bp Avr II-Hind III homologous arm and another 1829 bp Nde I-Hind III homologous arm were cloned from strain 17225 genome DNA covering both ends of the enterocin biosynthetic gene cluster. DNA fragments were ligated into pMD19-T simple and fragment sequences were identified by DNA sequencing. Two recycled DNA fragments were inserted into the delivery vector pYH7 [14] by Nde I-Hind III restriction sites to yield pWHU2343 (Supplementary Figure S1). Intergeneric conjugation of plasmid pWHU2343 into strain 172205 by E. coli ET12657/pUZ8002 were carried out as protocol described in Practical Streptomyces Genetics [15]. The donor ET12657/pUZ8002 containing plasmid and the recipient spores were mixed and spread on Mannitol-Soy-agar (MS) plates with 10 mM $MgCl_2$ and grown for 14 h at 28 °C. Then the plates were overlaid with 1 mL sterile water contained 4 μg/mL apramycin and 25 μg/mL nalidixic acid. Single colonies were transferred to a new MS plate with same antibiotics for further confirmation of antibiotic resistance. To screen the double-crossover mutants, single clones from no antibiotics plate were replicated on a MS plates with apramycin. Genome DNA of all candidates that had no apramycin resistance were extracted for PCR identification. Four pair of primers, enc-U, enc-D, enc-UD and enc-M, were used for screening (Supplementary Table S1), and a specific 1080 bp product for enc-UD was only amplified in mutant clones with absence of 21.6 kb gene cluster, but specific products for enc-U, enc-D and enc-M were only amplified in genome of wild-type clones. The mutant was also confirmed by detecting enterocin production in fermentation.

4.4. Extraction and Isolation

Strain 172205Δenc spores were inoculated into seed broth medium, cultured at 200 rpm, 28 °C for 3 days. Then seed broth was transferred to 200 of 1 L flasks consisted of 300 mL fermentation medium, shaken at 200 rpm for 7 days (media recipes in literature [12]). The broth was extracted by organic reagent as described [9] and evaporated to dryness (80 g). Samples and fractions were tested by HPLC fingerprint [9]. HPLC fingerprints were carried using the following gradient: H_2O (A)/MeOH (B): 0 min, 10% B; 15 min, 100% B; 20 min, 100% B; 21 min, 10% B; 30 min, 10% B; flow rate of 1 mL/min.

The crude extract was subjected to column chromatography on silica gel eluted by PE:CH_2Cl_2 (gradient from 1:0, 1:1 and 0:1, v:v) and CH_2Cl_2:MeOH (gradient from 100:1, 50:1, 5:1, 2:1 to methanol, v:v) to give A–F fractions. Importantly, the mix of crude extract and silica gel on column after elution was extracted by DMSO. DMSO layers were mixed with equal volume of NaCl saturated solution, and extracted again with ethyl acetate, then evaporated to fraction G. Fraction G was dissolved in DMSO and purified by HPLC (MeOH: H_2O = 75:25, flow rate 3 mL/min) to afford compound **1** (4 mg, t_R = 23.2 min). Fraction D was subject to silica gel column chromatography using cyclohexane: acetone (20:1 to 0:1 v:v) to afford five subfractions (D1–D5). Fraction D3 was purified by HPLC (MeCN: H_2O = 30:70) to afford compound **2** (15 mg, t_R = 16.9 min). Fraction D2 was purified by HPLC (MeOH: H_2O = 48:52) to afford compound **3** (5 mg, t_R = 30.7 min) and **4** (4 mg, t_R = 31.9 min). Fraction D5 was purified by HPLC (MeCN: H_2O = 20:80) to afford compound **5** (6 mg).

15R-17,18-dehydroxantholipin (**1**): dark red powder; $[\alpha]_D^{20}$ −168.85 (c 0.046, MeOH/$CHCl_3$ = 5:1); UV (MeOH) λ_{max} (log ε): 247 (4.34), 279 (4.23), 316 (4.08), 478 (3.80) nm; CD (c 0.041, $CHCl_3$) λ_{max} (Δε): 231 (−7.47), 249 (+5.09), 278 (−5.78), 314 (−1.29), 352 (−6.10), 485 (+1.41) nm; IR (KBr) v_{max} 3428, 2925, 1633, 1028 cm^{-1}; ^{1}H and ^{13}C NMR data, see Table 1; positive ion HRESIMS m/z 534.0587 [M + H]$^+$ (calcd for $C_{27}H_{17}ClNO_9$, 534.0586).

(3*E*,5*E*,7*E*)-3-methyldeca-3,5,7-triene-2,9-dione (**2**): yellow powder; UV (MeOH) λ_{max} (log ε): 225 (3.80), 324 (4.96) nm; IR (KBr) v_{max} 3430, 2955, 2930, 1709, 1664, 1361, 1253, 998, 604 cm^{-1}; ^{1}H and ^{13}C NMR data, see Table 1; positive ion HRESIMS *m/z* 179.1064 [M + H]$^+$ (calcd for $C_{11}H_{15}O_2$, 179.1067).

Qinlactone A (**3**): colorless oil; $[\alpha]_D^{19}$ +31.55 (c 0.727, MeOH); UV (MeOH) λ_{max} (log ε): 223 (4.07), 311 (4.40) nm; CD (c 0.013, MeOH) λ_{max} ($\Delta\varepsilon$): 200 (−0.6), 224 (+1.3), 316 (+0.4) nm; IR (KBr) v_{max} 3437, 2983, 2936, 1756, 1640, 1386, 1273, 1224, 1056, 995 cm^{-1}; ^{1}H and ^{13}C NMR data, see Table 2; positive ion HRESIMS *m/z* 279.1587 [M + H]$^+$ (calcd for $C_{16}H_{23}O_4$, 279.1591).

Qinlactone B (**4**): colorless oil; $[\alpha]_D^{19}$ −93.91 (c 0.553, MeOH); UV (MeOH) λ_{max} (log ε): 221 (4.11), 313 (4.46) nm; CD (c 0.011, MeOH) λ_{max} ($\Delta\varepsilon$): 201 (+1.2), 225 (−2.9), 310 (−3.8) nm; IR (KBr) v_{max} 3432, 2980, 2934, 1774, 1758, 1716, 1640, 1386, 1274, 1225, 1113, 1065, 996, 954 cm^{-1}; ^{1}H and ^{13}C NMR data, see Table 2; positive ion HRESIMS *m/z* 279.1587 [M + H]$^+$ (calcd for $C_{16}H_{23}O_4$, 279.1591).

Qinlactone C (**5**): light yellow oil; $[\alpha]_D^{20}$ −0.18 (c 0.552, MeOH); UV (MeOH) λ_{max} (log ε): 201 (3.81), 229 (3.78), 275 (4.04) nm; CD (c 0.055, MeOH) λ_{max} ($\Delta\varepsilon$): 216 (−3.4), 270 (+0.4) nm; IR (KBr) v_{max} 3415, 3194, 2986, 2942, 1758, 1678, 1401, 1285, 1205, 1137, 1066, 954, 837, 801, 723 cm^{-1}; ^{1}H and ^{13}C NMR data, see Table 2; positive ion HRESIMS *m/z* 313.1650 [M + H]$^+$ (calcd for $C_{16}H_{25}O_6$, 313.1646).

4.5. Effect of Compounds on Anti-Microbial and Antiproliferative Bioactivities

Antiproliferative activities against HeLa and MCF-7 cell lines were evaluated by 3-(4,5-dimethylthiazol-2-yl)-2,5-diphenyl tetrazolium bromide (MTT) assay as described [9]. Briefly, 6000 cells were plated into 96 well plate cultured with 90 μL DMEM (Dulbecco's Modified Eagle Medium) medium supplemented with 10% fetal bovine serum (FBS). After overnight culture, 10 μL compounds in 5% DMSO culture solutions with gradient final concentrations of 0.39, 0.78, 1.56, 3.13, 6.26, 12.5, 25 and 50 μg/mL were added into each well in triplicates, using positive control of paclitaxel. After 48 h incubation, 12 μL MTT solutions (final concentration of 0.5 mg/mL in PBS - phosphate buffered saline) were added and plates were further incubated for 4 h. Then, the medium was replaced gently by 100 μL DMSO. Plates were shaken and read by a Tecan Infinite M200 Pro reader at 570 nm, and the reference wavelength was 690 nm. The values of IC$_{50}$ were calculated by GraphPad Prism 7.0 by applying nonlinear regression with (inhibitor) versus normalized response.

Anti-microbial activities against *Escherichia coli* ATCC 25922, *Staphylococcus aureus* ATCC 51650 and *Candida albicans* ATCC 10231 were evaluated by microtiter broth dilution method as described [16,17] with some modifications. Briefly, 75 μL Lysogeny broth (LB) or yeast extract-peptone-dextrose (YPD) medium and 20 μL inoculums (5 × 10^5 CFU/mL, colony-forming unit/mL) was plated into each well in 96 well plate. Then 5 μL test compounds with gradient final concentrations of 0.78, 1.56, 3.13, 6.26, 12.5, 25, 50 and 100 μg/mL was added into each well with three copies, using the positive control of kanamycin (for bacteria) and nystatin (for fungus). Plates were shaken at 200 rpm and cultured at 30 °C for 20 h. At last, plates were examined for bacteria growth by turbidity in daylight. The MICs were defined as the lowest concentration at which no microbial growth could be detected.

4.6. ECD Calculation

The calculations were performed using DFT on Gaussian 03, and the calculation details were follow strictly as described in literature [18]. Briefly, the calculations were performed by using the density functional theory (DFT) as carried out in the Gaussian 03 [19]. The preliminary conformational distribution search was performed using Frog2 online version [20]. Further geometrical optimization was performed at the B3LYP/6-31G(d) level. Solvent effects of methanol solution were evaluated at the same DFT level by using the SCRF/PCM method [21]. TDDFT [22–24] at B3LYP/6-31G(d) was employed to calculate the electronic excitation energies and rotational strengths in methanol, except compound **1** with calculation in chloroform.

Supplementary Materials: The following are available online at http://www.mdpi.com/1660-3397/18/5/255/s1, Table S1: Oligonucleotide primers used in this study, Table S2: Deduced functions of ORFs in *xan*$_q$ biosynthetic pathway of strain 172205; Figure S1: Confirmation of enterocin gene cluster disruption by PCR, Figures S2–S8:

HERESIMS, IR, 1D and 2D spectra of compound **1**, Figures S9–S16: HERESIMS, IR, 1D and 2D spectra of compound **2**, Figures S17–S24: HERESIMS, IR, 1D and 2D spectra of compound **3**, Figures S25–S32: HERESIMS, IR, 1D and 2D spectra of compound **4**, Figures S33–S40: HERESIMS, IR, 1D and 2D spectra of compound **5**. Figure S41. Comparison of genetic organization of xan_q in strain 172205 and xan in *S. flavogriseus*.

Author Contributions: D.X. and K.H. designed the experiments; D.X. performed the experiments including fermentation, isolation and identification, as well as the bioassay test; E.T. helped and confirmed with the identification of part of compounds; F.K. performed the ECD calculations. D.X. wrote the paper, and the other authors revised the paper. All authors have read and agreed to the published version of the manuscript.

Funding: This work was partially supported by the National Key R&D Program of China (No. 2018YFC0311000), the National Natural Science Foundation of China (No. 31170467) and EU FP7 project PharmaSea (312184).

Conflicts of Interest: The authors declare no conflict of interest.

References

1. Xu, D.B.; Ye, W.W.; Han, Y.; Deng, Z.X.; Hong, K. Natural products from mangrove actinomycetes. *Mar. Drugs* **2014**, *12*, 2590–2613. [CrossRef] [PubMed]
2. Ziemert, N.; Alanjary, M.; Weber, T. The evolution of genome mining in microbes—A review. *Nat. Prod. Rep.* **2016**, *33*, 988–1005. [CrossRef] [PubMed]
3. Dan, V.M.; Vinodh, J.S.; Sandesh, C.J.; Sanawar, R.; Lekshmi, A.; Kumar, R.A.; Santhosh Kumar, T.R.; Marelli, U.K.; Dastager, S.G.; Pillai, M.R. Molecular networking and whole-genome analysis aid discovery of an angucycline that inactivates mTORC1/C2 and induces programmed cell death. *ACS Chem. Biol.* **2020**, *15*, 780–788. [CrossRef]
4. Almeida, E.L.; Kaur, N.; Jennings, L.K.; Carrillo Rincon, A.F.; Jackson, S.A.; Thomas, O.P.; Dobson, A.D.W. Genome mining coupled with OSMAC-based cultivation reveal differential production of surugamide A by the marine sponge isolate Streptomyces sp. SM17 when compared to its terrestrial relative S. albidoflavus J1074. *Microorganisms* **2019**, *7*, 394. [CrossRef]
5. Zerikly, M.; Challis, G.L. Strategies for the discovery of new natural products by genome mining. *Chembiochem* **2009**, *10*, 625–633. [CrossRef] [PubMed]
6. Bode, H.B.; Bethe, B.; Hofs, R.; Zeeck, A. Big effects from small changes: Possible ways to explore nature's chemical diversity. *Chembiochem* **2002**, *3*, 619–627. [CrossRef]
7. McAlpine, J.B.; Bachmann, B.O.; Piraee, M.; Tremblay, S.; Alarco, A.M.; Zazopoulos, E.; Farnet, C.M. Microbial genomics as a guide to drug discovery and structural elucidation: ECO-02301, a novel antifungal agent, as an example. *J. Nat. Prod.* **2005**, *68*, 493–496. [CrossRef]
8. Chiang, Y.M.; Ahuja, M.; Oakley, C.E.; Entwistle, R.; Asokan, A.; Zutz, C.; Wang, C.C.; Oakley, B.R. Development of genetic dereplication strains in *Aspergillus nidulans* results in the discovery of aspercryptin. *Angew. Chem. Int. Ed. Engl.* **2016**, *55*, 1662–1665. [CrossRef]
9. Xu, D.B.; Ma, M.; Deng, Z.X.; Hong, K. Genotype-driven isolation of enterocin with novel bioactivities from mangrove-derived *Streptomyces qinglanensis* 172205. *Appl. Microbiol. Biotechnol.* **2015**, *99*, 5825–5832. [CrossRef]
10. Terui, Y.; Yiwen, C.; Jun-ying, L.; Ando, T.; Yamamoto, H.; Kawamura, Y.; Tomishima, Y.; Uchida, S.; Okazaki, T.; Munetomo, E.; et al. Xantholipin, a novel inhibitor of HSP47 gene expression produced by *Streptomyces* sp. *Tetrahedron Lett.* **2003**, *44*, 5427–5430. [CrossRef]
11. Chen, Q.L.; Zhao, Z.H.; Lu, W.; Chu, Y.W. Bromoxantholipin: A novel polycyclic xanthone antibiotic produced by *Streptomyces flavogriseus* SIIA-A02191. *Chin. J. Antibiot.* **2011**, *36*, 566–570.
12. Zhang, W.; Wang, L.; Kong, L.; Wang, T.; Chu, Y.; Deng, Z.; You, D. Unveiling the post-PKS redox tailoring steps in biosynthesis of the type II polyketide antitumor antibiotic xantholipin. *Chem. Biol.* **2012**, *19*, 422–432. [CrossRef] [PubMed]
13. Hu, H.; Lin, H.P.; Xie, Q.; Li, L.; Xie, X.Q.; Hong, K. *Streptomyces qinglanensis* sp. nov., isolated from mangrove sediment. *Int. J. Syst. Evol. Microbiol.* **2012**, *62*, 596–600. [CrossRef] [PubMed]
14. Sun, Y.; He, X.; Liang, J.; Zhou, X.; Deng, Z. Analysis of functions in plasmid pHZ1358 influencing its genetic and structural stability in *Streptomyces lividans* 1326. *Appl. Microbiol. Biotechnol.* **2009**, *82*, 303–310. [CrossRef]
15. Kieser, T.; Bibb, M.J.; Buttner, M.J.; Chater, K.F.; Hopwood, D.A. *Practical Streptomyces Genetics*; The John Innes Foundation: Norwich, UK, 2000; pp. 249–252. ISBN 0-7084-0623-8.

16. Fu, P.; Kong, F.; Wang, Y.; Wang, Y.; Liu, P.; Zuo, G.; Zhu, W. Antibiotic metabolites from the coral-associated actinomycete *Streptomyces* sp. OUCMDZ-1703. *Chin. J. Chem.* **2013**, *31*, 100–104. [CrossRef]
17. Hong, K.; Gao, A.H.; Xie, Q.Y.; Gao, H.; Zhuang, L.; Lin, H.P.; Yu, H.P.; Li, J.; Yao, X.S.; Goodfellow, M.; et al. Actinomycetes for marine drug discovery isolated from mangrove soils and plants in China. *Mar. Drugs* **2009**, *7*, 24–44. [CrossRef]
18. Kong, F.D.; Fan, P.; Zhou, L.M.; Ma, Q.Y.; Xie, Q.Y.; Zheng, H.Z.; Zheng, Z.H.; Zhang, R.S.; Yuan, J.Z.; Dai, H.F.; et al. Penerpenes A-D, Four indole terpenoids with potent protein tyrosine phosphatase inhibitory activity from the marine-derived fungus *Penicillium* sp. KFD28. *Org. Lett.* **2019**, *21*, 4864–4867. [CrossRef]
19. Frisch, M. Gaussian 03 Rev. E. 01. 2004. Available online: http://www.gaussian.com/ (accessed on 15 April 2020).
20. Miteva, M.A.; Guyon, F.; Tuffery, P. Frog2: Efficient 3D conformation ensemble generator for small compounds. *Nucleic. Acids Res.* **2010**, *38*, W622–W627. [CrossRef]
21. Sai, C.M.; Li, D.H.; Xue, C.M.; Wang, K.B.; Hu, P.; Pei, Y.H.; Bai, J.; Jing, Y.K.; Li, Z.L.; Hua, H.M. Two pairs of enantiomeric alkaloid dimers from *Macleaya cordata*. *Org. Lett.* **2015**, *17*, 4102–4105. [CrossRef]
22. Miertus, S.; Tomasi, J. Approximate evaluations of the electrostatic free energy and internal energy changes in solution processes. *Chem. Phys.* **1982**, *65*, 239–245. [CrossRef]
23. Tomasi, J.; Persico, M. Molecular interactions in solution: An overview of methods based on continuous distributions of the solvent. *Chem. Rev.* **1994**, *94*, 2027–2094. [CrossRef]
24. Cammi, R.; Tomasi, J. Remarks on the use of the apparent surface charges (ASC) methods in solvation problems: Iterative versus matrix-inversion procedures and the renormalization of the apparent charges. *J. Comput. Chem.* **1995**, *16*, 1449–1458. [CrossRef]

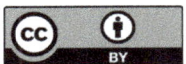

© 2020 by the authors. Licensee MDPI, Basel, Switzerland. This article is an open access article distributed under the terms and conditions of the Creative Commons Attribution (CC BY) license (http://creativecommons.org/licenses/by/4.0/).

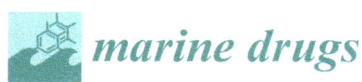

Article

Bioactive Indolyl Diketopiperazines from the Marine Derived Endophytic *Aspergillus versicolor* DY180635

Yi Ding, Xiaojing Zhu, Liling Hao, Mengyao Zhao, Qiang Hua and Faliang An *

State Key Laboratory of Bioreactor Engineering, East China University of Science and Technology, 130 Mei Long Road, Shanghai 200237, China; zjzsdy@163.com (Y.D.); 13761041863@163.com (X.Z.); holiday_hao1988@126.com (L.H.); myzhao@ecust.edu.cn (M.Z.); qhua@ecust.edu.cn (Q.H.)
* Correspondence: flan2016@ecust.edu.cn; Tel.: +86-21-6425-1185

Received: 3 June 2020; Accepted: 25 June 2020; Published: 28 June 2020

Abstract: Four new indolyl diketopiperazines, aspamides A–E (**1–4**) and two new diketopiperazines, aspamides F–G (**5–6**), along with 11 known diketopiperazines and intermediates were isolated from the solid culture of *Aspergillus versicolor*, which is an endophyte with the sea crab (*Chiromantes haematocheir*). Further chiral high-performance liquid chromatography resolution gave enantiomers (+)- and (−)-**4**, respectively. The structures and absolute configurations of compounds **1–6** were determined by the comprehensive analyses of nuclear magnetic resonance (NMR), high-resolution mass spectrometry (HR-MS), and electronic circular dichroism (ECD) calculation. All isolated compounds were selected for the virtual screening on the coronavirus 3-chymoretpsin-like protease (Mpro) of Severe Acute Respiratory Syndrome Coronavirus 2 (SARS-CoV-2), and the docking scores of compounds **1–2**, **5**, **6**, **8** and **17** were top among all screened molecules, may be helpful in fighting with Corona Virus Disease-19 (COVID-19) after further studies.

Keywords: endophyte fungus; *Aspergillus versicolor*; diketopiperazines; ECD calculation; enantiomers

1. Introduction

Endophytic fungi refer to harmless parasitic fungi that live in the internal organs of plants and animals without causing any adverse reactions. The host provides nutrients for endophytes, and endophytes produce bioactive substances, giving the host an advantage in survival competition [1]. Symbionts coexist with symptomless fish, sponges, algae, and soft corals that grow in a relatively harsh marine environment characterized by high salinity, scarce nutrients, and high osmotic and hydraulic pressures, which provides many environment-specific microorganisms that could coevolve with their hosts by undergoing the rapid and dynamic change of their genomes [2,3]. Thus, endophytic fungi are considered as a treasure trove of unique structural compounds and bioactive metabolites.

Indolyl diketopiperazines (IDKPs), cyclic dipeptides produced by the condensation of L-tryptophan and a second amino acid, were commonly isolated from fungi, especially from the genera *Aspergillus* and *Penicillium* [4,5]. IDKPs had drawn considerable attention from synthetic chemists, natural products researchers, and synthetic biologists for decades due to their significant biological activities, such as antiviral [6,7], anticancer [8–10], immunomodulatory [11,12], antioxidant [13], and α-glucosidase inhibitory activities [14]. Specifically, the vascular disrupting and tubulin-depolymerizing agent plinabulin, a synthetic analog based on the natural diketopiperazine (DKP) product halimide generated by the marine-derived *Aspergillus* sp. CNC-139, had entered the last stage of clinical study for the treatment of non-small-cell lung cancer [15,16]. Since the first IDKP alkaloid chaetomin isolated from the fungus *Chaetomium cochliodes* in the early 1940s, a series of DKPs and their biosynthesis clusters were reported [17–22]. In our continuous investigations of novel bioactive agents from the endophytic fungi [23,24], the endophytic strain *Aspergillus versicolor* DY180635 isolated from the sea crab was selected based on the bio-evaluation results. The ethyl acetate extracts of a rice solid culture of *A. versicolor* DY180635 showed 80% inhibition on the anti-inflammation model of the *Propionibacterium acnes*-induced THP-1 cells at the concentration of 0.1 mg/mL [25]. High-performance liquid chromatography (HPLC) analysis of the ethyl acetate extracts indicated the presence of IDKPs with a diode array detector (DAD) through ultraviolet characteristics at λ_{max} 236, 289, and 336 nm [26]. Thus, to discover structurally complex and/or bioactive DKPs, the spectroscopic-guided isolation was performed in this research.

Spectroscopic-guided isolation resulted in the identification of four new IDPKs, aspamides A–E (**1–4**) and two new DPKs, aspamides F–G (**5–6**), along with 11 known diketopiperazines and intermediates from the ethyl acetate (EtOAc) extracts of the solid culture of *A. versicolor* (Figure 1). The couple of epimers **1–2** were the first samples of brevianamides with an oxygenated aza-acetal structure at the proline motif. All isolated compounds were tested for anti-inflammation in *P. acnes*-induced THP-1 cells. Unfortunately, none showed active effect. With the appearance and spread of SARS-CoV-2 at the end of 2019, compounds **1–17** were selected for the virtual screening on the 3CL hydrolase (Mpro) of SARS-CoV-2, which had been exploited as a potential drug target to fight COVID-19 [27]. The docking scores of compounds **1–2, 5, 6, 8**, and **17** were top among all screened molecules (docking scores: −5.389, −4.772, −5.146, −4.962, −5.158), which may be helpful in fighting COVID-19 after further studies. Herein, we reported the isolation, structural identification, and bio-evaluation of isolated compounds.

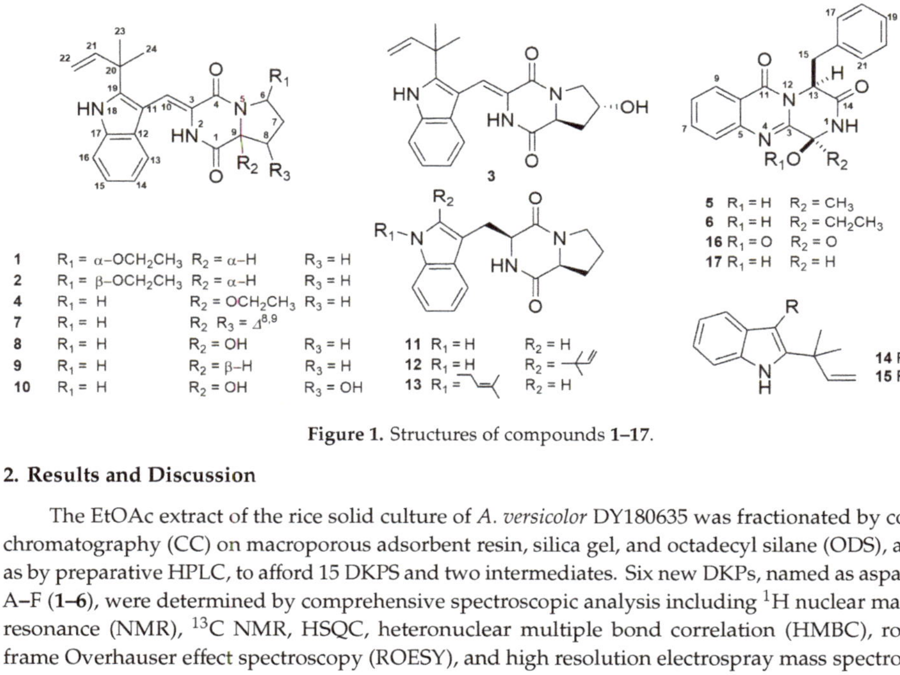

Figure 1. Structures of compounds **1–17**.

2. Results and Discussion

The EtOAc extract of the rice solid culture of *A. versicolor* DY180635 was fractionated by column chromatography (CC) on macroporous adsorbent resin, silica gel, and octadecyl silane (ODS), as well as by preparative HPLC, to afford 15 DKPS and two intermediates. Six new DKPs, named as aspamides A–F (**1–6**), were determined by comprehensive spectroscopic analysis including ^{1}H nuclear magnetic resonance (NMR), ^{13}C NMR, HSQC, heteronuclear multiple bond correlation (HMBC), rotating frame Overhauser effect spectroscopy (ROESY), and high resolution electrospray mass spectrometry (HRESIMS) spectra. By comparing the NMR and ESIMS data to the reported literatures in detail, 11 known compounds were determined as brevianamides K, N, and M (**7, 16, 17**) [28], brevianamide Q (**8**) [29], brevianamides V, U (**9–10**) [20], brevianamide F (**11**) [30], deoxybrevianamide E (**12**) [31], *N*-Prenyl-*cyclo*-L-tryptophyl-L-proline (**13**) [32], 2-(2-methyl-3-en-2-yl)-1*H*-indole-3-carbaldehyde (**14**) [33], and 2-(1,1-Dimethyl-allyl)-1*H*-indol-3-ylmercuric acetate (**15**) [34]. Herein, the details of the isolation, structural elucidation of these new compounds, and their bioactivities are described.

Aspamide A (**1**) was isolated as a yellowish powder. The UV spectrum with λ_{max} (logε) in methanol at 200 (6.13), 224 (6.13), 284 (5.46), and 341 (5.68) nm was indicative of indole functionality with an extended conjugation [26]. Its molecular formula was determined as $C_{23}H_{27}N_3O_3$ on the basis of high-resolution ESIMS (m/z 394.2117 [M + H]$^+$, calcd. for $C_{23}H_{28}N_3O_3$, 394.2125) and ^{13}C NMR data, requiring 12 degrees of unsaturation. The ^1H NMR, ^{13}C NMR, and heteronuclear multiple quantum correlation (HMQC) spectra (Table 1 and Figure S3 in Supporting Information) showed three methyl groups (δ_C 27.4, δ_H 1.45; δ_C 27.8, δ_H 1.49; δ_C 15.2, δ_H 1.13), three sp^3 methylenes (including one oxygenated methylene) (δ_C 29.6, δ_H 1.75, δ_H 1.97; δ_C 25.9, δ_H 2.13, δ_H 2.27; δ_C 63.6, δ_H 3.65), two sp^3 methine carbon signals (including one oxygen-bearing carbon) (δ_C 56.5, δ_H 4.57; δ_C 86.7, δ_H 5.59), six sp^2 methines, one sp^2 methylene, seven sp^2, and one sp^3 non-protonated carbon. The NMR data and UV absorptions were close to those of brevianamide V [20], with the exception that there was an additional oxygenated aza-acetal structure located at the proline motif (δ_C 86.7, δ_H 5.59; δ_C 63.6, δ_H 3.65; δ_C 15.2, and δ_H 1.13).

Further information about the structure was derived from heteronuclear multiple bond correlation (HMBC) spectra analyses (Figure S4). The key HMBC correlations (Figure 2A) from OCH$_2$CH$_3$-6 (δ_H 3.65) to C-6 (δ_C 86.7), H-6 (δ_H 5.59) to C-9 (δ_C 56.5), H-9 (δ_H 4.57) to C-8 (δ_C 25.9) and C-1 (δ_C 165.9), and H-8α (δ_H 2.27) to C-9 were observed. These data suggested that an oxethyl group was located at C-6 and confirmed the oxygenated aza-acetal structure at the proline motif, which was previous unpresented in the brevianamide analogues. Thus, the planar structure of **1** was determined as shown in Figure 1.

In order to determine the relative configuration of **1**, the rotating frame Overhauser effect spectroscopy (ROESY, Figure S5) experiment was performed. The ROESY correlation (Figure 2B) between NH-2 (δ_H 9.01) and H-13 (δ_H 7.29) revealed the Z configuration about $\Delta^{3,10}$, and the ROESY signals between H-8β (δ_H 2.13) and H-6, and between H-8α (δ_H 2.27) and H-9 suggested that H-6 and H-9 were *trans* form. The absolute configuration of **1** was assigned as (6R,9S) by comparing the experimental and calculated electronic circular dichroism (ECD) values obtained using Time-dependent Density functional theory (TD-DFT) at the B3LYP/6–31+g (d, p) level (Figure 2C).

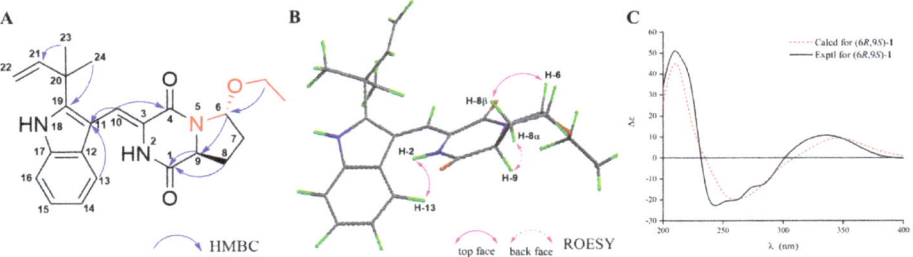

Figure 2. The key heteronuclear multiple bond correlation (HMBC) (**A**) and rotating frame Overhauser effect spectroscopy (ROESY) (**B**) correlations, and experimental and calculated electronic circular dichroism (ECD) spectra (**C**) of compound **1**.

Aspamide B (**2**) was obtained as a yellowish powder. Its molecular formula was determined as $C_{23}H_{27}N_3O_3$ on the basis of HRESIMS (m/z 394.2120 [M + H]$^+$, calcd. for $C_{23}H_{28}N_3O_3$, 394.2125) and ^{13}C NMR data, corresponding to 12 degrees of unsaturation. By comparing the ^1H, ^{13}C, and HMQC data (Table 1, Figure S11) of **2** with those of **1**, it was discovered that **2** possessed the identical planar structure as that of **1**. Further analyses of the 2D NMR data of **2**, the key HMBC correlations from H-6 (δ_H 5.35) to OCH$_2$CH$_3$-6 (δ_C 64.3) and C-9 (δ_C 58.7), as well as H-9 (δ_H 4.44) to C-1 (δ_C 166.8) revealed that the oxethyl group was located at C-6. Furthermore, the difference between H-6 (δ_H 5.35, dd, J = 2.8, 1.7 Hz) in **2** and H-6 (δ_H 5.59, dd, J = 5.7, 1.7 Hz) in **1** indicated that **2** was the C-6 epimer of **1**. Furthermore, the same ECD cotton effects (Figure 3C) of **2** compared to **1** indicated that the absolute configuration of C-9 in **2** was consistent with that in **1**. This result suggested that within the used spectral window, the ECD cotton effects were mainly caused by the chiral center of C-9 in both compounds **1** and **2**, and it could also be confirmed by the experimental ECD data of (+)-brevianamide V and (−)-brevianamide V [35]. Thus, the absolute configuration of compound **2** was ascertained as (6S,9S).

Aspamide C (**3**) was obtained as a yellowish powder. The molecular formula was established as $C_{21}H_{23}N_3O_3$ by HRESIMS (m/z 366.1807 [M + H]$^+$, calcd. for $C_{21}H_{24}N_3O_3$, 366.1812), indicating 12 degrees of unsaturation. The UV and NMR spectra were very similar to those of compound **1**. A comparison of the NMR data for **3** with **1**, together with characteristic HMBC signals (Figure 3A), suggested that the oxethyl group was replaced by a second OH in **3**. However, the OH group was not located at C-6, which was the same as the **1**, to form the aza-acetal structure for which the chemical shift of oxygenated methylene (δ_C 66.6) was far below the shift of C-6 (δ_C 86.7) in **1**. Thus, the second OH was distributed to C-7, and the planar structure of **3** was determined as shown in Figure 1. The ROESY correlation (Figure S20) between NH-2 (δ_H 8.93) and H-13 (δ_H 7.29) confirmed the *cis* form of the double bond between C-3 and C-10. Furthermore, the ROESY signals (Figure 3B) between H-8β (δ_H 1.98) and H-7 (δ_H 4.35), and between H-8α (δ_H 2.12) and H-9 (δ_H 4.65) revealed that H-7 and H-9 were *trans* form. Finally, the absolute configuration of **3** was determined as (7R,9S) by comparison of the experimental ECD curve of **3** with that of **1** (Figure 3C).

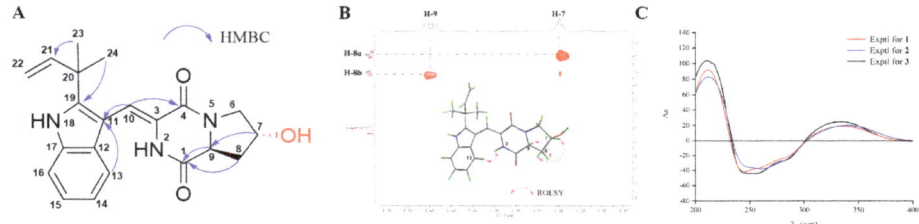

Figure 3. The key HMBC correlations (**A**) and partial enlarged view of ROESY spectra (**B**) of **3**, and experimental ECD spectra (**C**) of compounds **1–3**.

Table 1. ^{1}H (600 MHz) and ^{13}C (150 MHz) NMR data of **1–3** in DMSO-d_6.

No.	1		2		3	
	δ_C	δ_H, Mult. (J in Hz)	δ_C	δ_H, Mult. (J in Hz)	δ_C	δ_H, Mult. (J in Hz)
1	165.9	-	166.8	-	166.2	-
2	-	9.01, s	-	9.43, s	-	8.93, s
3	125.3	-	125.9	-	126.2	-
4	158.9	-	161.1	-	158.4	-
6a	86.7	5.59, dd (5.7, 1.7)	85.4	5.35, dd (2.8, 1.7)	54.4	3.32, m
6b	-	-	-	-	-	3.75, dd (12.7, 4.5)
7a	29.6	1.75, dddd (13.4, 8.4, 5.0, 1.7)	30.7	1.92, m	66.6	4.35, t (4.5)
7b		1.97, m		-		
8a	25.9	2.13, dddd (12.2, 9.7, 6.7, 5.0)	24.5	1.92, m	37.6	1.98, ddd (12.7, 11.5, 4.5)
8b		2.27, m		2.10, m		2.12, dd (12.7, 6.0)
9	56.5	4.57, dd (8.9, 6.7)	58.7	4.44, m	57.0	4.65, dd (11.5, 6.0)
10	111.9	6.98, s	113.2	7.05, s	110.7	6.92, s
11	103.9	-	104.3	-	103.8	-
12	125.9	-	125.8	-	126.0	-
13	119.6	7.29, d (8.0)	119.7	7.23, d (8.0)	119.4	7.29, d (8.0)
14	119.4	6.99, m	119.3	6.99, ddd (8.0, 7.0, 1.2)	119.3	7.00, m

Table 1. Cont.

No.	1 δ_C	1 δ_H, Mult. (J in Hz)	2 δ_C	2 δ_H, Mult. (J in Hz)	3 δ_C	3 δ_H, Mult. (J in Hz)
15	120.7	7.08, ddd (8.0, 7.0, 1.2)	120.7	7.07, ddd (8.0, 7.0, 1.2)	120.7	7.08, ddd (8.0, 7.0, 1.2)
16	111.5	7.41, d (8.0)	111.6	7.41, m	111.4	7.41, d (8.0)
17	135.1	-	135.1	-	135.1	-
18	-	11.06, s	-	11.06, s	-	11.03, s
19	144.3	-	144.7	-	144.0	-
20	39.0	-	39.1	-	39.0	-
21	145.1	6.07, dd (17.4, 10.5)	145.1	6.09, dd (17.1, 10.8)	145.2	6.08, dd (17.3, 10.5)
22	111.7	5.05, m	111.7	5.06, m	111.6	5.04, m
23	27.4	1.45, s	27.5	1.47, s	27.4	1.46, s
24	27.8	1.49, s	27.9	1.51, s	27.7	1.50, s
6-OEt	63.6	3.65, m	64.3	3.60, m	-	-
	15.2	1.13, t (7.1)	15.4	1.09, t (7.1)	-	-

The racemic (±)-aspamide D (**4**) was isolated as colorless gum with the molecular formula of $C_{23}H_{27}N_3O_3$ from an HRESIMS peak at m/z 394.2120 [M + H]$^+$ (calcd. for $C_{23}H_{28}N_3O_3$, 394.2125). Its NMR data and UV absorption were similar to compound **1**. Comparing to **1**, the major change was that two sp^3 methines were replaced by one sp^3 methylene and one sp^3 non-protonated carbon, suggesting that the oxethyl group was connected to C-9 rather to the C-6. Additionally, the key HMBC signals (Figure 4) from OCH$_2$CH$_3$-9 (δ_H 3.53) to C-9 (δ_C 91.0), H-6 (δ_H 3.62) to C-4 (δ_C 159.4) and C-9, and H-8a (δ_H 2.02) to C-1 (δ_C 163.1) confirmed the aforementioned planar structure. There was no Cotton effect observed on its ECD spectra (Figure S29), which in accordance with the racemic (±)-brevianamide X [35], indicating that **4** might be a pair of enantiomers. Furthermore, the chiral HPLC resolution of **4** contributed to the separation of a pair of enantiomers (+)-**4** and (−)-**4**, which exhibited nearly mirror-image ECD spectra (Figure 5). The absolute configurations of (+)-**4** and (−)-**4** were discriminably determined as 9R and 9S by comparing the experimental and calculated ECD data obtained using TD-DFT at the B3LYP/6-31+g (d, p) level (Figure 5). Correspondingly, we named (+)-**4** and (−)-**4** as (+)-aspamide D and (−)-aspamide D, respectively.

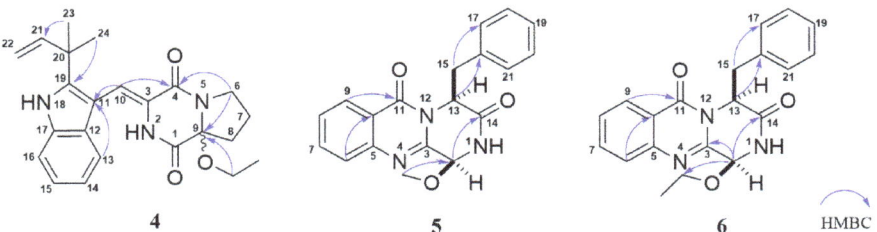

Figure 4. The key HMBC correlations of compounds **4**–**6**.

Aspamide F (**5**) was obtained as a brown powder with the molecular formula of $C_{19}H_{17}N_3O_3$ from an HRESIMS peak at m/z 336.1336 [M + H]$^+$ (calcd. for $C_{19}H_{18}N_3O_3$, 336.1343), requiring 13 indices of hydrogen deficiency. The ^{1}H NMR, ^{13}C NMR, and HMQC spectra (Table 2 and Figure S35) suggested the presence of one oxygenated methyl group, one sp^3 methylene, two sp^3 methines carbon signals (including one oxygen-bearing carbon), nine sp^2 methines, and six sp^2 non-protonated carbons. These NMR data of **5** were similar to those of brevianamide M [28], except for the different chemical shifts for C-2 and C-3 due to the presence of a methoxy at C-2 in **5**, implying that **5** was an analogue of brevianamide M with a methoxy at C-2. Additionally, the key HMBC correlations (Figure 4) from OCH$_3$-2 (δ_H 3.53) to C-2 (δ_C 83.9), from H-2 (δ_H 5.27) to C-3 (δ_C 146.9)/C-14 (δ_C 170.0), and from H-13

(δ_H 5.53) to C-15 (δ_C 40.0)/C-16 (δ_C 135.9) confirmed the planner structure of **5** as shown in Figure 4. The absolute configuration of **5** was determined as (2S,13S) via comparing the ECD curve (Figure 6) of **5** with the brevianamide M (**17**).

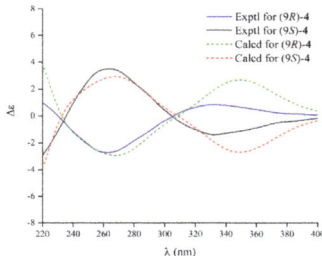

Figure 5. Experimental and calculated ECD spectra of **4**.

Table 2. ^{1}H (600 MHz) and ^{13}C (150 MHz) NMR data of **4–6** (**4** in DMSO-d_6, **5–6** in CDCl$_3$).

No.	4 δ	4 δ$_H$, Mult. (J in Hz)	5 δ$_C$	5 δ$_H$, Mult. (J in Hz)	6 δ$_C$	6 δ$_H$, Mult. (J in Hz)
1	163.1	-	-	-	-	-
2	-	9.43, s	83.9	5.27, d (4.7)	78.3	6.40, d (4.3)
3	125.5	-	146.9	-	151.1	-
4	159.4	-	-	-	-	-
5	-	-	146.7	-	139.0	-
6	45.1	3.62, dd (8.6, 5.8)	127.8	7.74, d (8.0)	122.9	8.23, d, (8.0)
7a	19.5	1.92, m	134.9	7.79, t (8.0)	136.7	7.91, t (8.0)
7b		1.96, m				
8a	32.4	2.02, m	128.0	7.53, t (8.0)	129.7	7.66, t (8.0)
8b		2.33, m				
9	91.0	-	127.0	8.24, d (8.0)	127.9	8.23, d, (8.0)
10	112.7	7.02, s	120.8	-	119.1	-
11	103.9	-	160.3	-	157.4	-
12	126.3	-	-	-	-	-
13	119.1	7.21, d (8.0)	57.4	5.53, dd (8.8, 6.5)	58.1	5.54, t (7.8)
14	119.0	7.00, m	170.0	-	167.6	-
15	120.7	7.09, m	40.0	3.43, m	39.9	3.48, m
16	111.6	7.43, d (8.0)	135.9	-	134.9	-
17	135.1	-	129.8	7.29, m	129.7	7.24, m
18		11.10, s	128.6	7.28, m	128.8	7.24, m
19	144.4	-	127.0	7.24, m	127.7	7.20, m
20	39.0	-	128.6	7.28, m	128.8	7.24, m
21	145.2	6.09, ddd (17.1, 10.8, 1.6)	129.8	7.29, m	129.7	7.24, m
22	111.7	5.06, m	-	-	-	-
23	27.4	1.47, s	-	-	-	-
24	27.8	1.50, s	-	-	-	-
9-OEt	59.2	3.53, qd (7.0, 3.9)	-	-	-	-
-	15.2	1.22, td (7.0, 1.5)	-	-	-	-
2-OMe/	-	-	56.0	3.53, s	66.2	4.04, dt (9.0, 7.0)
2-OEt	-	-	-	-	15.4	4.11, dt (9.0, 7.0)
						1.35, t (7.0)

Aspamide G (**6**) was isolated as a brown powder. The molecular formula was determined as $C_{20}H_{19}N_3O_3$ by HRESIMS (m/z 350.1498 [M + H]$^+$, calcd. for $C_{20}H_{20}N_3O_3$, 350.1499), which was 14 Dalton more than **5**. The ^{13}C NMR data of **6** showed a close resemblance to those of **5**, except for an additional oxygenated sp^3 methylene, suggesting that there was an ethoxy group located at C-2 in **6**. The key HMBC signal (Figure 4) from H-2 (δ_H 6.40) to OCH$_2$-2 (δ_C 66.2) verified that **6** was an analogue of brevianamide M (**17**) with an ethoxy motif at C-2. In addition, similar Cotton effects at 212, 220, and 237 nm in the ECD spectra (Figure 6) of **6** suggested that **6** and **17** had the same counterpart absolute configurations. Thus, the absolute configuration of **6** was assigned as (2S,13S), and it was elucidated as 6-ethoxy-aspamide F.

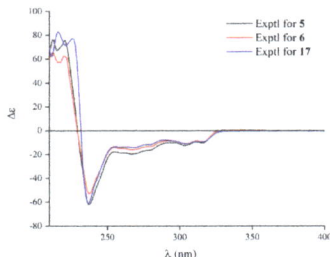

Figure 6. Experimental ECD spectra of **5**, **6**, and **17**.

All isolated compounds were tested for their anti-inflammatory activities in *P. acnes*-induced THP-1 cells; unfortunately, none of the compounds showed moderate anti-inflammatory properties. Aiming to give our contribution to the COVID-19 research, all compounds were selected for the virtual screening on the 3CL hydrolase (Mpro) of SARS-CoV-2, which had been exploited as a potential drug target to fight COVID-19 [27]. The docking scores of compounds **1–2**, **5**, **6**, **8** and **17** were top among all screened molecules (docking scores: −5.389, −4.772, −5.146, −4.962, −5.158), and the score of ritonavir [36] (a potent inhibitor in vitro of human immunodeficiency virus type 1 protease) was −7.039, which suggested that these compounds may be helpful in fighting COVID-19 after further studies.

3. Materials and Methods

3.1. General Experimental Procedures

Optical rotations were recorded on a JASCO P-1020 polarimeter (JASCO Corporation, Tokyo, Japan) in MeOH at 25 °C. UV spectra were measured using a Shimadzu UV-1800 spectrophotometer (Shimadzu Corporation, Tokyo, Japan). High-resolution electrospray ionization (HR-ESI-MS) were obtained with an Agilent 6529B Q-TOF instrument (Agilent Technologies, Santa Clara, CA, USA). ECD spectra were carried out with Chirascan circular dichroism spectrometers (Applied Photophysics Ltd., Leatherhead, UK). Both 1D and 2D NMR spectra were acquired on a Bruker AVIII-400 and Bruker AVIII-600 NMR spectrometers with tetramethylsilane (TMS) as an internal standard (Bruker, Karlsruhe, Germany). Preparative high-performance liquid chromatography (Pre-HPLC) was performed utilizing a Shimadzu LC-20 system (Shimadzu, Tokyo, Japan) equipped with a Shim-pack RP-C18 column (20 × 250 mm i.d., 10 μm, Shimadzu, Tokyo, Japan) with a flow rate at 10 mL/min at 25 °C, which was recorded by a binary channel UV detector at 210 nm and 254 nm. The analytical chiral HPLC used was a JASCO LC-2000 system equipped with a Daicel Chiralpak AD-H column (4.6 mm × 250 mm, 5 μm) and a CD-2095 chiral detector at 280 nm. The mobile phase was *n*-hexane/isopropanol (80:20, *v*/*v*) used at a flow rate of 0.5 mL/min. Column chromatography (CC) was performed with silica gel (200–300 mesh, Qingdao Marine Chemical Inc., Qingdao, China) and ODS (50 μm, YMC, Kyoto, Japan) on a Flash Chromatograph System (SepaBen machine, Santai Technologies, Changzhou, China). Thin-layer chromatography (TLC) was performed using precoated silica gel GF254 plates (Qingdao Marine Chemical Inc., Qingdao, China).

3.2. Fungal Material

The endophytic DY180635 was isolated from a sample of crab (*Chiromantes haematocheir*), which was collected from the intertidal zone of Zhoushan, Zhejiang, China, in June 2018. It was incubated on a potato dextrose agar (PDA) plate at 28 °C. The strain DY180635 was identified using ITS rDNA sequence analysis by RuiDi (Shanghai, China) and its DNA sequence using BLAST was compared to the GenBank data. The result of BLAST searching was closest to that of *Aspergillus versicolor* NRRL 238 (GenBank accession number NG_067623) with 99% sequence identity. The nucleotide sequences of the ITS gene (accession number MT361076) of *A. versicolor* DY180635 were deposited in GenBank. A reference culture is stored in State Key Laboratory of Bioreactor Engineering laboratory of Shanghai at −80 °C.

3.3. Fermentation, Extraction, and Isolation

The fungus was incubated on potato dextrose agar (PDA) medium at 28 °C for approximately 2–3 days; then it was cut into three agar pieces (nearly the size of 0.5 × 0.5 × 0.5 cm) and transferred into a 500 mL Erlenmeyer flask, containing 200 mL of potato dextrose broth (PDB). The flasks were cultured for 2 days at 28 °C on a rotary shaker at 180 rpm for inoculation. The seed cultures were added to the 200 × 1 L flasks containing rice medium (110 g rice, 120 mL deionized water), which was previously sterilized at 121 °C for 25 min. All flasks were incubated at 28 °C for four weeks.

Following incubation, the solid rice cultures were extracted three times by EtOAc to give a crude extract (489.0 g); the crude extract was suspended in water and then partitioned with EtOAc to give an EtOAc soluble fraction (185.2 g) after the solvent was removed to dryness under reduced pressure. The EtOAc fraction was further separated on macroporous adsorbent resin with a stepped gradient elution with EtOH-H_2O (30, 50, 70 and 100%). The 50% fraction was sequentially separated by silica gel with petroleum ether-EtOAc (5:1 to 0:1) to give four subfractions (A–D) using the TLC. The subfraction B (9.0 g) was sequentially loaded onto silica gel CC (petroleum ether-EtOAc, 5:1) and preparative HPLC (MeCN-H_2O, 50:50, 10.0 mL/min) to yield compounds **1** (10.4 mg, t_R 34.9 min), **2** (6.4 mg, t_R 27.1 min), **4** (5.9 mg, t_R 33.5 min), and **6** (8.7 mg, t_R 23.2 min). Subfraction C (15.0 g) was further separated by an ODS column (MeCN-H_2O, 40:60) and repeated preparative HPLC with MeCN-H_2O (50:50, 10 mL/min) to give compounds **3** (4.6 mg, t_R 8.8 min) and **5** (4.7 mg, t_R 17.1 min).

Aspamide A (**1**): yellowish powder; $[\alpha]_D^{25}$ + 120.0 (c 0.05, MeOH); ECD (5 mg/L, MeOH) λ_{max} ($\Delta\varepsilon$) 212 (92.18), 245 (−41.48) 335 (19.29) nm; UV (MeOH) λ_{max} (logε) 200 (6.13), 224 (6.13), 284 (5.46), 341 (5.68) nm; ^{1}H and ^{13}C NMR (DMSO-d_6), see Table 1; positive HR-ESI-MS *m/z* 394.2117 [M + H]$^+$, (calcd. for $C_{23}H_{28}N_3O_3$, 394.2125).

Aspamide B (**2**): yellowish powder; $[\alpha]_D^{25}$ + 112.0 (c 0.05, MeOH); ECD (5 mg/L, MeOH) λ_{max} ($\Delta\varepsilon$) 212 (83.31), 261 (−37.91), 340 (20.41) nm; UV (MeOH) λ_{max} (logε) 200 (6.18), 224 (6.18), 283 (5.45), 345 (5.73) nm; ^{1}H and ^{13}C NMR (DMSO-d_6), see Table 1; positive HR-ESI-MS *m/z* 394.2120 [M + H]$^+$, (calcd. for $C_{23}H_{28}N_3O_3$, 394.2125).

Aspamide C (**3**): yellowish powder; $[\alpha]_D^{25}$ + 125.0 (c 0.05, MeOH); ECD (5 mg/L, MeOH) λ_{max} ($\Delta\varepsilon$) 211 (103.75), 255 (−44.38), 334 (24.79) nm; UV (MeOH) λ_{max} (logε) 200 (6.20), 224 (6.19), 284 (5.56), 337 (5.75) nm; ^{1}H and ^{13}C NMR (DMSO-d_6), see Table 1; positive HR-ESI-MS *m/z* 366.1807 [M + H]$^+$, (calcd. for $C_{21}H_{24}N_3O_3$, 366.1812).

(±)-Aspamide D (**4**): colorless gum; $[\alpha]_D^{25}$ + 5.0 (c 0.05, MeOH); UV (MeOH) λ_{max} (logε) 200 (6.07), 224 (6.06), 283 (5.33), 346 (5.60) nm; ^{1}H and ^{13}C NMR (DMSO-d_6), see Table 2; positive HR-ESI-MS *m/z* 394.2122 [M + H]$^+$, (calcd. for $C_{23}H_{28}N_3O_3$, 394.2125).

Aspamide F (**5**): brown powder; $[\alpha]_D^{25}$ + 40.0 (c 0.05, MeOH); ECD (5 mg/L, MeOH) λ_{max} ($\Delta\varepsilon$) 212 (65.33), 220 (62.98), 237 (−52.79) nm; UV (MeOH) λ_{max} (logε) 206 (5.95), 224 (6.15), 270 (5.25),

278 (5.23) nm; ^{1}H and ^{13}C NMR (CDCl$_3$), see Table 2; positive HR-ESI-MS *m/z* 336.1336 [M + H]$^+$, (calcd. for C$_{19}$H$_{18}$N$_3$O$_3$, 336.1343).

Aspamide G (**6**): brown powder; $[\alpha]_D^{25}$ + 56.0 (*c* 0.05, MeOH); ECD (5 mg/L, MeOH) λ_{max} ($\Delta\varepsilon$) 212 (76.04), 221 (75.42), 237 (-62.18) nm; UV (MeOH) λ_{max} (logε) 205 (5.92), 222 (5.88), 270 (5.16), 278 (5.13) nm; ^{1}H and ^{13}C NMR (CDCl$_3$), see Table 2; positive HR-ESI-MS *m/z* 350.1498 [M + H]$^+$, (calcd. for C$_{20}$H$_{20}$N$_3$O$_3$, 350.1499).

3.4. ECD Calculation

The relative configuration of **1** was established initially according to its ROESY NMR spectra. Monte Carlo conformational searches were carried out by means of the Spartan's 14 software using the Merck molecular force field (MMFF). The conformers with Boltzmann population of over 1% were chosen for ECD calculations, and then the conformers were initially optimized at the B3LYP/6-31G(d,p) level in gas. The theoretical calculation of ECD was conducted in MeOH using Time-dependent Density functional theory (TD-DFT) at the B3LYP/6-31+G(d,p) level for all conformers. Rotatory strengths for a total of 100 excited states were calculated. ECD spectra were generated using the program SpecDis 1.6 (University of Würzburg, Würzburg, Germany) and GraphPad Prism 5 (University of California San Diego, USA) from dipole-length rotational strengths by applying Gaussian band shapes with sigma = 0.3 eV. And UV-shift values of all configurations were −10 nm. The spectra of enantiomers were produced directly by mirror inversions.

3.5. Virtual Screening Against COVID-19 Main Protease

3.5.1. Protein and Ligand Preparation

The 3CL hydrolase (Mpro) of SARS-CoV-2 had been exploited as a potential drug target to fight COVID-19 [27]. Thus, the virtual screening was conducted by using the SARS-CoV-2 enzyme (PDB ID 6LU7) obtained from the Protein Data Bank (PDB, http://www.rcsb.org/pdb), and the structure was optimized by using the protein preparation wizard module in Maestro software package (Schrodinger LLC, NY, USA). Specifically, the water and heteroatom were removed, the polar hydrogens were added to the protein to the protonation state, the entire structure was assumed as a neutral pH, and the energy of the structure was minimized by using an OPLS2005 force field. The docking grid of 20 Å size was generated over the co-crystallized ligand. All compounds **1**–**17** were implemented by Ligprep software, and the structure energy was minimized using OPL2005 force field.

3.5.2. Virtual Screening

Virtual screening was performed by the Schrodinger glide docking module, and the standard-precision (SP) docking was designated to get accurate results [37]. The results were measured by docking score, and only the compounds with scores in the top half were subjected to the extra-precision (XP) docking.

3.6. Cell Culture and Cell Viability Assay

The human monocytic cell line, THP-1 (Cell Bank of China Science Academy, Shanghai, China) and *P. acnes* (ATCC6919, Xiangfu biotech, Shanghai, China), were used for the anti-inflammatory assay. THP-1 cells were cultured in RPMI1640 medium with 10% fetal bovine serum (FBS, Gibco, NY, USA) in a humidified incubator (37 °C, 5% CO$_2$). *P. acnes* bacteria were incubated in Cooked Meat Medium, containing cooked beef granules (Rishui biotechnology, Qingdao, China) in an anaerobic environment. The THP-1 cells were stimulated by the *P. acnes*, which was harvested at the exponential phase. The viability of THP-1 cells was evaluated by the MTT assay, specifically, seeding the THP-1 cells in 96-well plates at a density of 2×10^5 cells/well and treated with serially diluted compounds for 36 h (37 °C, 5% CO$_2$). After that, we added 20 μL MTT regent (5 mg/mL, Genetimes Technology Inc.,

Shanghai, China) to each well and incubated the samples at 37 °C for 4 h. Removing the supernatant, the formazan crystals were fully solubilized in DMSO (150 µL), and the absorbance was measured at 570 nm and 630 nm.

4. Conclusions

Chemical investigation of a marine-derived fungus *Aspergillus versicolor* DY180635 led to the isolation and identification of four new IDPKs, aspamides A–E (**1–4**) and two new DPKs, aspamides F–G (**5–6**), along with 11 known diketopiperazines and intermediates. Further chiral high-performance liquid chromatography resolution gave enantiomers (+)- and (−)-**4**, respectively. The structures and absolute configurations of compounds **1–6** were determined by the comprehensive analyses of NMR, HRESIMS, and ECD calculation. Compounds **1–17** were selected for the virtual screening on the 3CL hydrolase (Mpro) of SARS-CoV-2, and compounds **1–2, 5, 6, 8** and **17** possessed top docking scores and thus may be helpful in fighting COVID-19 after further studies.

Supplementary Materials: The following are available online at: http://www.mdpi.com/1660-3397/18/7/338/s1, Figures S1–S46: ^{1}H, ^{13}C, HSQC, HMBC, ROESY, UV, ECD, and HRESIMS spectra of the new compounds **1–6**, Tables S1–S6: Computational data of **1** and **4**.

Author Contributions: Y.D. performed the isolation, purification and identification of all compounds. X.Z. tested the anti-inflammatory activities. L.H. and M.Z. supervised the laboratory work. Q.H. edited the manuscript. F.A. supervised the laboratory work, designed the experiments and edited the manuscript. All authors have read and agree to the published version of the manuscript.

Funding: This work was funded by the National Key R&D Program of China (2018YFC1706200, 2019YFC0312504), and the National Natural Science Foundation of China (41876189, 81703388). This work was also supported by State Key Laboratory of Bioreactor Engineering. Authors thank Prof. Lixin Zhang (State Key Laboratory of Bioreactor Engineering, East China University of Science and Technology) for assistance in the virtual screening on the Mpro of SARS-CoV-2.

Conflicts of Interest: The authors declare no conflict of interest.

References

1. Strobel, G.; Daisy, B.; Castillo, U.; Harper, J. Natural products from endophytic microorganisms. *J. Nat. Prod.* **2004**, *67*, 257–268. [CrossRef]
2. Blunt, J.W.; Copp, B.R.; Keyzers, R.A.; Munro, M.H.G.; Prinsep, M.R. Marine natural products. *Nat. Prod. Rep.* **2017**, *34*, 235–294. [CrossRef] [PubMed]
3. Bugni, T.S.; Ireland, C.M. Marine-derived fungi: A chemically and biologically diverse group of microorganisms. *Nat. Prod. Rep.* **2004**, *21*, 143–163. [CrossRef]
4. Ma, Y.M.; Liang, X.A.; Kong, Y.; Jia, B. Structural diversity and biological activities of indole diketopiperazine alkaloids from fungi. *J. Agric. Food Chem.* **2016**, *64*, 6659–6671. [CrossRef] [PubMed]
5. Borthwick, A.D. 2,5-Diketopiperazines: Synthesis, reactions, medicinal chemistry, and bioactive natural products. *Chem. Rev.* **2012**, *112*, 3641–3716. [CrossRef] [PubMed]
6. Wang, W.L.; Lu, Z.Y.; Tao, H.W.; Zhu, T.J.; Fang, Y.C.; Gu, Q.Q.; Zhu, W.M. Isoechinulin-type alkaloids, variecolorins A-L, from halotolerant *Aspergillus variecolor*. *J. Nat. Prod.* **2007**, *70*, 1558–1564. [CrossRef]
7. Cai, S.X.; Sun, S.W.; Peng, J.X.; Kong, X.L.; Zhou, H.N.; Zhu, T.J.; Gu, Q.Q.; Li, D.H. Okaramines S-U, three new indole diketopiperazine alkaloids from *Aspergillus taichungensis* ZHN-7-07. *Tetrahedron* **2015**, *71*, 3715–3719. [CrossRef]
8. Wang, F.Z.; Fang, Y.C.; Zhu, T.J.; Zhang, M.; Lin, A.Q.; Gu, Q.Q.; Zhu, W.M. Seven new prenylated indole diketopiperazine alkaloids from holothurian-derived fungus *Aspergillus fumigatus*. *Tetrahedron* **2008**, *64*, 7986–7991. [CrossRef]
9. Tsukamoto, S.; Kato, H.; Samizo, M.; Nojiri, Y.; Onuki, H.; Hirota, H.; Ohta, T. Notoamides F–K, prenylated indole alkaloids isolated from a marine-derived *Aspergillus* sp. *J. Nat. Prod.* **2008**, *71*, 2064–2067. [CrossRef]
10. Kozlovsky, A.G.; Vinokurova, N.G.; Adanin, V.M. Diketopiperazine alkaloids from the fungus *Penicillium piscarium* westling. *Appl. Biochem. Microbiol.* **2000**, *36*, 271–275. [CrossRef]

11. Ravikanth, V.; Niranjan Reddy, V.L.; Ramesh, P.; Prabhakar Rao, T.; Diwan, P.V.; Khar, A.; Venkateswarlu, Y. An immunosuppressive tryptophan-derived alkaloid from *Lepidagathis cristata*. *Phytochemistry* **2001**, *58*, 1263–1266. [CrossRef]
12. Fujimoto, H.; Sumino, M.; Okuyama, E.; Ishibashi, M. Immunomodulatory constituents from an Ascomycete. *J. Nat. Prod.* **2004**, *67*, 98–102. [CrossRef]
13. Kuramochi, K.; Ohnishi, K.; Fujieda, S.; Nakajima, M.; Saitoh, Y.; Watanabe, N.; Takeuchi, T.; Nakazaki, A.; Sugawara, F.; Arai, T.; et al. Synthesis and biological activities of neoechinulin A derivatives: New aspects of structure-activity relationships for neoechinulin A. *Chem. Pharm. Bull.* **2008**, *56*, 1738–1743. [CrossRef] [PubMed]
14. Fan, Z.; Sun, Z.H.; Liu, Z.; Chen, Y.C.; Liu, H.X.; Li, H.H.; Zhang, W.M. Dichotocejpins A-C: New diketopiperazines from a deep-sea-derived fungus *Dichotomomyces cejpii* FS110. *Mar. Drugs* **2016**, *14*, 1–9. [CrossRef] [PubMed]
15. Mohanlal, R.W.; Lloyd, K.; Huang, L. Plinabulin, a novel small molecule clinical stage IO agent with anti-cancer activity, to prevent chemo-induced neutropenia and immune related AEs. *J. Clin. Oncol.* **2018**, *36*, 126. [CrossRef]
16. Gomes, N.G.M.; Lefranc, F.; Kijjoa, A.; Kiss, R. Can some marine-ferived fungal metabolites become actual anticancer agents? *Mar. Drugs* **2015**, *13*, 3950–3991. [CrossRef]
17. Geiger, W.B.; Conn, J.E.; Waksman, S.A. Chaetomin, a new antibiotic substance produced by *Chaetomium cochliodes*: II. Isolation and Concentration. *J. Bacteriol.* **1944**, *48*, 531–536. [CrossRef]
18. Tian, W.; Sun, C.; Zheng, M.; Harmer, J.R.; Yu, M.; Zhang, Y.; Peng, H.; Zhu, D.; Deng, Z.; Chen, S.L.; et al. Efficient biosynthesis of heterodimeric C^3-aryl pyrroloindoline alkaloids. *Nat. Commun.* **2018**, *9*, 4428. [CrossRef]
19. Ye, Y.; Du, L.; Zhang, X.W.; Newmister, S.A.; McCauley, M.; Alegre-Requena, J.V.; Zhang, W.; Mu, S.; Minami, A.; Fraley, A.E.; et al. Fungal-derived brevianamide assembly by a stereoselective semipinacolase. *Nat. Catal.* **2020**. [CrossRef]
20. Song, F.; Liu, X.; Guo, H.; Ren, B.; Chen, C.; Piggott, A.M.; Yu, K.; Gao, H.; Wang, Q.; Liu, M.; et al. Brevianamides with antitubercular potential from a marine-derived isolate of *Aspergillus versicolor*. *Org. Lett.* **2012**, *14*, 4770–4773. [CrossRef]
21. James, E.D.; Knuckley, B.; Alqahtani, N.; Porwal, S.; Ban, J.; Karty, J.A.; Viswanathan, R.; Lane, A.L. Two distinct cyclodipeptide synthases from a marine *Actinomycete* catalyze biosynthesis of the same diketopiperazine natural product. *ACS Synth. Biol.* **2016**, *5*, 547–553. [CrossRef] [PubMed]
22. Haines, B.E.; Nelson, B.M.; Grandner, J.M.; Kim, J.; Houk, K.N.; Movassaghi, M.; Musaev, D.G. Mechanism of permanganate-promoted dihydroxylation of complex diketopiperazines: Critical roles of counter-cation and ion-pairing. *J. Am. Chem. Soc.* **2018**, *140*, 13375–13386. [CrossRef]
23. Ding, Y.; An, F.L.; Zhu, X.J.; Yu, H.Y.; Hao, L.L.; Lu, Y.H. Curdepsidones B-G, six depsidones with anti-inflammatory activities from the marine-derived fungus *Curvularia* sp. IFB-Z10. *Mar. Drugs* **2019**, *17*, 266. [CrossRef]
24. Liu, W.H.; Ding, Y.; Ji, X.; An, F.L.; Lu, Y.H. Curvulaide A, a bicyclic polyketide with anti-anaerobic bacteria activity from marine-derived *Curvularia* sp. *J. Antibiot.* **2019**, *72*, 111–113. [CrossRef]
25. Guo, M.M.; Lu, Y.; Yang, J.P.; Zhao, X.; Lu, Y.H. Inhibitory effects of *Schisandra chinensis* extract on acne-related inflammation and UVB-induced photoageing. *Pharm. Biol.* **2016**, *54*, 2987–2994. [CrossRef] [PubMed]
26. Dillman, R.L.; Cardellina, J.H. Aromatic secondary metabolites from the sponge *Tedania ignis*. *J. Nat. Prod.* **1991**, *54*, 1056–1061. [CrossRef]
27. Jin, Z.M.; Du, X.Y.; Xu, Y.C.; Deng, Y.Q.; Liu, M.Q.; Zhao, Y.; Zhang, B.; Li, X.F.; Zhang, L.K.; Peng, C.F.; et al. Structure of M^{pro} from COVID-19 virus and discovery of its inhibitors. *Nature* **2020**, *582*, 289–293. [CrossRef] [PubMed]
28. Li, G.Y.; Yang, T.; Luo, Y.G.; Chen, X.Z.; Fang, D.M.; Zhang, G.L. Brevianamide J, a new indole alkaloid dimer from fungus *Aspergillus versicolor*. *Org. Lett.* **2009**, *11*, 3714–3717. [CrossRef]
29. Li, G.Y.; Li, L.M.; Yang, T.; Chen, X.Z.; Fang, D.M.; Zhang, G.L. Four new alkaloids, brevianamides O-R, from the fungus *Aspergillus versicolor*. *Helv. Chim. Acta* **2010**, *93*, 2075–2080. [CrossRef]
30. Liu, Y.X.; Ma, S.G.; Wang, X.J.; Zhao, N.; Qu, J.; Yu, S.S.; Dai, J.G.; Wang, Y.H.; Si, Y.K. Diketopiperazine alkaloids produced by the endophytic fungus *Aspergillus fumigatus* from the Stem of *Erythrophloeum fordii* Oliv. *Helv. Chim. Acta* **2012**, *95*, 1401–1408. [CrossRef]

31. Schkeryantz, J.M.; Woo, J.C.G.; Siliphaivanh, P.; Depew, K.M.; Danishefsky, S.J. Total synthesis of gypsetin, deoxybrevianamide E, brevianamide E, and tryprostatin B: Novel constructions of 2,3-disubstituted indoles. *J. Am. Chem. Soc.* **1999**, *121*, 11964–11975. [CrossRef]
32. Sanz-Cervera, J.F.; Stocking, E.M.; Usui, T.; Osada, H.; Williams, R.M. Synthesis and evaluation of microtubule assembly inhibition and cytotoxicity of prenylated derivatives of cyclo-L-Trp-L-Pro. *Bioorg. Med. Chem.* **2000**, *8*, 2407–2415. [CrossRef]
33. May Zin, W.W.; Buttachon, S.; Dethoup, T.; Pereira, J.A.; Gales, L.; Inácio, Â.; Costa, P.M.; Lee, M.; Sekeroglu, N.; Silva, A.M.S.; et al. Antibacterial and antibiofilm activities of the metabolites isolated from the culture of the mangrove-derived endophytic fungus *Eurotium chevalieri* KUFA 0006. *Phytochemistry* **2017**, *141*, 86–97. [CrossRef] [PubMed]
34. Pirrung, M.C.; Fujita, K.; Park, K. Organometallic routes to 2,5-dihydroxy-3-(indol-3-yl)-benzoquinones. Synthesis of demethylasterriquinone B4. *J. Org. Chem.* **2005**, *70*, 2537–2542. [CrossRef]
35. Liu, W.; Wang, L.P.; Wang, B.; Xu, Y.C.; Zhu, G.L.; Lan, M.M.; Zhu, W.M.; Sun, K.L. Diketopiperazine and diphenylether derivatives from marine algae-derived *Aspergillus versicolor* OUCMDZ-2738 by epigenetic activation. *Mar. Drugs* **2019**, *17*, 6. [CrossRef]
36. Markowitz, M.; Saag, M.; Powderly, W.G.; Hurley, A.M.; Hsu, A.; Valdes, J.M.; Henry, D.; Sattler, F.; La Marca, A.; Leonard, J.M.; et al. A preliminary study of ritonavir, an inhibitor of HIV-1 protease, to treat HIV-1 infection. *N. Engl. J. Med.* **1995**, *333*, 1534–1539. [CrossRef]
37. Halgren, T.A.; Murphy, R.B.; Friesner, R.A.; Beard, H.S.; Frye, L.L.; Pollard, W.T.; Banks, J.L. Glide: A new approach for rapid, accurate docking and scoring. 2. Enrichment factors in database screening. *J. Med. Chem* **2004**, *47*, 1750–1759. [CrossRef]

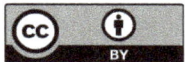 © 2020 by the authors. Licensee MDPI, Basel, Switzerland. This article is an open access article distributed under the terms and conditions of the Creative Commons Attribution (CC BY) license (http://creativecommons.org/licenses/by/4.0/).

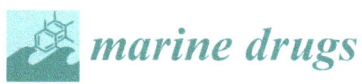

Article

Bioactive Bianthraquinones and Meroterpenoids from a Marine-Derived *Stemphylium* sp. Fungus

Ji-Yeon Hwang [1], Sung Chul Park [1], Woong Sub Byun [1], Dong-Chan Oh [1], Sang Kook Lee [1], Ki-Bong Oh [2,*] and Jongheon Shin [1,*]

1. Natural Products Research Institute, College of Pharmacy, Seoul National University, San 56-1, Sillim, Gwanak, Seoul 151-742, Korea; yahyah7@snu.ac.kr (J.-Y.H.); sungchulpark@snu.ac.kr (S.C.P.); sky_magic@naver.com (W.S.B.); dongchanoh@snu.ac.kr (D.-C.O.); sklee61@snu.ac.kr (S.K.L.)
2. Department of Agricultural Biotechnology, College of Agriculture and Life Science, Seoul National University, San 56-1, Sillim, Gwanak, Seoul 151-921, Korea
* Correspondence: ohkibong@snu.ac.kr (K.-B.O.); shinj@snu.ac.kr (J.S.); Tel.: +82-2-880-4646 (K.-B.O.); +82-2-880-2484 (J.S.)

Received: 22 July 2020; Accepted: 19 August 2020; Published: 21 August 2020

Abstract: Three new bianthraquinones, alterporriol Z1–Z3 (**1**–**3**), along with three known compounds of the same structural class, were isolated from the culture broth of a marine-derived *Stemphylium* sp. fungus. Based upon the results of spectroscopic analyses and ECD measurements, the structures of new compounds were determined to be the 6-6'- (**1** and **2**) and 1-5'- (**3**) C–C connected *pseudo*-dimeric anthraquinones, respectively. Three new meroterpenoids, tricycloalterfurenes E–G (**7**–**9**), isolated together with the bianthraquinones from the same fungal culture broth, were structurally elucidated by combined spectroscopic methods. The relative and absolute configurations of these meroterpenoids were determined by modified Mosher's, phenylglycine methyl ester (PGME), and computational methods. The bianthraquinones significantly inhibited nitric oxide (NO) production and suppressed inducible nitric oxide synthase (iNOS) and cyclooxygenase-2 (COX-2) expression in LPS-stimulated RAW 264.7 cells.

Keywords: bianthraquinones; meroterpenoids; marine-derived fungus; anti-inflammatory activity; *Stemphylium* sp.

1. Introduction

Polyketides are a representative class of fungal metabolites [1,2]. These compounds possess a vast range of structural diversity resulting in several subgroups such as anthraquinones, naphthoquinones, benzophenones, xanthones, flavonoids, macrolides, and tropolones [3,4]. Among these, anthraquinones are biosynthetically derived from an octaketide chain formed by the incorporation of one acetyl-CoA and seven malonyl-CoA units [5–7]. Although widely distributed in fungi, anthraquinone derivatives occur far frequently in the genera of *Alternaria*, *Aspergillus*, *Fusarium*, *Stemphylium*, and *Trichoderma* [8]. Anthraquinones typically contain various substituents (methyl, hydroxyl, methoxyl, or more complex substituents), often attributed to characteristic colors by their properties and positions at the aromatic core moiety [9,10].

A frequently encountered structural variation of fungal anthraquinones is the dimerization through a C–C bond formation between two similar units [3]. The dimerization patterns for these bianthraquinones are also diversified through both homo- and hetero- bond formation, providing additional structural variation to the anthraquinones. To date, a vast number of fungal examples were reported including alterporriols, icterinoidin, rubellin, and skyrin [3,11]. In addition to their monomeric precursors, bianthraquinones often co-occur with biosynthetically related compounds of the polyketide pathway [4,12]. Wide structural diversity, in conjunction with significant bioactivities such as antibacterial, anti-inflammatory, antituberculosis, and cytotoxic activities, designates bianthraquinones as an important group of fungal polyketides [3,8,11,13].

Meanwhile, tricycloalternarenes (TCAs) are a structural class of fungal meroterpenoids [14]. Structurally, these are closely related to the ACTG toxins with differences at the isoprenoid side chain and the substitution pattern at the C-ring of TCAs [15]. Biosynthetically, these meroterpenoids are proposed to be generated from a hybrid shikimate–isoprenoid route [16]. Exclusively found in *Alternaria* and *Guignardia*, tricycloalternarene-type meroterpenoids are regarded as one of the key chemical characteristics of these fungal genera [17,18]. These compounds were also reported to exhibit diverse bioactivities, including antimicrobial, cytotoxic, and NF-κB-inhibitory [19,20].

During the course of a search for bioactive compounds from marine-derived fungi, we isolated a strain (strain number FJJ006) of *Stemphylium* sp. from an unidentified sponge specimen collected off the coast of the island of Jeju-do, Korea. LC-ESIMS and LC-UV analyses of the culture broth of this strain showed the presence of several compounds with various profiles, prompting extensive chemical investigation. The large-scale cultivation, sequentially followed by extraction, solvent-partitioning, and chromatographic separations, afforded six new and three known compounds (Figure 1). Here, we report the structures of bianthraquinone alterporriols Z1–Z3 (**1**–**3**) and meroterpenoid tricycloalterfurenes E–G (**7**–**9**). This is first time isolating not only the tricycloalternarene-type meroterpenoids but also their co-occurrence with polyketide-derived anthracenes from the fungus *Stemphylium*. Compounds **1** and **2** exhibited moderate anti-inflammatory activity in LPS-stimulated RAW 264.7 cells.

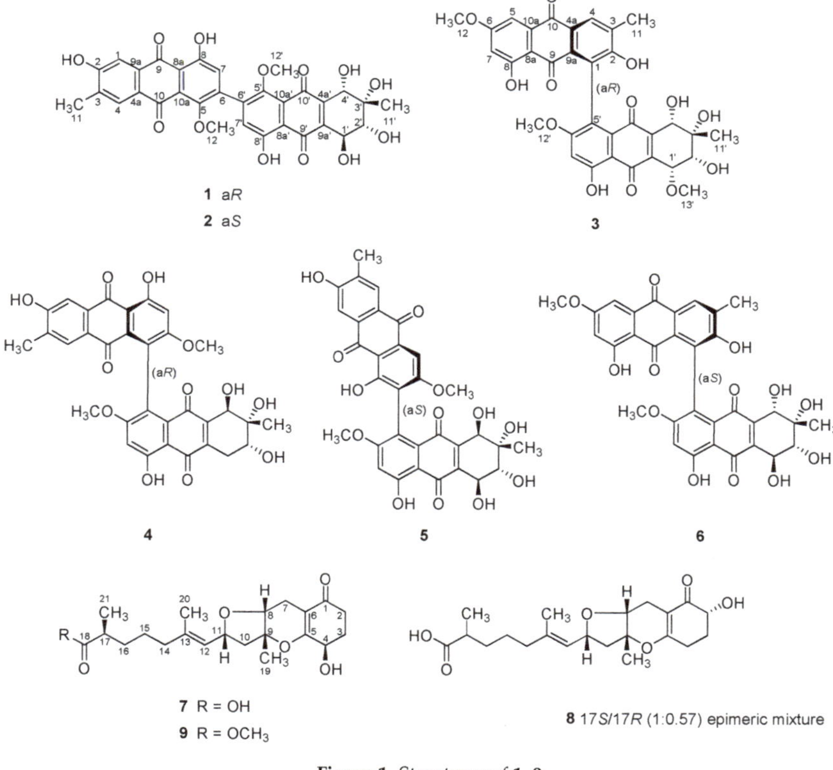

Figure 1. Structures of **1**–**9**.

2. Results and Discussion

Compound **1** was an orange amorphous powder which was analyzed to have the molecular formula of $C_{32}H_{26}O_{13}$, with 20 unsaturation degrees, by HRFABMS analysis ([M + H]$^+$ m/z 619.1449, calcd $C_{32}H_{27}O_{13}$, 619.1446). The ^{13}C NMR data of this compound showed signals of four carbonyl (δ_C 190.5, 188.7, 185.7, 183.5) and twenty deshielded methine and quaternary carbons (δ_C 166.9–104.6). Aided by the HSQC data, the chemical shifts of corresponding methine protons at δ_H 7.65, 7.51, 6.81, and 6.78 in the ^{1}H NMR data revealed the presence of aromatic moieties (Table 1). Since these NMR features were accounted for 14 unsaturation degrees, **1** must be a hexacyclic compound.

Table 1. ^{13}C and ^{1}H NMR data of compounds **1–3** in CD$_3$OD.

No.	1 [a]		2 [b]		3 [c]	
	δ_C, Type	δ_H (J in Hz)	δ_C, Type	δ_H (J in Hz)	δ_C, Type	δ_H (J in Hz)
1	111.7, CH	7.51, d (0.5)	111.8, CH	7.51, d (0.5)	129.0, C	
2	164.0, C		163.7, C		165.5, C [d]	
3	133.8, C		133.8, C		134.5, C	
4	131.2, CH	7.65, d (0.5)	131.3, CH	7.65, d (0.5)	130.5, CH	8.00, s
4a	126.8, C		127.1, C		131.2, C	
5	165.8, C		166.2, C		106.9, CH	7.20, d (2.5)
6	125.3, C		125.7, C		167.1, C	
7	104.6, CH	6.78, s	104.3, CH	6.80, s	105.9, CH	6.52, d (2.5)
8	166.9, C		167.1, C		166.0, C	
8a	111.9, C		111.7, C		112.1, C	
9	188.7, C		188.6, C		191.0, C	
9a	134.7, C		134.6, C		132.8, C	
10	183.5, C		183.5, C		182.3, C	
10a	133.4, C		132.8, C		137.8, C	
11	16.6, CH$_3$	2.23, s	16.6, CH$_3$	2.23, s	17.9, CH$_3$	2.21, s
12	56.9, CH$_3$	3.69, s	56.9, CH$_3$	3.70, s	56.3, CH$_3$	3.89, s
1'	70.6, CH	4.73, d (7.5)	70.6, CH	4.73, d (7.4)	75.2, CH	4.58, d (4.7)
2'	75.2, CH	3.79, d (7.5)	75.2, CH	3.76, d (7.4)	70.7, CH	3.93, d (4.7)
3'	74.6, C		74.7, C		75.4, C	
4'	70.1, CH	4.26, s	70.2, CH	4.26, s	70.6, CH	4.39, s
4a'	143.8, C		143.9, C		144.7, C	
5'	166.3, C		166.5, C		130.7, C	
6'	123.4, C		123.9, C		166.8, C	
7'	104.6, CH	6.81, s	104.6, CH	6.82, s	104.5, CH	6.79, s
8'	166.1, C		166.4, C		165.9, C	
8a'	111.0, C		111.0, C		110.9, C	
9'	190.5, C		190.6, C		189.6, C	
9a'	143.9, C		143.7, C		141.0, C	
10'	185.7, C		185.5, C		185.7, C	
10a'	130.8, C		130.7, C		n.d. [e]	
11'	22.3, CH$_3$	1.33, s	22.3, CH$_3$	1.32, s	21.6, CH$_3$	1.33, s
12'	57.0, CH$_3$	3.70, s	57.0, CH$_3$	3.71, s	56.8, CH$_3$	3.71, s
13'					62.8, CH$_3$	3.77, s

[a–c] Measured at 150/600, 100/400, and 200/800 MHz for ^{13}C/^{1}H NMR, respectively. [d] Assigned by HMBC data. [e] Not detected.

A combination of ^{13}C and ^{1}H NMR and HSQC data diagnosed the remaining NMR signals as an oxy-quaternary carbon (δ_C 74.6) and three oxymethine (δ_C/δ_H 75.2/3.79, 70.6/4.73, and 70.1/4.26), two oxymethyl (δ_C/δ_H 57.0/3.70 and 56.9/3.69), and two methyl (δ_C/δ_H 22.3/1.33 and 16.6/2.23) groups. Aided by the literature study, the overall spectroscopic features suggested **1** to be a bianthraquinone consisting of each one unit of anthraquinone and tetrahydroanthraquinone.

Having the information above, the structure determination of **1** was mostly accomplished by extensive H–C long-range analyses for this proton-deficient compound (Figure 2). Firstly, long-range correlations of two aromatic protons at δ_H 7.51 (H-1) and 7.65 (H-4) and a benzylic methyl proton at δ_H 2.23 (H$_3$-11) with neighboring carbons not only constructed a 2-hydroxy-3-methylbenzene moiety (C-1-C-4, C-4a, and C-9a) but also placed two carbonyls at δ_C 188.7 (C-9) and 183.5 (C-10) *ortho*-substituted to the benzene. Similarly, combined HMBC and LR-HSQMBC correlations of the protons at δ_H 6.78 (H-7) and 3.69 (H$_3$-12) with neighboring carbons revealed the presence of an 8-hydroxy-5-methoxybenzene moiety (C-5-C-8, C-8a, and C-10a). The linkage between C-8a and C-9 was also secured by crucial H-7/C-9 correlation. Although it was not evidenced by HMBC data, the carbon chemical shifts of C-10 (δ_C 183.5) and C-10a (δ_C 133.4), in conjunction with the MS-derived unsaturation degree, directly linked these carbons, thus, constructing an anthraquinone moiety for **1**.

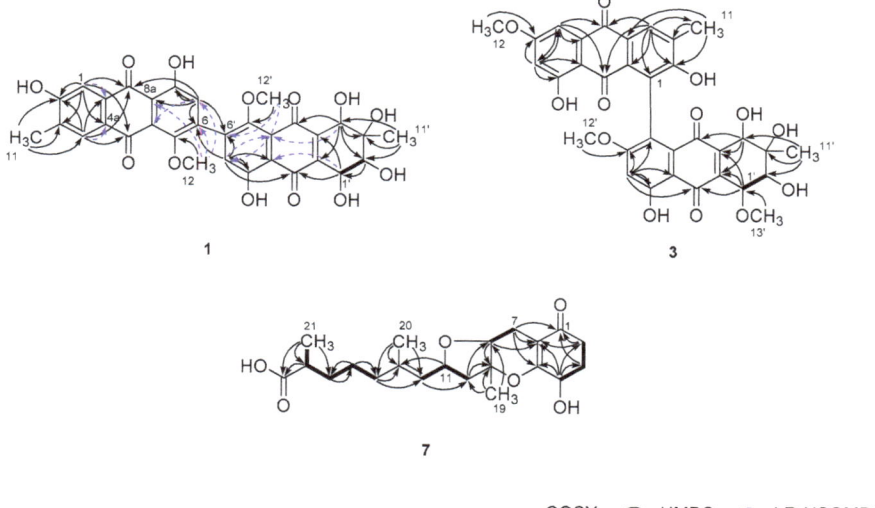

Figure 2. Key correlations of COSY (bold), HMBC (arrow), and LR-HSQMBC (J_{CH} = 2 Hz, dashed arrow) experiments for compounds **1**, **3**, and **4**.

Meanwhile, ^{1}H–^{1}H COSY data showed direct spin coupling (*J* = 7.5 Hz) between oxymethine protons at δ_H 4.73 (H-1′) and 3.79 (H-2′) (Figure 2). Subsequently, HMBC correlations of these protons and an isolated oxymethine and a methyl proton at δ_H 4.26 (H-4′) and 1.33 (H-11′), respectively, with the olefinic and hydroxyl-bearing carbons, defined a 3-methyl-2,3,4,5-tetrahydroxy cyclohexene-type moiety (C-1′–C-4′, C-4a′, and C-9a′). The attachment of two carbonyl carbons at δ_C 190.5 (C-9′) and 185.7 (C-10′) at the cyclohexene unit was also accomplished by their HMBC correlations with H-4′ and H-1′, respectively.

The HMBC correlations of an aromatic and a methoxy proton at δ_H 6.81 (H-7′) and 3.70 (H$_3$-12′), respectively, with aromatic carbons, revealed an 8′-hydroxy-5′-methoxybenzene (C-5′–C-8′, C-8a′, and C-10a′), analogous to the C-5–C-10a unit. Subsequently, further connection to the diketo-bearing cyclohexene unit constructing a tetrahydroanthraquinone moiety was also accomplished by the HMBC and LR-HSQMBC correlations between these. Since the anthraquinone and tetrahydroanthraquinone moieties had open ends at C-6 and C-6′, respectively, C–C linkage between these carbons was anticipated. The crucial evidence was provided by the HMBC data, in which long-range correlations were found at H-7/C-6′ and H-7′/C-6. Thus, the planar structure of **1** was determined as a bianthraquinone analogous to alterporriols [3]. Although significant numbers of bianthraquinones were reported from diverse fungi, those having a 6-6′ C–C linkage are rather rare. To the best of our knowledge, alterporriol K–M are the only previous examples having the same type of C–C linkage [21].

The structure of **1**, designated as alterporriol Z1, possessed four stereogenic centers at C-1′–C-4′ at the aliphatic ring and a chiral axis at C-6/C-6′, requiring configurational determination. Firstly, relative configurations at the aliphatic ring were assigned by proton–proton coupling constants and NOESY analyses (Figure 3). The large coupling (J = 7.5 Hz) between H-1′ and H-2′ oriented both protons axial to the cyclohexene ring that was supported by the NOESY cross peak at H-2′/1′-OH. Then, the neighboring 11′-CH$_3$ group was equatorially oriented by the cross peak H-2′/H$_3$-11′. Although both H-4′ and 4′-OH protons showed spatial proximity with H$_3$-11′, the NOESY cross peak at H-2′/H-4′ was crucial to the axial orientation of H-4′ (Supplementary Materials, Figure S9 and Table S2). Thus, the overall relative configurations were assigned as 1′S^*, 2′R^*, 3′S^*, and 4′S^*. The absolute configurations at these centers were approached by computational methods and are described later.

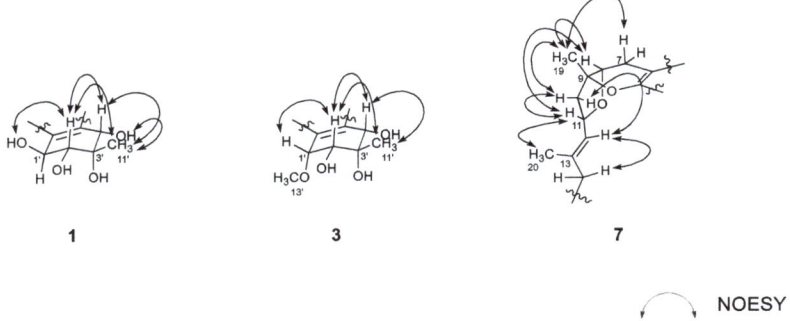

Figure 3. Key correlations of NOESY (arrow) experiments for compounds **1**, **3**, and **7**.

The configuration at the C-6/C-6′ chiral axis was assigned by ECD measurements. As shown in Figure 4, the measured ECD profile of **1** showed significant Cotton effects at 269 (Δε 35.79) and 285 (Δε −36.06) nm, assigning an aR configuration at the C-6/C-6′ axis. Although this interpretation was supported by the same configuration at structurally related alterporriols A and L [21,22], a question would arise from the possible contribution of ECD by the C-1′–C-4′ stereogenic centers. That is, the absolute configurations at these centers would remarkably influence overall ECD profiles. Conversely, depending on the results, it would be also possible to deduce the absolute configurations of stereogenic centers at the cyclohexene moiety. To clarify this, ECD data were calculated for the aR atropisomeric contribution with two possible absolute configurations at the stereogenic centers. The results were that these profiles were very similar to each other at both wavelengths and intensity of Cotton effects, regardless of the configurations at the cyclohexene moiety (Figure 5). Thus, the aR configuration was unambiguously assigned for the chiral axis.

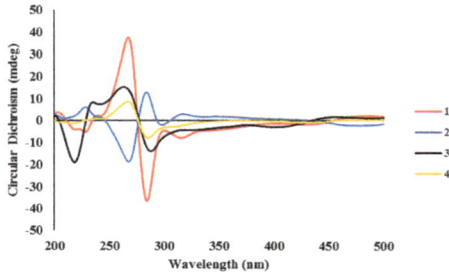

Figure 4. Experimental ECD spectra of compounds **1–4**.

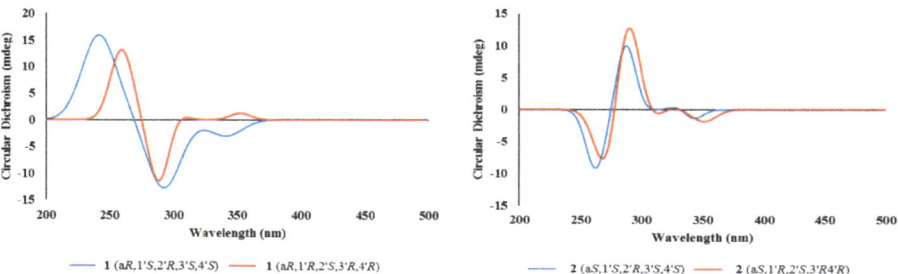

Figure 5. Calculated ECD spectra of compounds **1** and **2**.

Having fixed axial chirality, the absolute configurations at C-1'–C-4' were subsequently approached by DP4 calculations. However, two models derived from the opposite configurations expected very similar ^{13}C and ^{1}H NMR data from each other (Supplementary Materials, Figure S52 and Table S1), which was consistent with the results of ECD analysis. Thus, the absolute configurations of the cyclohexene moiety remained unassigned [23]. Overall, the structure of alterporriol Z1 (**1**) was determined to be a bianthraquinone of the alterporriol class.

The molecular formula of alterporriol Z2 (**2**) was established to be $C_{32}H_{26}O_{13}$, identical to **1**, by HRFABMS analysis ([M + H]$^+$ m/z 619.1454, calcd for $C_{32}H_{27}O_{13}$, 619.1446). A comparison of the ^{13}C and ^{1}H NMR data of this compound with those of **1** revealed a very close structural similarity between them (Table 1). Subsequently, the extensive 1D and 2D NMR analyses of **2** deduced the same planar structure and relative configurations of the aliphatic ring as those of 1. Accordingly, the structural difference was traced to the chiral axis at C-6–C-6', in which the measured ECD spectrum of **2** showed a quasi-mirror profile from **1** (Figure 4). The noticeably reduced intensities of Cotton effects would be attributed from the stereogenic center-bearing cyclohexene moiety. However, the calculated ECD data of **2** were virtually identical to each other, regardless of absolute configurations at the cyclohexene stereogenic centers, eradicating the possibility of the reversal of measured ECD by these factors (Figure 5). Thus, the structure of alterporriol Z2 (**2**) was defined as an atropisomer of alterporriol Z1 (**1**).

A minor constituent of alterporriol Z3 (**3**) was isolated as a dark red amorphous solid that was analyzed for the molecular formula of $C_{33}H_{28}O_{13}$ by HRFABMS analysis ([M + Na]$^+$ m/z 655.1430, calcd for $C_{33}H_{28}O_{13}Na$, 655.1422). The ^{13}C and ^{1}H NMR data of this compound were similar to those of **1** and **2**, indicating the same bianthraquinone nature (Table 1). An extensive examination of these data, in conjunction with a literature and database search, revealed that **3** had close structural similarity with a congener alterporriol N (**6**) [23]. The most conspicuous difference in NMR data was the presence of an additional methoxy group at δ_C/δ_H 62.8/3.77 in **3**.

Given this information, the planar structure of **3** was determined by HMBC analyses. Despite the limited amount of obtained materials, almost all carbons and protons except for unprotonated C-10a' were adequately assigned by HSQC and HMBC correlations (Figure 2). In this way, **3** was defined as consisting of an anthraquinone and a tetrahydroanthraquinone moiety, as with other compounds. The newly appeared methoxy group (C-13') was also attached at C-1' by COSY correlation at H-1'/H-2' and HMBC correlation at H$_3$-13'/C-1'. Due to the lack of neighboring protons, the C–C linkage was not directly evidenced by HMBC data. However, the diagnostic chemical shifts of the unprotonated C-1 and C-5' carbons at δ_C 129.0 and 130.7, respectively, were indicative of the linkage between the anthraquinone and tetrahydroanthraquinone moiety at these carbons.

The configurations at cyclohexene and C-1/C-6' chiral axis of **3** were assigned using the same methods as in **1** and **2**. Firstly, the small coupling constants (J = 4.7 Hz) between the vicinal H-1' and H-2' indicated the orientations of these to be either axial–equatorial or equatorial–equatorial to the cyclohexene ring. Then, the NOESY data showed mutual cross peaks among H-2', H-4', and H$_3$-11', placing these at the same phase of the cyclohexene ring (Figure 3). Therefore, the former two oxymethine protons were axially oriented, while the C-11' methyl group was equatorially oriented to the ring system. Aided with the additional cross peak with H-2', the H-1' oxymethine proton was also equatorially oriented. Thus, the overall relative configurations were assigned as 1'R^*, 2'R^*, 3'S^*, and 4'S^*. The absolute configuration of the C-1/C-6' chiral axis of **3** was also assigned by ECD measurement. As shown in Figure 4, the ECD data of this compound were similar to **1**, assigning the same aR configuration. Thus, the structure of alteroporriol Z3 (**3**) was defined as a new bianthraquinone of the alterporriol class.

In addition to **1**–**3**, the crude extract of *Stemphylium* sp. contained three known bianthraquinones (**4**–**6**). Based upon the results of combined spectroscopic analyses, these were identified as alterporriols F (**4**) [24], G (**5**) [25], and N (**6**) [23], respectively. The spectroscopic data of these compounds were in good accordance with those in the literature. Among these, the configuration of C-5/C-5' chiral axis of **4**, previously unassigned, was determined to be aR by the ECD measurement in this work (Figure 4).

In addition to bianthraquinones, the culture broth of *Stemphylium* sp. contained three new meroterpenoids. The molecular formula of compound **7**, a brown amorphous solid, was deduced to be $C_{21}H_{30}O_6$ with seven unsaturation degrees, by HRFABMS analysis ([M + H]$^+$ m/z 379.2118, calcd for $C_{21}H_{31}O_6$, 379.2115). The ^{13}C NMR data of this compound showed signals of three significantly deshielded carbons (δ_C 200.4, 180.9, and 170.4) and three olefinic carbons (δ_C 139.7, 127.5, and 107.5). The odd numbers of the latter carbons were indicative of a highly differentiated double bond possibly consisting of a deshielded carbon (δ_C 170.4) and a shielded carbon (δ_C 107.5). Between two carbonyl carbons, the conspicuous one (δ_C 200.4) was readily assigned as a ketone, while the other one (δ_C 180.9) was thought to be either a carboxylic acid or an ester group by a strong absorption band at 1755 cm^{-1} in the IR data. Aided by the ^{1}H NMR and HSQC data, the remaining 15 carbons in the ^{13}C NMR data were diagnosed to be one oxy-quaternary (δ_C 85.8), three oxymethine (δ_C 78.1, 74.5, and 66.8), one methine (δ_C 40.8), seven methylene (δ_C 46.8, 40.2, 34.5, 33.6, 30.5, 26.3, and 19.8), and three methyl (δ_C 20.1, 17.7, and 16.4) carbons (Table 2). Overall, preliminary examination of the spectroscopic data suggested **7** to be a tricyclic compound possessing two carbonyl groups and two double bonds.

Table 2. ^{13}C and ^1H NMR Data of compounds **7–9** in CD$_3$OD.

No.	7 [a]		8 [a]		9 [b]	
	δ_C, type	δ_H (J in Hz)	δ_C, type	δ_H (J in Hz)	δ_C, type	δ_H (J in Hz)
1	200.4, C		199.9, C		200.4, C	
2	33.6, CH$_2$	2.62, m 2.32, ddd (16.9, 6.9, 4.9)	72.4, CH	4.07, dd (12.6, 4.9)	33.6, CH$_2$	2.62, m 2.32, ddd (17.0, 6.8, 5.1)
3	30.5, CH$_2$	2.18, m 1.97, m	30.7, CH$_2$	2.24, m 1.83, m	30.5, CH$_2$	2.19, m 1.97, m
4	66.8, CH	4.30, t (5.1)	28.8, CH$_2$	2.58, m 2.44, m	66.8, CH	4.29, t (5.3)
5	170.4, C		170.8, C		170.4, C	
6	107.5, C		105.6, C		107.5, C	
7	19.8, CH$_2$	2.59, d (17.8) 2.22, dd (17.7, 4.2)	19.8, CH$_2$	2.68, d (17.8) 2.20, dd (17.7, 4.2)	19.8, CH$_2$	2.59, d (17.8) 2.22, dd (17.7, 4.2)
8	78.1, CH	3.95, dd (4.3, 1.2)	77.9, CH	3.95, dd (4.3, 1.2)	78.1, CH	3.95, dd (4.5, 1.3)
9	85.8, C		85.7, C		85.8, C	
10	46.8, CH$_2$	2.42, dd (13.6, 9.4) 2.07, dd (13.6, 3.9)	46.9, CH$_2$	2.39, m 2.00, dd (13.7, 3.7)	46.8, CH$_2$	2.42, dd (13.7, 9.5) 2.07, dd (13.6, 3.9)
11	74.5, CH	4.80, td (9.0, 3.9)	74.5, CH	4.80, td (9.0, 3.9)	74.4, CH	4.79, m
12	127.5, CH	5.17, br d (8.8)	127.5, CH	5.17, br d (8.8)	127.7, CH	5.17, br d (8.5)
13	139.7, C		139.7, C		139.6, C	
14	40.2, CH$_2$	1.99, m	40.3, CH$_2$	1.98, m	40.1, CH$_2$	1.98, m
15	26.3, CH$_2$	1.42, m	26.5, CH$_2$	1.42, m	26.1, CH$_2$	1.39, m
16	34.5, CH$_2$	1.59, m 1.38, m	34.9, CH$_2$	1.58, m 1.35, m	34.4, CH$_2$	1.58, m 1.38, m
17	40.8, CH	2.37, dq (13.8, 7.0)	41.6, CH	2.37, m	40.5, CH	2.46, m
18	180.9, C		182.1, C		178.9, C	
19	20.1, CH$_3$	1.35, s	19.9, CH$_3$	1.30, s	20.1, CH$_3$	1.35, s
20	16.4, CH$_3$	1.65, s	16.4, CH$_3$	1.64, s	16.3, CH$_3$	1.65, s
21	17.7, CH$_3$	1.11, d (7.0)	18.0, CH$_3$	1.11, d (7.0)	17.5, CH$_3$	1.11, d (7.0)
22					52.1, OCH$_3$	3.65, s

[a], [b] Measured at 100/800 and 100/500 MHz for $^{13}C/^1H$, respectively.

The planar structure of **7** was determined by combined ^1H–^1H COSY and HMBC analyses (Figure 2). That is, COSY data revealed a linear assembly of an oxymethine and two methylene groups (δ_C/δ_H 33.6/2.62 and 2.32, 30.5/2.18 and 1.97, and 66.8/4.30, C-2–C-4). Then, the HMBC correlations of these protons with neighboring carbons not only placed a ketone (δ_C 200.4, C-1) and a tetra-substituted double bond (δ_C 170.4 and 107.5, C-6 and C-5) at the adjacent locations, but also constructed a 4-oxygenated cyclohexanone moiety (C-1–C-6, ring A): H-4/C-2, C-3, C-5, and C-6, H$_2$-3/C-1, and H$_2$-2/C-1 and C-6. The COSY data also found a direct linkage between methylene and oxymethine (δ_C/δ_H 19.8/2.59 and 2.22 and 78.1/3.95, C-7 and C-8). Subsequently, their attachment at C-6 of ring A was secured by the HMBC of H$_2$-7 with ring carbons: H$_2$-7/C-1, C-5, and C-6. Similarly, a quaternary carbon (δ_C 85.8, C-9) and a methyl group (δ_C/δ_H 20.1/1.35, C-19) were linearly connected at C-8 by a number of key HMBC correlations: H-8/C-9 and H$_3$-19/C-8 and C-9.

The COSY data revealed the presence of another linear spin system consisting of each one of methylene, oxymethine, and olefinic methine (δ_C/δ_H 46.8/2.42 and 2.07, 74.5/4.80, and 127.5/5.17, C-10–C-12; Figure 2). The accomplishment of a full olefin (with δ_C 139.7, C-13) as well as the attachment of a vinyl methyl group (δ_C/δ_H 16.4/1.65, C-20) was made by HMBC correlations: H-11/C-13 and H$_3$-20/C-12 and C-13. The linkage of this moiety at the C-9 quaternary carbon was also secured by HMBC data: H$_3$-19/C-10 and H$_2$-10/C-8 and C-9.

Based on the COSY data, the remaining proton signals were found to form a linear assembly of three methylenes, a methine, and a methyl group (δ_C/δ_H 40.2/1.99 (2H); 26.3/1.42 (2H); 34.5/1.59 and 1.38, 40.8/2.37; and 17.7/1.11, C-14–C-17, and C-21). Subsequently, the attachments of this moiety at C-13 and a carbonyl group (δ_C 180.9, C-18) were secured by a series of HMBC correlations: H$_3$-20/C-14;

H$_2$-14/C-12; and C-13, H-17/C-18, and H$_3$-21/C-18. Thus, the framework of **7** was constructed as a C$_{21}$ meroterpenoid of the tricycloalterfurene class.

The 2D NMR-based structure elucidation of **7** assigned, in addition to the C-1 ketone, six oxygenated positions at C-4, C-5, C-8, C-9, C-11, and C-18, accounting for two rings inherent from the mass data. A literature study suggested cyclic ether linkages at C-5/C-9 and C-8/C-11 constructing a dihydropyran (ring B) and a tetrahydrofuran (ring C), respectively, while the remaining carbons were functionalized as the 4-hydroxy and 21-carboxylic acid group. The comparison of ^{13}C and ^{1}H NMR data of **7** were in good accordance with tricycloalterfurene A [15], supporting this interpretation. Crucial evidence was provided in the process for relative and absolute configurations and described later.

The configurations at the stereogenic centers of **7** were initially approached by NOESY data (Figure 3). The 13*E* configuration was assigned by cross peaks at H-11/H$_3$-20 and H-12/H$_2$-14 as well as the diagnostic carbon chemical shifts of C-20 (δ_C 16.4) and C-14 (δ_C 40.2). The NOESY data also placed H-7β (δ_H 2.22), H-8, H$_3$-19, H-10β (δ_H 2.42), and H-11 at one phase of the B/C ring plane by a series of cross peaks: H-7β/H$_3$-19, H-8/H$_3$-19, H-8/H-11, H$_3$-19/H-10β, and H-10β/H-11. To have these cross peaks, the B/C ring juncture must have a *cis* orientation. Overall, relative configurations at the stereogenic centers were assigned as 8*R**, 9*R**, and 11*R**.

The configurations at the remotely placed C-4 and C-17 stereogenic centers were independently assigned by modified Mosher's and phenylglycine methyl ester (PGME) methods, respectively. That is, the treatments of **7** with (*R*)- and (*S*)-α-methoxy-α-(trifluoromethyl)-phenylacetyl chloride (MTPA-Cl) produced corresponding (*S*)- and (*R*)-MTPA esters, **7-4*S*** and **7-4*R***, respectively. The resulting Δδ ($\delta_S - \delta_R$) values between these esters assigned the 4*R* absolute configuration (Figure 6). Similarly, **7** was also converted to (*S*)- and (*R*)-PGME amides, **7-18*S*** and **7-18*R*** by treatments with (*S*)- and (*R*)-PGME, respectively. Subsequently, the Δδ ($\delta_S - \delta_R$) values between the amides clearly assigned the 17*S* configuration (Figure 7). As described earlier, the productions of 4-esters and 17-amides by these reactions unambiguously confirmed the presence of 4-hydroxy and 18-carboxylic acid groups.

Figure 6. Δδ values [Δδ = $\delta_S - \delta_R$] obtained for (*S*)- and (*R*)-MTPA esters of **7** and **8**.

Figure 7. Δδ values [Δδ = $\delta_S - \delta_R$] obtained for (*S*)- and (*R*)-PGME amide derivatives of **7** and **8**.

Finally, given the absolute configurations at the remote stereogenic centers, those at rings B and C were determined by computational methods. As shown in Figure 7, the measured ECD profile of **7** matched well with the calculated one, with 8*R*, 9*R*, and 11*R* configurations in both wavelength and intensity of the absorption maximum at 258 nm. Overall, the absolute configurations of **7** were determined to be 4*R*, 8*R*, 9*R*, 11*R*, and 17*S* by combined NOESY, chemical derivatization, and computational methods. Thus, the structure of **7**, designated as tricycloalterfurene E, was determined to be a tricyclic meroterpenoid.

The molecular formula of compound **8** was deduced to be $C_{21}H_{30}O_6$, identical to **7**, by HRFABMS analysis ([M + H]$^+$ m/z 379.2120, calcd for $C_{21}H_{31}O_6$, 379.2115). The spectroscopic data of this compound were also very similar to those of **7**, suggesting the same tricyclic meroterpenoid nature. However, detailed examination of its ^{13}C and ^{1}H NMR and HSQC data revealed noticeable differences in the signals of carbons and protons at the hydroxyl-bearing cyclohexanone moiety (ring A) (Table 2). Although ^{1}H-^{1}H COSY data showed the presence of the same linear assembly of a hydroxyl-methine and two methylene protons as **7**, the HMBC data revealed grossly different proton–carbon correlations. That is, the C-1 ketone (δ_C 199.9) was correlated with hydroxyl-methine (δ_H 4.07) and methylene (δ_H 2.24 and 1.83) protons. The latter methylene protons were additionally correlated to the C-6 (δ_C 105.6) and C-5 (δ_C 170.8) olefinic carbons. Therefore, **8** was structurally defined to be a regioisomer of **7** bearing a hydroxyl group at C-2.

The relative and absolute configurations of **8** were pursued stepwise as for **7**. First, the NOESY data of this compound showed identical proton–proton spatial proximities to **7**, revealing the same relative configurations at rings B and C. Then, the absolute configuration at C-2 was also assigned as *R* by modified Mosher's method (Figure 6). Strikingly, however, the ^{1}H NMR spectra of PGME-amides of **8** from treatments with (*S*)- and (*R*)-PGME were virtually identical to each other and consisted of pairing proton signals. A detailed examination indeed revealed that **5** was a mixture of two 17-epimers with a ratio of 1:0.57. Based upon the proton intensity, the PGME analysis also concluded the 17*S* and 17*R* configuration for the major and minor constituents, respectively. The analytical and spectroscopic behaviors of **8** as not an epimeric mixture but a single compound would be attributed from the far remote location of C-17 from other stereogenic centers. Having this, the absolute configurations of **8** were also assigned by ECD measurements. As shown in Figure 8, the measured ECD profile of **8** was very similar to that of **7**, defining the same absolute configurations for the ring portion between these compounds. This interpretation was firmly supported by the calculated ECD data of **8** with fixed absolute configurations and epimeric ratio (1:0.57), which were almost identical to the measured one. Thus, the structure of **8**, designated as tricycloalterfurene F, was determined to be an epimeric mixture of tricyclic meroterpene carboxylic acids.

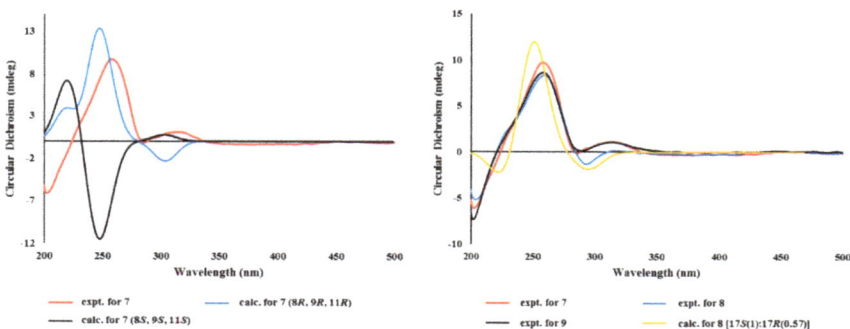

Figure 8. Experimental and calculated ECD spectra of compounds **7–9**.

The molecular formula of tricycloalterfurene G (**9**) was established as $C_{22}H_{32}O_6$ by HRFABMS analysis ([M + Na]$^+$ m/z 415.2104, calcd for $C_{22}H_{32}O_6Na$, 415.2091). The ^{13}C and ^{1}H NMR data of this compound were very similar to those of **7**, with appearance of a methoxy group (δ_C/δ_H 52.1/3.65) as the most noticeable difference (Table 2). This methyl group was placed at the C-18 carboxylic group by combined 2D NMR data, including crucial HMBC correlation between the methoxy proton and carboxylic carbon (δ_C 178.9). After deducing the same NOESY-based relative configurations as **7**, the experimental ECD profiles of **9** were also very similar to those of **7**, assigning the same absolute configurations between these (Figure 8). Thus, the structure of tricycloalterfurene G (**9**) was defined to be an ester derivative of tricycloalterfurene E (**7**).

The obtained bianthraquinones (**1–6**) and meroterpenoids (**7–9**) were assayed for their cytotoxicity. However, all of these were inactive (IC_{50} » 20 µM) against a number of human cancer cell-lines: A549 (lung cancer), HCT116 (colon cancer), MDA-MB-231 (breast cancer), PC3 (prostate cancer), SK-Hep1 (liver cancer), and SNU638 (stomach cancer). In addition, these compounds were inactive (MIC > 128 µg/mL) against diverse human pathogenic bacterial strains *Enterococcus faecalis* (ATCC19433), *Enterococcus faecium* (ATCC19434), *Klebsiella pneumoniae* (ATCC10031), *Proteus hauseri* (NBRC3851), *Salmonella enterica* (ATCC14028), and *Staphylococcus arueus* (ATCC6538p). These compounds were also inactive (IC_{50} > 145 µM) against microbial key enzymes sortase A (SrtA) and isocitrate lyase (ICL).

In our further assay using bianthraquinones, the anti-inflammatory activities were indirectly evaluated by ability to suppress lipopolysaccharide (LPS)-induced nitric oxide (NO) production in RAW 264.7 mouse macrophages. As shown in Figure 9, compounds **1**, **2**, and **4–6** showed moderate anti-inflammatory activity with IC_{50} values of 11.6 ± 0.7, 16.1 ± 1.1, 9.6 ± 1.6, 8.4 ± 0.4, and 10.7 ± 0.6 µM, respectively, while 3 was inactive. No measurable cytotoxicity was observed against mouse macrophages at these concentrations (Supplementary Materials, Figure S55). To further elucidate the inhibitory mechanism on NO production, the effect of compounds on the protein expression levels of iNOS and COX-2, the key inflammatory mediators, was evaluated. As shown in Figure 10, protein levels of iNOS and COX-2 in RAW 264.7 cells incubated with LPS for 18 h increased in comparison to quiescent cells, but this was significantly down-regulated by treatment of the compounds (20 µM) 30 min prior to LPS exposure. These findings showed that the bianthraquinones would be potential candidates for the anti-inflammatory related study.

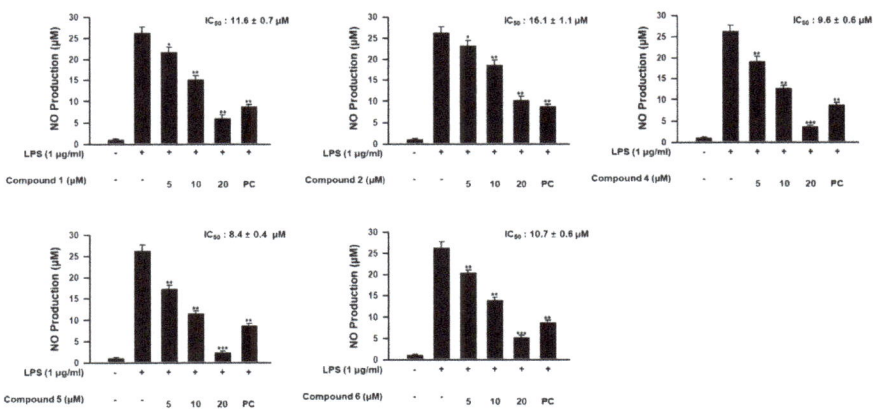

Figure 9. Concentration-dependent effect of **1**, **2**, and **4–6** on lipopolysaccharide (LPS)-stimulated NO production in RAW 264.7 cells. * $p < 0.05$, ** $p < 0.01$, and *** $p < 0.001$ indicate significant differences relative to the vehicle-treated control group.

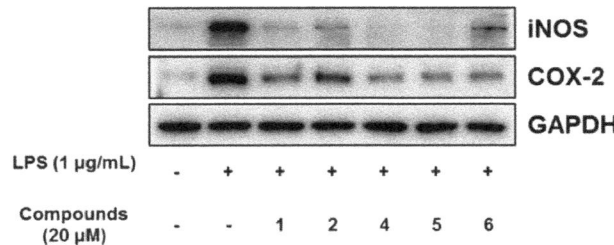

Figure 10. Effect of compounds **1**, **2**, and **4**–**6** on LPS-induced protein expressions of iNOS and COX-2 in RAW 264.7 cells. The cells were treated with 20 μM of compounds for 30 min prior to LPS (1 μg/mL) treatment and incubated for 18 h. Protein expression levels were determined by Western blotting analysis. Glyceraldehyde-3-phosphate dehydrogenase (GAPDH) was used as the internal standard.

3. Materials and Methods

3.1. General Experimental Procedures

Optical rotations were measured on a JASCO P1020 polarimeter (Jasco, Tokyo, Japan) using a 1 cm cell. UV spectra were acquired with a Hitachi U-3010 spectrophotometer (Hitachi High-Technologies, Tokyo, Japan). ECD spectra were recorded on an Applied Photophysics Chirascan plus CD spectrometer. IR spectra were recorded on a JASCO 4200 FT-IR spectrometer (Jasco, Tokyo, Japan) using a ZnSe cell. ^{1}H and ^{13}C NMR spectra were measured in CD$_3$OD and THF-d_8 solutions on Bruker Avance -500, -800 instruments (Billerica, MA, USA) and JEOL -400, -600 instruments (Peabody, MA, USA). High resolution FAB mass spectrometric data were obtained at the Korea Basic Science Institute (Daegu, Korea), and were acquired using a JEOL JMS 700 mass spectrometer (Jeol, Tokyo, Japan) with *meta*-nitrobenzyl alcohol (NBA) as the matrix. Semi-preparative HPLC separations were performed on a Spectrasystem p2000 equipped with a Spectrasystem RI-150 refractive index detector. All solvents used were spectroscopic grade or distilled from glass prior to use.

3.2. Fungal Material

The fungal strain *Stemphylium* sp. (strain number FJJ006) was isolated from an unidentified sponge collected using SCUBA at a depth of 30 m off the coast of Jeju-do (Island), Korea, on 29 September 2014. The sponge specimen was macerated and diluted using sterile seawater. One milliliter of the diluted sample was processed utilizing the spread plate method in YPG agar media (5 g of yeast extract, 5 g of peptone, 10 g of glucose, 0.15 g of penicillin G, 0.15 g of streptomycin sulfate, 24.8 g of Instant Ocean, and 16 g of agar in 1 L of distilled water) plates. The plates were incubated at 28 °C for 5 days. The strain was identified using standard molecular biology protocols by DNA amplification and sequencing of the ITS region. Genomic DNA extraction was performed using Intron's i-genomic BYF DNA Extraction Mini Kit according to the manufacturer's protocol. The nucleotide sequence of FJJ006 was deposited in the GenBank database under accession number KU519425. The 18S rDNA sequence of this strain exhibited 99% identity (577/579) with that of *Stemphylium* sp. PNYZ13070801 (GenBank accession number KJ481209).

3.3. Fermentation

The fungal strain was cultured on a solid YPG medium (5 g of yeast extract, 5 g of peptone, 10 g of glucose, 24.8 g of Instant Ocean, and 16 g of agar in 1 L of distilled water) for 7 days. An agar plug (1 × 1 cm) was inoculated for 7 days in a 250 mL flask that contained 100 mL of YPG medium. Then, 10 mL of each culture was transferred to a 2.8 L Fernbach flask containing semi-solid rice medium (200 g of rice, 0.5 g of yeast extract, 0.5 g of peptone, and 12.4 g of Instant Ocean in 500 mL of distilled water). In total, 2000 g of rice media were prepared and cultivated for 35 days at 28 °C, agitating once every week.

3.4. Extraction and Isolation

The entire culture was macerated and extracted with MeOH (1 L × 3 for each flask). The solvent was evaporated in vacuo to afford a brown organic extract (5.8 g). The extract was separated by C_{18} reversed-phase vacuum flash chromatography using sequential mixtures of H_2O and MeOH (seven fractions of H_2O-MeOH, gradient from 60:40 to 0:100), acetone, and finally, EtOAc as the eluents. Based on the results of ^1H NMR analysis, the fractions eluted with H_2O-MeOH 50:50 (550 mg), 40:60 (300 mg), and 20:80 (670 mg) were chosen for further separation. The fraction that eluted with H_2O-MeOH (50:50) was separated by semi-preparative reversed-phase HPLC (YMC-ODS-A column, 250 × 10 mm, 5 µm; gradient from H_2O-MeCN (90:10) to (50:50), 1.8 mL/min), to yield compound 9 (t_R = 52.6 min). The H_2O-MeOH (40:60) fraction from vacuum flash chromatography was separated by semi-preparative reversed-phase HPLC (H_2O-MeCN, (80:20) to (30:70), 2.0 mL/min) to afford, in the order of elution, compounds 1 (t_R = 44.8 min), 2 (t_R = 45.4 min), 4 (t_R = 50.8 min), 6 (t_R = 51.4 min), 7 (t_R = 59.4 min), and 8 (t_R = 61.3 min). The H_2O-MeOH (20:80) fraction from vacuum flash chromatography was separated by semi-preparative reversed-phase HPLC (H_2O-MeCN, (65:35) to (25:75), 2.0 mL/min), affording compounds 3 (t_R = 51.2 min) and 5 (t_R = 40.6 min). The overall isolated amounts of 1–9 were 7.0, 3.0, 0.7, 3.0, 3.2, 3.2, 6.5, 8.2, and 2.8 mg, respectively.

Alterporriol Z1 (1): orange amorphous solid, $[\alpha]_{25}^{D}$ +1.8 (c 0.10, MeOH); UV (MeOH) λ_{max} (log ε) 223 (3.97), 275 (3.86), 430 (3.36) nm; ECD (c 1.62 × 10^{-4} M, MeOH) λ_{max} (Δε), 220 (−4.02), 229 (−5.06), 269 (35.79), 285 (−36.06), 317 (−7.91) nm; IR (ZnSe) v_{max} 3544, 2970, 1622, 1593, 1372 cm^{-1}; ^1H and ^{13}C NMR data, see Table 1; HRFABMS m/z 619.1449 [M + H]$^+$ (calcd for $C_{32}H_{27}O_{13}$, 619.1446).

Alterporriol Z2 (2): orange amorphous solid, $[\alpha]_{25}^{D}$ −2.5 (c 0.10, MeOH); UV (MeOH) λ_{max} (log ε) 227 (3.79), 274 (3.68), 432 (3.09) nm; ECD (c 1.62 × 10^{-4} M, MeOH) λ_{max} (Δε), 228 (6.18), 267 (−18.63), 284 (12.77), 317 (3.02) nm; IR (ZnSe) v_{max} 3412, 2973, 2938, 1638, 1580, 1397, 1293 cm^{-1}; ^1H and ^{13}C NMR data, see Table 1; HRFABMS m/z 619.1454 [M + H]$^+$ (calcd for $C_{32}H_{27}O_{13}$, 619.1446).

Alterporriol Z3 (3): dark red amorphous solid, $[\alpha]_{25}^{D}$ +13.5 (c 0.20, MeOH); UV (MeOH) λ_{max} (log ε) 212 (3.83), 278 (3.70), 420 (3.27) nm; ECD (c 1.58 × 10^{-4} M, MeOH) λ_{max} (Δε), 218 (−18.94), 235 (8.44), 263 (15.31), 287 (−13.9) nm; IR (ZnSe) v_{max} 3416, 3120, 2973, 2931, 1638, 1605, 1322 cm^{-1}; ^1H and ^{13}C NMR data, see Table 1; HRFABMS m/z 655.1430 [M + Na]$^+$ (calcd for $C_{33}H_{28}O_{13}Na$, 655.1422).

Tricycloalterfurene E (7): brown amorphous solid, $[\alpha]_{25}^{D}$ +88.2 (c 0.20, MeOH); UV (MeOH) λ_{max} (log ε) 220 (3.53), 262 (3.48) nm; ECD (c 2.65 × 10^{-4} M, MeOH) λ_{max} (Δε), 258 (9.73), 313 (1.06) nm; IR (ZnSe) v_{max} 3546, 3347, 2930, 2854, 1748, 1610, 1538, 1371 cm^{-1}; ^1H and ^{13}C NMR data, see Table 2; HRFABMS m/z 379.2118 [M + H]$^+$ (calcd for $C_{21}H_{31}O_6$, 379.2115).

Tricycloalterfurene F (8): brown amorphous solid, $[\alpha]_{25}^{D}$ +74.0 (c 0.20, MeOH); UV (MeOH) λ_{max} (log ε) 225 (3.42), 258 (3.35) nm; ECD (c 2.65 × 10^{-4} M, MeOH) λ_{max} (Δε), 259 (8.39), 315 (0.17) nm; IR (ZnSe) v_{max} 3593, 3350, 2928, 2860, 1757, 1674, 1617, 1514, 1221 cm^{-1}; ^1H and ^{13}C NMR data, see Table 2; HRFABMS m/z 379.2120 [M + H]$^+$ (calcd for $C_{21}H_{31}O_6$, 379.2115).

Tricycloalterfurene G (9): brown amorphous solid, $[\alpha]_{25}^{D}$ +58.4 (c 0.20, MeOH); UV (MeOH) λ_{max} (log ε) 211 (3.49) nm; ECD (c 2.55 × 10^{-4} M, MeOH) λ_{max} (Δε), 258 (8.67), 315 (1.07) nm; IR (ZnSe) v_{max} 3603, 3356, 2933, 2860, 1742, 1602, 1536, 1371 cm^{-1}; ^1H and ^{13}C NMR data, see Table 2; HRFABMS m/z 415.2104 [M + Na]$^+$ (calcd for $C_{22}H_{32}O_6Na$, 415.2091).

3.5. Preparations of the (S)- and (R)-MTPA Esters of Compounds 7 and 8

To a solution of compound 7 (0.6 mg, 1 µM) in dry pyridine (500 µL), (S)-MTPA chloride (10 µL, 5.2 µM) and DMAP (0.5 mg) were successively added. After stirring for 3 h at 40 °C under N_2, the reaction mixture was concentrated under reduced pressure, and the residue was purified by reversed-phase HPLC (YMC-ODS column, 4.6 × 250 mm; H$_2$O-MeCN, 73:27) to give 7-4R (0.3 mg), the (R)-MTPA ester of 7. Compound 7-4S (0.3 mg), the (S)-MTPA ester of 7, was prepared from (R)-MTPA chloride in a similar fashion. Compounds 8-2S and 8-2R (0.3 mg each), the (S)- and (R)-MTPA esters of 5, respectively, were also prepared using this method.

3.5.1. (S)-MTPA Ester of 7 (7-4S)

White amorphous solid; ^{1}H NMR (CD$_3$OD, 800 MHz) δ_H 7.574–7.566 (2H, m, MTPA-Ar), 7.457–7.435 (3H, m, MTPA-Ar), 5.864 (1H, dd, J = 6.5, 5.0 Hz, H-4), 5.227 (1H, dq, J = 8.7, 1.1 Hz, H-12), 4.789 (1H, td, J = 9.1, 3.8 Hz, H-11), 3.903 (1H, dd, J = 4.6, 1.5 Hz, H-8), 3.633 (3H, s, H-22), 3.574 (3H, s, MTPA-OMe), 2.591 (1H, d, J = 18.2 Hz, H-7α), 2.512 (1H, dd, J = 8.2, 5.2 Hz, H-2α), 2.488 (1H, m, H-2β), 2.474 (1H, m, H-3α), 2.371 (1H, m, H-17), 2.346 (1H, m, H-10α), 2.238 (1H, m, H-3β), 2.192 (1H, ddd, J = 18.1, 4.5, 1.0 Hz, H-7β), 2.022 (2H, m, H-14), 1.945 (1H, dd, J = 13.7, 3.7 Hz, H-10β), 1.654 (3H, d, J = 1.1 Hz, H-20), 1.612 (1H, m, H-16α), 1.428 (2H, m, H-15), 1.411 (1H, m, H-16β), 1.122 (3H, d, J = 7.0 Hz, H-21), 1.015 (3H, s, H-19); LRESIMS m/z 609.2 [M + H]$^+$.

3.5.2. (R)-MTPA Ester of 7 (7-4R)

White amorphous solid; ^{1}H NMR (CD$_3$OD, 800 MHz) δ_H 7.575–7.567 (2H, m, MTPA-Ar), 7.459–7.431 (3H, m, MTPA-Ar), 5.804 (1H, t, J = 4.9 Hz, H-4), 5.231 (1H, dq, J = 8.7, 1.0 Hz, H-12), 4.819 (1H, m, H-11), 3.979 (1H, dd, J = 4.5, 1.4 Hz, H-8), 3.633 (3H, s, H-22), 3.579 (3H, s, MTPA-OMe), 2.619 (1H, d, J = 18.3 Hz, H-7α), 2.463 (1H, m, H-17), 2.443 (1H, m, H-10α), 2.371 (1H, dd, J = 6.2, 5.0 Hz, H-2α), 2.343 (1H, dd, J = 8.9, 4.9 Hz, H-2β), 2.300 (1H, m, H-3α), 2.253 (1H, dd, J = 18.6, 4.3 Hz, H-7β), 2.149 (1H, m, H-3β), 2.029 (1H, dd, J = 13.7, 3.9 Hz, H-10β), 2.003 (2H, m, H-14), 1.654 (3H, d, J = 1.0 Hz, H-20), 1.603 (1H, m, H-16α), 1.414 (2H, m, H-15), 1.402 (1H, m, H-16β), 1.295 (3H, s, H-19), 1.109 (3H, d, J = 7.0 Hz, H-21); LRESIMS m/z 609.2 [M + H]$^+$.

3.5.3. (S)-MTPA Ester of 8 (8-2S)

White amorphous solid; ^{1}H NMR (CD$_3$OD, 800 MHz) δ_H 7.680–7.668 (2H, m, MTPA-Ar), 7.428–7.416 (3H, m, MTPA-Ar), 5.581 (1H, dd, J = 13.1, 5.3 Hz, H-2), 5.149 (1H, dq, J = 8.6, 1.1 Hz, H-12), 4.798 (1H, td, J = 9.0, 3.9 Hz, H-11), 3.966 (1H, dd, J = 4.6, 1.3 Hz, H-8), 3.615 (3H, s, H-22), 3.551 (3H, s, MTPA-OMe), 2.742 (1H, t, J = 14.8 Hz, H-4α), 2.655 (1H, dd, J = 17.8, 1.1 Hz, H-7α), 2.526 (1H, dd, J = 17.2, 4.1 Hz, H-4β), 2.441 (1H, m, H-17), 2.413 (1H, m, H-10α), 2.316 (1H, m, H-3α), 2.232 (1H, m, H-7β), 2.209 (1H, m, H-3β), 2.023 (1H, dd, J = 13.7, 3.9 Hz, H-10β), 1.971 (2H, m, H-14), 1.636 (3H, s, H-20), 1.571 (1H, m, H-16α), 1.381 (2H, m, H-15), 1.372 (1H, m, H-16β), 1.339 (3H, s, H-19), 1.095 (3H, d, J = 7.0 Hz, H-21); LRESIMS m/z 609.2 [M + H]$^+$.

3.5.4. (R)-MTPA Ester of 8 (8-2R)

White amorphous solid; ^{1}H NMR (CD$_3$OD, 800 MHz) δ_H 7.671–7.659 (2H, m, MTPA-Ar), 7.422–7.408 (3H, m, MTPA-Ar), 5.611 (1H, dd, J = 12.8, 5.3 Hz, H-2), 5.133 (1H, br d, J = 8.6 Hz, H-12), 4.800 (1H, td, J = 9.0, 3.9 Hz, H-11), 3.973 (1H, d, J = 4.5 Hz, H-8), 3.655 (3H, s, MTPA-OMe), 3.603 (3H, s, H-22), 2.705 (1H, m, H-4α), 2.682 (1H, dd, J = 17.9, 1.2 Hz, H-7α), 2.480 (1H, d, J = 17.2 Hz, H-4β), 2.428 (1H, m, H-17), 2.409 (1H, m, H-10α), 2.243 (1H, m, H-7β), 2.165 (1H, m, H-3α), 2.067 (1H, dd, J = 12.4, 5.3 Hz, H-3β), 2.017 (1H, dd, J = 13.7, 3.9 Hz, H-10β), 1.956 (2H, m, H-14), 1.634 (3H, s, H-20), 1.555 (1H, m, H-16α), 1.368 (2H, m, H-15), 1.359 (1H, m, H-16β), 1.340 (3H, s, H-19), 1.082 (3H, d, J = 7.0 Hz, H-21); LRESIMS m/z 609.2 [M + H]$^+$.

3.6. Preparations of the (S)- and (R)-PGME Amides of Compounds 7 and 8

To a dry DMF solution (500 µL) of compound 7 (0.6 mg, 1.6 µM) and (S)-PGME (1.4 mg, 7.4 µM), PyBOP (3.8mg, 7.4 µM), HOBT (1.0mg, 7.4 µM), and N-methylmorpholine (100 µL) were added.

After stirring the mixture for 3 h at room temp, a 5% HCl solution and EtOAc were added to the reaction mixture. The EtOAc layer was subsequently washed with saturated NaHCO$_3$ solution and brine. The organic layer was dried over anhydrous Na$_2$SO$_4$. After removing the solvent under vacuum, the residue was purified by reversed-phase HPLC (YMC-ODS column, 4.6 × 250 mm; H$_2$O-MeOH, 35:65) to give (S)-PGME amide 7-18S (0.3 mg). Compound 7-18R (0.4 mg), the (R)-PGME amide of 7, was prepared from (R)-PGME in a similar fashion. Compounds 8-18S and 8-18R (0.3 mg each), the (S)- and (R)-PGME amides of 5, respectively, were also prepared using this method.

3.6.1. (S)-PGME Amide of 7 (7-18S)

Brown amorphous solid; ^{1}H NMR (CD$_3$OD, 800 MHz) δ_H 7.371–7.329 (5H, m, PGME-Ar), 5.427 (1H, s, PGME-H-1), 5.202 (1H, dq, J = 8.6, 1.1 Hz, H-12), 4.802 (1H, td, J = 9.0, 4.1 Hz, H-11), 4.299 (1H, t, J = 5.1 Hz, H-4), 3.945 (1H, dd, J = 4.6, 1.6 Hz, H-8), 3.681 (3H, s, PGME-OMe), 2.612 (1H, m, H-2α), 2.592 (1H, d, J = 17.8 Hz H-7α), 2.456 (1H, m, H-17), 2.419 (1H, dd, J = 13.7, 9.4 Hz, H-10α), 2.309 (1H, ddd, J = 16.9, 6.9, 4.8 Hz, H-2β), 2.230 (1H, dd, J = 18.0, 4.6 Hz, H-7β), 2.169 (1H, m, H-3α), 2.090 (1H, dd, J = 13.7, 4.1 Hz, H-10β), 2.005 (2H, m, H-14), 1.964 (1H, m, H-3β), 1.669 (3H, d, J = 1.2 Hz, H-20), 1.589 (1H, m, H-16α), 1.454 (2H, m, H-15), 1.354 (3H, s, H-19), 1.332 (1H, m, H-16β), 1.049 (3H, d, J = 6.9 Hz, H-21); LRESIMS m/z 526.3 [M + H]$^+$.

3.6.2. (R)-PGME Amide of 7 (7-18R)

Brown amorphous solid; ^{1}H NMR (CD$_3$OD, 800 MHz) δ_H 7.361–7.318 (5 H, m, PGME-Ar), 5.466 (1H, s, PGME-H-1), 5.126 (1H, dq, J = 8.6, 1.1 Hz, H-12), 4.763 (1H, td, J = 9.1, 4.2 Hz, H-11), 4.253 (1H, t, J = 5.1 Hz, H-4), 3.933 (1H, dd, J = 4.6, 1.6 Hz, H-8), 3.697 (3H, s, PGME-OMe), 2.603 (1H, m, H-2α), 2.587 (1H, d, J = 17.6 Hz H-7α), 2.460 (1H, m, H-17), 2.393 (1H, dd, J = 13.7, 9.4 Hz, H-10α), 2.284 (1H, ddd, J = 16.9, 6.9, 4.9 Hz, H-2β), 2.224 (1H, dd, J = 18.0, 4.7 Hz, H-7β), 2.151 (1H, m, H-3α), 2.044 (1H, dd, J = 13.7, 4.1 Hz, H-10β), 1.957 (1H, m, H-3β), 1.918 (2H, m, H-14), 1.576 (3H, d, J = 1.2 Hz, H-20), 1.532 (1H, m, H-16α), 1.345 (3H, s, H-19), 1.321 (1H, m, H-16β), 1.288 (2H, m, H-15), 1.108 (3H, d, J = 6.9 Hz, H-21); LRESIMS m/z 526.3 [M + H]$^+$.

3.6.3. (S)-PGME Amide of 8 (8-18S)

Major isomer; brown amorphous solid; ^{1}H NMR (CD$_3$OD, 800 MHz) δ_H 7.373–7.331 (5H, m, PGME-Ar), 5.429 (1H, s, PGME-H-1), 5.200 (1H, br d, J = 8.4 Hz, H-12), 4.799 (1H, td, J = 9.0, 4.1 Hz, H-11), 4.067 (1H, dd, J = 12.7, 5.2 Hz, H-2), 3.944 (1H, dd, J = 4.8, 1.3 Hz, H-8), 3.683 (3H, s, PGME-OMe), 2.674 (1H, d, J = 17.8 Hz H-7α), 2.572 (1H, m, H-4α), 2.465 (1H, m, H-17), 2.446 (1H, m, H-4β), 2.396 (1H, m, H-10α), 2.238 (1H, m, H-3α), 2.207 (1H, m, H-7β), 2.026 (1H, m, H-10β), 2.007 (2H, m, H-14), 1.823 (1H, m, H-3β), 1.668 (3H, d, J = 0.9 Hz, H-20), 1.596 (1H, m, H-16α), 1.462 (2H, m, H-15), 1.341 (1H, m, H-16β), 1.308 (3H, s, H-19), 1.048 (3H, d, J = 6.8 Hz, H-21); LRESIMS m/z 526.3 [M + H]$^+$.

3.6.4. (R)-PGME Amide of 8 (8-18R)

Major isomer; brown amorphous solid; ^{1}H NMR (CD$_3$OD, 800 MHz) δ_H 7.367–7.324 (5H, m, PGME-Ar), 5.473 (1H, s, PGME-H-1), 5.111 (1H, br d, J = 8.7 Hz, H-12), 4.759 (1H, td, J = 9.0, 4.0 Hz, H-11), 4.060 (1H, dd, J = 12.4, 5.2 Hz, H-2), 3.933 (1H, dd, J = 4.8, 1.0 Hz, H-8), 3.695 (3H, s, PGME-OMe), 2.667 (1H, d, J = 18.0 Hz H-7α), 2.566 (1H, m, H-4α), 2.462 (1H, m, H-17), 2.445 (1H, m, H-4β), 2.370 (1H, m, H-10α), 2.232 (1H, m, H-3α), 2.206 (1H, m, H-7β), 1.975 (1H, m, H-10β), 1.919 (2H, m, H-14), 1.815 (1H, m, H-3β), 1.574 (3H, d, J = 0.5 Hz, H-20), 1.546 (1H, m, H-16α), 1.328 (1H, m, H-16β), 1.304 (2H, m, H-15), 1.300 (3H, s, H-19), 1.108 (3H, d, J = 6.8 Hz, H-21); LRESIMS m/z 526.3 [M + H]$^+$.

3.7. ECD Calculations

The ground-state geometries were optimized with density functional theory (DFT) calculations, using Turbomole with the basis set def-SVP for all atoms and the functional B3-LYP. The ground states were further confirmed by the harmonic frequency calculation. The calculated ECD data corresponding to the optimized structures were obtained with the time-dependent density-functional theory (TD-DFT) at the B3-LYP functional. The ECD spectra were simulated by overlapping Gaussian functions for each transition, where σ is the width of the band at $1/e$ height. Values ΔE_i and R_i were the excitation energies and rotatory strengths, respectively, for transition i. In the current work, the value was 0.10 eV.

$$\Delta \in (E) = \frac{1}{2.297 \times 10^{-39}} \frac{1}{\sqrt{2\pi}\sigma} \sum_i^A \Delta E_i R_i e^{[-(E-\Delta E_i)^2/(2\sigma)^2]} \tag{1}$$

3.8. DP4 Analysis

Conformational searches were performed using MacroModel software (Version 9.9, Schrödinger LLC, New York, NY, USA) interfaced in Maestro (Version 9.9, Schrödinger LLC) with a mixed torsional/low-mode sampling method. Conformers within 10 kJ/mol found in the MMFF force field were regarded and the geometry of the conformers was optimized at the B3-LYP/6-31G++ level in the gas phase. Ground state geometry optimization of each conformer was carried out by density functional theory (DFT) modeling with TurbomoleX 4.3.2 software. The basis set for the calculation was def-SVP for all atoms, and the level of theory was B3-LYP at the functional level in the gas phase. The calculated chemical shift values were averaged by the Boltzmann populations and utilized for DP4 analysis.

3.9. Cytotoxic, Antibacterial, and Enzyme-Inhibitory Activities Assays

Cytotoxicity assay was performed in accordance with the published protocols [26]. The antimicrobial and SrtA and ICL-inhibitory assays were performed according to previously described methods [27–29].

3.10. RAW 264.7 Cell Culture

A RAW 264.7 murine macrophage cell line was purchased from American Type Cell Culture (Rockville, MD, USA). Cells were cultured in DMEM with 10% fetal bovine serum and antibiotic−antimycotics (i.e., penicillin G sodium, 100 units/mL; streptomycin, 100 µg/mL; amphotericin B, 250 ng/mL) at 37 °C in a humidified incubator with 5% carbon dioxide. All reagents used for cell culture were purchased from Gibco® Invitrogen Corp. (Grand Island, NY, USA).

3.11. Nitrite Production Measurement

The concentration of nitrite in the cultured media was used as a measure of NO production. The assay was performed as previously described [30]. RAW 264.7 cells were plated at a density of 5×10^5 per well in a 24-well culture plate and incubated in a 37 °C humidified incubator with 5% CO_2 in air for 18 h. The incubated cells were pretreated with phenol-red-free medium containing various concentrations of tested compounds for 30 min, followed by 1 µg/mL of LPS treatment for 18 h more. Aliquots of the supernatant from each well (100 µL) were transferred to a 96-well plate, and nitrite concentration was measured using Griess reagent. After the Griess reaction, MTT solution (final concentration of 500 µg/mL) was added to each well and further incubated for 4 h at 37 °C. Each medium was discarded, and dimethyl sulfoxide was added to each well to dissolve generated formazan. The absorbance was measured at 570 nm, and percent survival was determined by comparison with LPS treated control group. All reagents used in the nitrite production measurement were purchased from Sigma-Aldrich (St. Louis, MO, USA).

3.12. Western Blotting Analysis

The Western blotting analysis was performed as previously described [31]. Briefly, the samples with cell lysates were boiled for 10 min at 100 °C. The concentrations of proteins in the cell lysates were quantified using the bicinchoninic acid method. Equal amounts of protein were subjected to 8%–10%

sodium dodecyl sulfate-polyacrylamide gel electrophoresis and transferred to polyvinylidene fluoride membranes (Millipore, Bedford, MA, USA) activated with 100% methanol. The membranes were blocked using 5% BSA in a mixture of Tris-buffered saline and Tween 20 (1×), and subsequently probed with the following antibodies: anti-iNOS, COX-2, and GAPDH (Cell Signaling Technology, Beverly, MA, USA). The blots were visualized using an enhanced chemiluminescence detection kit (Intron Biotechnology, Sungnam, Korea) and an ImageQuant LAS-4000 Imager (Fujifilm Corp., Tokyo, Japan).

4. Conclusions

Three new bianthraquinones, alterporriol Z1–Z3 (1–3), along with three known compounds (4–6) of the same structural class, were isolated from the culture broth of a marine-derived *Stemphylium* sp. fungus. Based upon the results of combined spectroscopic analyses and ECD measurements, the structures of new compounds were determined to be the 6-6'- (1 and 2) and 1-5'- (3) C-C connected *pseudo*-dimeric anthraquinones, respectively. The absolute configuration of the chiral axis of 4 was also assigned similarly. In addition, three new meroterpenoids, tricycloalterfurenes E–G (7–9), isolated from the same fungal culture broth, were structurally elucidated by combined spectroscopic methods. The relative and absolute configurations of these meroterpenoids were determined by modified Mosher's, PGME, and computational methods. Although none of these compounds were active against cytotoxic and antibacterial assays, the bianthraquinones (except 3) exhibited significantly inhibited nitric oxide (NO) production and suppressed the expression of iNOS and COX-2 in LPS-stimulated RAW 264.7 cells.

Supplementary Materials: The following are available online at http://www.mdpi.com/1660-3397/18/9/436/s1. Figures S1–S45: HRFABMS, 1D and 2D NMR spectra of 1–3 and 7–9, Figures S46–S49: ^{1}H NMR spectrum of (*S*), (*R*)-MTPA Ester of 7–8, Figures S50-S53: ^{1}H NMR spectrum of (*S*), (*R*)-PGME Amide of 7–8, Figure S54: The results of DP4 probability analysis of 1, Figure S55: The viability of RAW 264.7 cells was measured using the MTT assay, Table S1: Experimental (Exp.) and calculated (Cal.) chemical shift values of enantiomers A and B on aliphatic ring part of 1, Table S2: ^{1}H NMR Data of 1 in THF-d_8.

Author Contributions: J.-Y.H. and S.C.P. carried out isolation and structural elucidation; W.S.B. and S.K.L. performed the anti-inflammatory activity bioassay; K.-B.O. performed antimicrobial and enzyme inhibition bioassays; J.S. and D.-C.O. reviewed and evaluated all data; J.S. and K.-B.O. supervised the research work and prepared the paper. All authors have read and agreed to the published version of the manuscript.

Funding: This study was supported by the National Research Foundation (NRF, grant no. 2018R1A4A1021703) funded by the Ministry of Science, ICT, & Future Planning, Korea.

Conflicts of Interest: The authors declare no conflict of interest.

References

1. Cox, R.J.; Simpson, T.J. Fungal type I polyketide synthases. *Methods Enzymol.* **2009**, *459*, 49–78. [CrossRef]
2. Cox, R.J. Polyketides, proteins and genes in fungi: Programmed nano-machines begin to reveal their secrets. *Org. Biomol. Chem.* **2007**, *5*, 2010–2026. [CrossRef]
3. Fouillaud, M.; Venkatachalam, M.; Girard-Valenciennes, E.; Caro, Y.; Dufosse, L. Anthraquinones and derivatives from marine-derived fungi: Structural diversity and selected biological activities. *Mar. Drugs* **2016**, *14*, 64. [CrossRef] [PubMed]
4. Hussain, H.; Al-Sadi, A.M.; Schulz, B.; Steinert, M.; Khan, A.; Green, I.R.; Ahmed, I. A fruitful decade for fungal polyketides from 2007 to 2016: Antimicrobial activity, chemotaxonomy and chemodiversity. *Future Med. Chem.* **2017**, *9*, 1631–1648. [CrossRef] [PubMed]
5. Stoessl, A.; Unwin, C.H.; Sthothers, J.B. On the biosynthesis of some polyketide metabolites in *Alternaria solani*: ^{13}C and ^{2}Hmr studies. *Can. J. Chem.* **1983**, *61*, 372–377. [CrossRef]
6. Bringmann, G.; Irmer, A.; Feineis, D.; Gulder, T.A.M.; Fiedler, H.-P. Convergence in the biosynthesis of acetogenic natural products from plants, fungi, and bacteria. *Phytochemistry* **2009**, *70*, 1776–1786. [CrossRef]
7. Caro, Y.; Anamale, L.; Fouillaud, M.; Laurent, P.; Petit, T.; Dufosse, L. Natural hydroxyanthraquinoid pigments as potent food grade colorants: An overview. *Nat. Prod. Bioprospect.* **2012**, *2*, 174–193. [CrossRef]

8. Ge, X.; Sun, C.; Feng, Y.; Wang, L.; Peng, J.; Che, Q.; Gu, Q.; Zhu, T.; Li, D.; Zhang, G. Anthraquinone derivatives from a marine-derived fungus *Sporendonema casei* HDN16-802. *Mar. Drugs* **2019**, *17*, 334. [CrossRef]
9. Gessler, N.N.; Egorova, A.S.; Belozerskaia, T.A. Fungal anthraquinones. *Appl. Biochem. Microbiol.* **2013**, *49*, 85–99. [CrossRef]
10. Fouillaud, M.; Caro, Y.; Venkatachalam, M.; Grondin, I.; Dufossé, L. Anthraquinones. In *Phenolic Compounds in Food Characterization and Analysis*; Nollet, L.M.L., Gutierrez-Uribe, J.A., Eds.; CRC Press: Boca Raton, FL, USA, 2018; pp. 130–170.
11. Griffiths, S.; Mesarich, C.H.; Saccomanno, B.; Vaisberg, A.; Wit, P.J.G.M.; Cox, R.; Collemare, J. Elucidation of cladofulvin biosynthesis reveals a cytochrome P450 monooxygenase required for anthraquinone dimerization. *Proc. Natl. Acad. Sci. USA* **2016**, *113*, 6851–6856. [CrossRef]
12. Bräse, S.; Encinas, A.; Keck, J.; Nising, C.F. Chemistry and biology of mycotoxins and related fungal metabolites. *Chem. Rev.* **2009**, *109*, 3903–3990. [CrossRef] [PubMed]
13. Malik, E.M.; Muller, C.E. Anthraquinones as pharmacological tools and drugs. *Med. Res. Rev.* **2016**, *36*, 705–748. [CrossRef] [PubMed]
14. Geris, R.; Simpson, T.J. Meroterpenoids produced by fungi. *Nat. Prod. Rep.* **2009**, *26*, 1063–1094. [CrossRef] [PubMed]
15. Shi, Z.Z.; Miao, F.P.; Fang, S.T.; Liu, X.H.; Yin, X.L.; Ji, N.Y. Sesteralterin and tricycloalterfurenes A–D: terpenes with rarely occurring frameworks from the marine-alga-epiphytic fungus *Alternaria alternata* k21-1. *J. Nat. Prod.* **2017**, *80*, 2524–2529. [CrossRef]
16. Zhang, G.J.; Wu, G.W.; Zhu, T.J.; Kurtán, T.; Mándi, A.; Jiao, J.J.; Li, J.; Qi, X.; Gu, Q.Q.; Li, D.H. Meroterpenoids with diverse ring systems from the sponge-associated fungus *Alternaria* sp. JJY-32. *J. Nat. Prod.* **2013**, *76*, 1946–1957. [CrossRef] [PubMed]
17. Bai, Z.Q.; Lin, X.P.; Wang, J.F.; Zhou, X.F.; Liu, J.; Yang, B.; Yang, X.W.; Liao, S.R.; Wang, L.S.; Liu, Y.H. New meroterpenoids from the endophytic fungus *Aspergillus flavipes* AIL8 derived from the mangrove plant *Acanthus ilicifolius*. *Mar. Drugs* **2015**, *13*, 237–248. [CrossRef]
18. Lou, J.; Fu, L.; Peng, Y.; Zhou, L. Metabolites from *Alternaria* fungi and their bioactivities. *Molecules* **2013**, *18*, 5891–5935. [CrossRef]
19. Shen, L.; Tian, S.-J.; Song, H.-L.; Chen, X.; Guo, H.; Wan, D.; Wang, Y.-R.; Wang, F.-W.; Liu, L.-J. Cytotoxic tricycloalternarene compounds from endophyte *Alternaria* sp. W-1 associated with *Laminaria japonica*. *Mar. Drugs* **2018**, *16*, 402. [CrossRef]
20. Zhang, H.; Zhao, Z.; Chen, J.; Bai, X.; Wang, H. Tricycloalternarene analogs from a symbiotic fungus *Aspergillus* sp. D and their antimicrobial and cytotoxic effects. *Molecules* **2018**, *23*, 855. [CrossRef]
21. Huang, C.-H.; Pan, J.-H.; Chen, B.; Yu, M.; Huang, H.-B.; Zhu, X.; Lu, Y.-J.; She, Z.-G.; Lin, Y.-C. Three bianthraquinone derivatives from the mangrove endophytic fungus *Alternaria* sp. ZJ9-6B from the South China Sea. *Mar. Drugs* **2011**, *9*, 832–843. [CrossRef]
22. Zhou, X.-M.; Zheng, C.-J.; Chen, G.-Y.; Song, X.-P.; Han, C.-R.; Li, G.-N.; Fu, Y.-H.; Chen, W.-H.; Niu, Z.-G. Bioactive anthraquinone derivatives from the mangrove-derived fungus *Stemphylium* sp. 33231. *J. Nat. Prod.* **2014**, *77*, 2021–2028. [CrossRef] [PubMed]
23. Debbab, A.; Aly, A.H.; Edrada-Ebel, R.; Wray, V.; Pretsch, A.; Pescitelli, G.; Kurtan, T.; Proksch, P. New anthracene derivatives—Structure elucidation and antimicrobial activity. *Eur. J. Org. Chem.* **2012**, *2012*, 1351–1359. [CrossRef]
24. Phuwapraisirisan, P.; Rangsan, J.; Siripong, P.; Tip-pyang, S. New antitumour fungal metabolites from *Alternaria porri*. *Nat. Prod. Res.* **2009**, *23*, 1063–1071. [CrossRef] [PubMed]
25. Debbab, A.; Aly, A.H.; Edrada-Ebel, R.; Wray, V.; Müller, W.E.G.; Totzke, F.; Zirrgiebel, U.; Schächtele, C.; Kubbutat, M.H.G.; Lin, W.H.; et al. Bioactive metabolites from the endophytic fungus *Stemphylium globuliferum* isolated from *Mentha pulegium*. *J. Nat. Prod.* **2009**, *72*, 626–631. [CrossRef] [PubMed]
26. Kwon, O.-S.; Kim, C.-K.; Byun, W.S.; Oh, J.; Lee, Y.-J.; Lee, H.-S.; Sim, C.J.; Oh, D.-C.; Lee, S.K.; Oh, K.-B.; et al. Cyclopeptides from the Sponge *Stylissa flabelliformis*. *J. Nat. Prod.* **2018**, *81*, 1426–1434. [CrossRef]
27. Lee, H.-S.; Lee, T.-H.; Yang, S.H.; Shin, H.J.; Shin, J.; Oh, K.-B. Sesterterpene sulfates as isocitrate lyase inhibitors from tropical sponge *Hippospongia* sp. *Bioorg. Med. Chem. Lett.* **2007**, *17*, 2483–2486. [CrossRef]
28. Oh, K.-B.; Kim, S.-H.; Lee, J.; Cho, W.-J.; Lee, T.; Kim, S. Discovery of diarylacrylonitriles as a novel series of small molecule sortase A inhibitors. *J. Med. Chem.* **2004**, *47*, 2418–2421. [CrossRef]

29. Oh, K.-B.; Lee, J.H.; Chung, S.-C.; Shin, J.; Shin, H.J.; Kim, H.-K.; Lee, H.-S. Antimicrobial activities of the bromophenols from the red alga *Odonthalia corymbifera* and some synthetic derivatives. *Bioorg. Med. Chem. Lett.* **2008**, *18*, 104–108. [CrossRef]
30. Hong, S.-H.; Ban, Y.H.; Byun, W.S.; Kim, D.; Jang, Y.-J.; An, J.S.; Shin, B.; Lee, S.K.; Shin, J.; Yoon, Y.J.; et al. Camporidines A and B: antimetastatic and anti-inflammatory polyketide alkaloids from a gut bacterium of *Camponotus kiusiuensis*. *J. Nat. Prod.* **2019**, *82*, 903–910. [CrossRef]
31. Byun, W.S.; Kim, W.K.; Han, H.J.; Chung, H.-J.; Jang, K.; Kim, H.S.; Kim, S.; Kim, D.; Bae, E.S.; Park, S.; et al. Targeting histone methyltransferase DOT1L by a novel psammaplin A analog inhibits growth and metastasis of triple-negative breast cancer. *Mol. Ther. Oncolytics* **2019**, *15*, 140–152. [CrossRef]

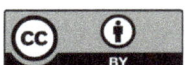

© 2020 by the authors. Licensee MDPI, Basel, Switzerland. This article is an open access article distributed under the terms and conditions of the Creative Commons Attribution (CC BY) license (http://creativecommons.org/licenses/by/4.0/).

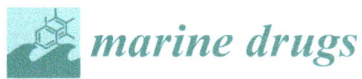

Article

Rare Chromone Derivatives from the Marine-Derived *Penicillium citrinum* with Anti-Cancer and Anti-Inflammatory Activities

Yi-Cheng Chu [1], Chun-Hao Chang [2], Hsiang-Ruei Liao [3], Ming-Jen Cheng [4], Ming-Der Wu [4], Shu-Ling Fu [1,*] and Jih-Jung Chen [5,6,*]

1. Institute of Traditional Medicine, School of Medicine, National Yang-Ming University, Taipei 112, Taiwan; xbox88888@ym.edu.tw
2. Institute of Biopharmaceutical Sciences, Pharmaceutical Sciences, National Yang-Ming University, Taipei 112, Taiwan; howard860212@ym.edu.tw
3. Graduate Institute of Natural Products, College of Medicine, Chang Gung University, Taoyuan 333, Taiwan; liaoch@mail.cgu.edu.tw
4. Bioresource Collection and Research Center (BCRC), Food Industry Research and Development Institute (FIRDI), Hsinchu 300, Taiwan; cmj@firdi.org.tw (M.-J.C.); wmd@firdi.org.tw (M.-D.W.)
5. Faculty of Pharmacy, School of Pharmaceutical Sciences, National Yang-Ming University, Taipei 112, Taiwan
6. Department of Medical Research, China Medical University Hospital, China Medical University, Taichung 404, Taiwan
* Correspondence: slfu@ym.edu.tw (S.-L.F.); chenjj@ym.edu.tw (J.-J.C.); Tel.: +886-2-2826-7177 (S.-L.F.); +886-2-2826-7195 (J.-J.C.); Fax: +886-2-2822-5044 (S.-L.F.); +886-2-2823-2940 (J.-J.C.)

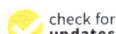

Citation: Chu, Y.-C.; Chang, C.-H.; Liao, H.-R.; Cheng, M.-J.; Wu, M.-D.; Fu, S.-L.; Chen, J.-J. Rare Chromone Derivatives from the Marine-Derived *Penicillium citrinum* with Anti-Cancer and Anti-Inflammatory Activities. *Mar. Drugs* 2021, 19, 25. https://doi.org/10.3390/md19010025

Received: 17 November 2020
Accepted: 5 January 2021
Published: 8 January 2021

Publisher's Note: MDPI stays neutral with regard to jurisdictional claims in published maps and institutional affiliations.

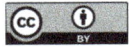

Copyright: © 2021 by the authors. Licensee MDPI, Basel, Switzerland. This article is an open access article distributed under the terms and conditions of the Creative Commons Attribution (CC BY) license (https://creativecommons.org/licenses/by/4.0/).

Abstract: Three new and rare chromone derivatives, epiremisporine C (**1**), epiremisporine D (**2**), and epiremisporine E (**3**), were isolated from marine-derived *Penicillium citrinum*, together with four known compounds, epiremisporine B (**4**), penicitrinone A (**5**), 8-hydroxy-1-methoxycarbonyl-6-methylxanthone (**6**), and isoconiochaetone C (**7**). Among the isolated compounds, compounds **2–5** significantly decreased fMLP-induced superoxide anion generation by human neutrophils, with IC_{50} values of 6.39 ± 0.40, 8.28 ± 0.29, 3.62 ± 0.61, and 2.67 ± 0.10 µM, respectively. Compounds **3** and **4** exhibited cytotoxic activities with IC_{50} values of 43.82 ± 6.33 and 32.29 ± 4.83 µM, respectively, against non-small lung cancer cell (A549), and Western blot assay confirmed that compounds **3** and **4** markedly induced apoptosis of A549 cells, through Bcl-2, Bax, and caspase 3 *signaling* cascades.

Keywords: *Penicillium citrinum*; chromone derivatives; anti-inflammatory activity; anti-cancer activity

1. Introduction

There are many natural products isolated from marine-derived fungi. These compounds are important source of biologically effective secondary metabolites, which are very interesting and important for drug discovery. In particular, a large number of natural products with biological activities are found in the genus *Penicillium*, which has diverse biological activities such as antibacterial, antifungal, antitumor, and antiviral activities [1–18]. Diverse dihydroisocoumarins [4], citrinin [15], benzopyrans [17], benzophenones [18] and their derivatives were isolated from *Penicillium citrinum* in the past studies. Many of these isolated compounds showed anti-bacterial [4,17,18], anti-fungal [15], and anti-cancer [18] activities.

Human neutrophils are known to play a critical role in the pathogenesis of various inflammatory diseases [19,20]. In response to different stimuli, activated neutrophils secrete a series of cytotoxins, such as superoxide anion ($O_2^{\bullet -}$), granule proteases, and bioactive lipids [19,21,22]. Suppression of inappropriate activation of neutrophils by drugs was proposed as a way to combat inflammatory diseases [23].

According to statistics from Taiwan's Ministry of Health and Welfare, cancer remained the top killer in Taiwan for many years [24]. The apoptosis-related proteins, such as Bcl-2,

Bax, and caspase-3, regulate cancer cell apoptosis or survival, which was confirmed to be related to many cancers and diseases [25–27]. In a preliminary screening, the methanolic extract of *P. citrinum* showed anti-inflammatory and anti-cancer activities in vitro. The current chemical investigation of this fungus led to the isolation of three new chromone derivatives, epiremisporine C (**1**), epiremisporine D (**2**), and epiremisporine E (**3**), along with four known compounds. The structural elucidation of **1–3** and anti-inflammatory and anti-cancer properties of **1–7** are described herein.

2. Results and Discussion

2.1. Fermentation, Extraction, and Isolation

In this study, the marine-derived fungal strain *Penicillium citrinum* (BCRC 09F0458) was cultured in solid-state culturing conditions, in order to enrich the diversity of the fungal secondary metabolites. Chromatographic isolation and purification of the *n*-BuOH-soluble fraction of an EtOH extract of *Penicillium citrinum* on a silica gel column and preparative thin-layer chromatography (TLC) obtained three new (**1–3**) and four known compounds (**4–7**) (Figure 1).

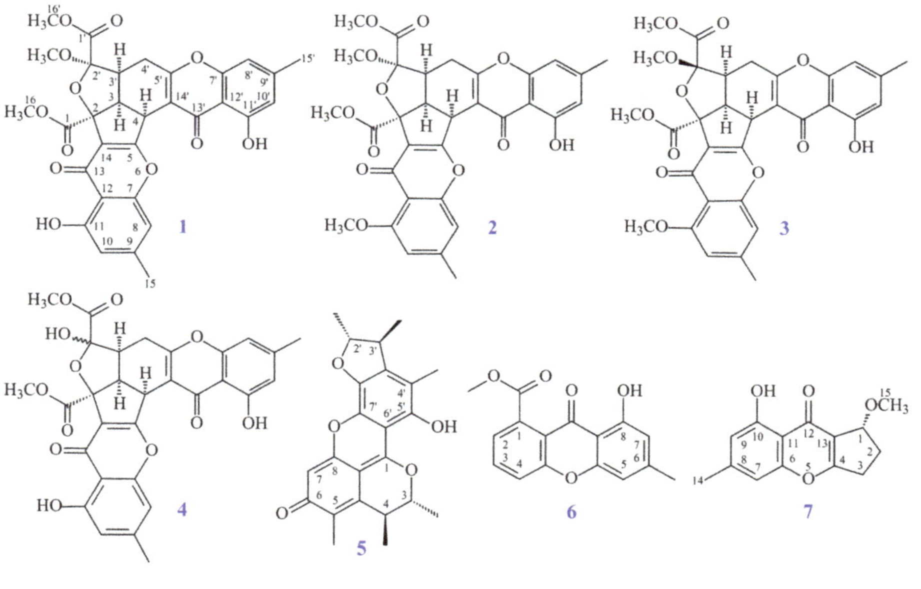

Figure 1. The chemical structures of compounds **1–7** isolated from *Penicillium citrinum*.

2.2. Structural Elucidation

Compound **1** was isolated as a yellowish amorphous powder. Its molecular formula $C_{31}H_{26}O_{12}$, was determined on the basis of the positive HR-ESI-MS ion at *m/z* 613.13200 [M + Na]$^+$ (calcd. 613.13219) and supported by the ^{1}H- and ^{13}C- NMR data. The IR spectrum showed the presence of hydroxyl (3428 cm^{-1}), ester carbonyl (1744 cm^{-1}), and conjugated carbonyl (1655 cm^{-1}) groups. The ^{1}H- and ^{13}C-NMR data of **1** showed the presence of two hydroxy groups, two methyl groups, three methoxy groups, two pairs of meta-coupling aromatic protons, two methylene protons, and three methine protons. The signals at δ 12.11 and 12.30 exhibited two chelated hydroxyl groups with the carbonyl group. Comparison of the ^{1}H and ^{13}C NMR data of **1** with those of epiremisporine B [16] suggested that their structures were closely related, except that the 2′-methoxyl group of **1** replaced the 2′-hydroxy group of epiremisporine B [16]. This was supported by both

HMBC correlations between OMe-2' (δ_H 3.50) and C-2' (δ_C 111.1) and ROESY correlations between OMe-2' (δ_H 3.50) and H-3' (δ_H 2.86). The relative configuration of **1** was elucidated on the basis of ROESY experiments. The ROESY cross-peaks between H-3/H-4, H-3/H-3', H-3/H$_\alpha$-4', OMe-2'/H-3', and H-3/H-16 suggested that H-3, H-4, H-3', OMe-2', and COOMe-2 are α-oriented, and COOMe-2' is β-oriented. To further confirm the relative configuration of **1**, a computer-assisted 3D structure was obtained by using the molecular-modeling program CS CHEM 3D Ultra 16.0, with MM2 force-field calculations for energy minimization. The calculated distances between H-3/H-4 (2.210 Å), H-3/H-3' (2.491 Å), OMe-2'/H-3' (2.305 Å), and H-3/H-16 (2.371 Å) were all less than 4 Å (Figure 2). This was consistent with the well-defined ROESY observed for each of these H-atom pairs. The absolute configuration of **1** was evidenced by the CD Cotton effects at 332.5 ($\Delta\varepsilon$ +8.81), 293.0 ($\Delta\varepsilon$ −1.23), 258.5 ($\Delta\varepsilon$ +15.60), 239.5 ($\Delta\varepsilon$ −4.12), and 206.5 ($\Delta\varepsilon$ +4.09) nm, in analogy with those of epiremisporine B [16]. The ^{1}H- and ^{13}C-NMR resonances were fully assigned by the ^{1}H–^{1}H COSY, HSQC, ROESY, and HMBC experiments (Figure 3). On the basis of the above data, the structure of **1** was elucidated, as shown in Figure 1, and named epiremisporine C.

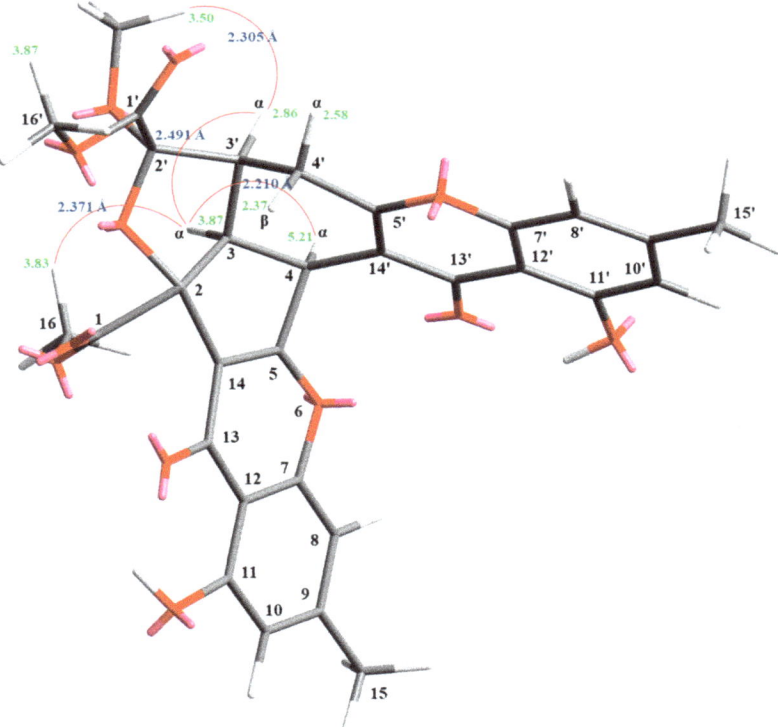

Figure 2. Selected ROESY correlations and relative configuration of **1**.

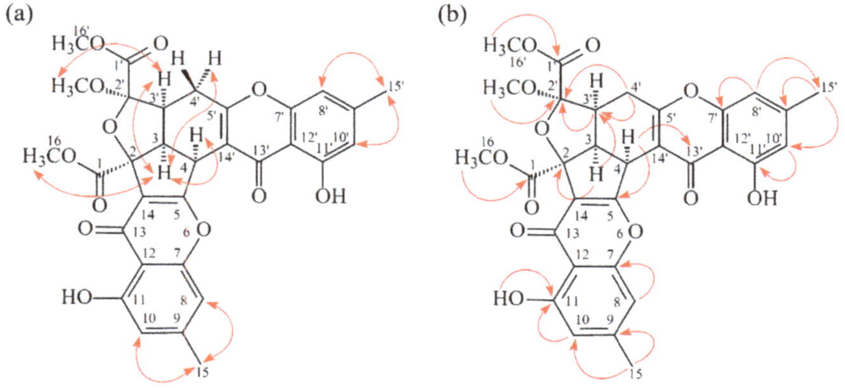

Figure 3. Key ROESY (**a**) and HMBC (**b**) correlations of **1**.

Compound **2** was obtained as an amorphous powder. The ESI–MS demonstrated the quasi-molecular ion [M + Na]$^+$ at m/z 627, implying a molecular formula of $C_{32}H_{28}O_{12}$, which was confirmed by the HR-ESI-MS (m/z 627.12902 [M + Na]$^+$, calcd. 627.14784) and by the ^{1}H- and ^{13}C-NMR data. The IR spectrum showed the presence of hydroxyl (3480 cm^{-1}), ester carbonyl (1763 cm^{-1}), and conjugated carbonyl (1657 cm^{-1}) groups. The signal at δ 12.36 exhibited a chelated hydroxyl group with the carbonyl group. Comparison of the ^{1}H and ^{13}C NMR data of **2** with those of epiremisporine C (**1**), suggested that their structures were closely related, except that the 11-methoxyl group of **2** replaced the 11-hydroxy group of **1**. This was supported by both HMBC correlations between OMe-11 (δ$_H$ 3.91) and C-11 (δ$_C$ 160.0) and ROESY correlations between OMe-11 (δ$_H$ 3.91) and H-10 (δ$_H$ 6.58). The relative configuration of **2** was elucidated on the basis of ROESY experiments. The ROESY cross-peaks between H-3/H-4, H-3/H-3′, H-3/H$_α$-4′, OMe-2′/H-3′, and H-3/H-16 suggested that H-3, H-4, H-3′, OMe-2′, and COOMe-2 were α-oriented, and COOMe-2′ was β-oriented. To further confirm the relative configuration of **2**, a computer-assisted 3D structure was obtained by using the molecular-modeling program CS CHEM 3D Ultra 16.0, with MM2 force-field calculations for energy minimization. The calculated distances between H-3/H-4 (2.200 Å), H-3/H-3′ (2.484 Å), OMe-2′/H-3′ (2.306 Å), and H-3/H-16 (2.329 Å) were all less than 4 Å (Figure 4). This was consistent with the well-defined ROESY observed for each of these H-atom pairs. Compound **2** showed similar CD Cotton effects [330.5 (Δε +5.39), 290.5 (Δε −6.24), 262.5 (Δε +19.72), 238.5 (Δε −2.06), and 207.0 (Δε +13.72) nm] compared with **1** and epiremisporine B [16]. Thus, **2** possessed a 2S,3R,2′R,3′S-configuration. On the basis of the above data, the structure of **2** was elucidated, as shown in Figure 1, and named epiremisporine D, which was further confirmed by the ^{1}H-^{1}H COSY, ROESY (Figure 5a), DEPT, HSQC, and HMBC (Figure 5b) experiments.

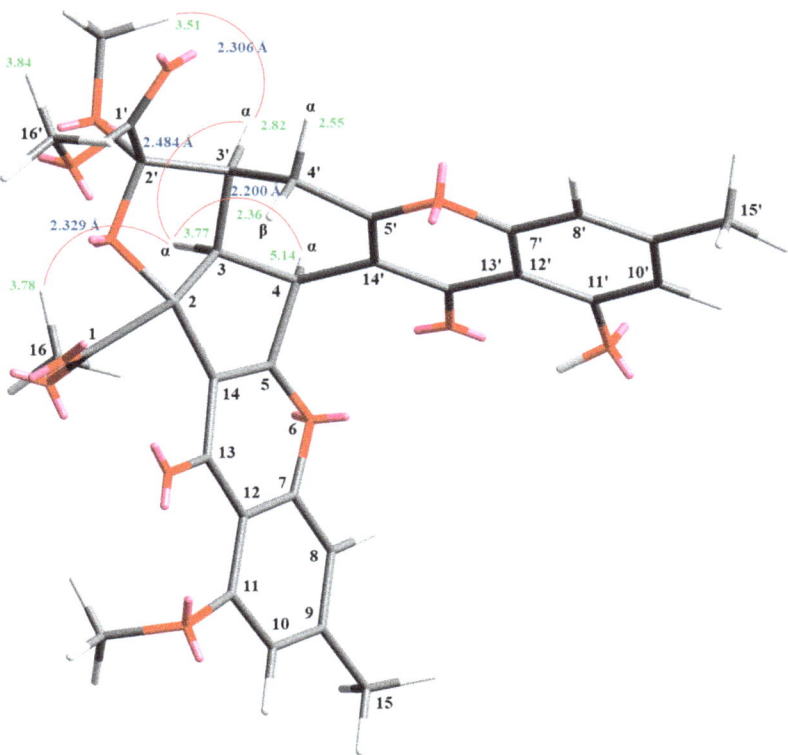

Figure 4. Selected ROESY correlations and relative configuration of **2**.

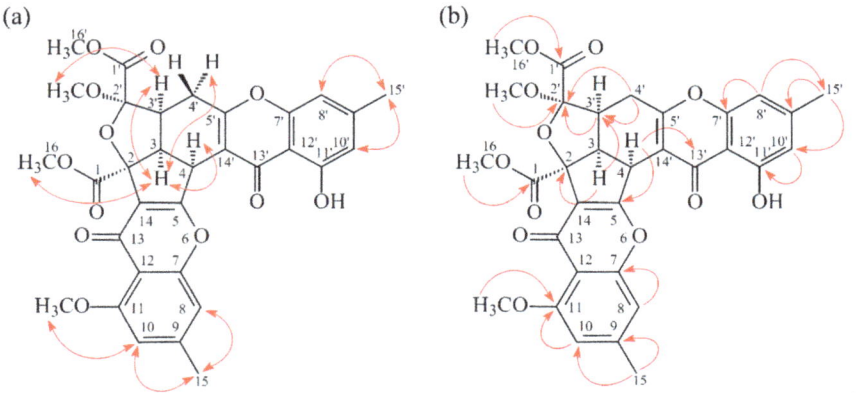

Figure 5. Key ROESY (**a**) and HMBC (**b**) correlations of **2**.

Compound **3** was isolated as an amorphous powder. The ESI–MS demonstrated the quasi-molecular ion [M + Na]$^+$ at m/z 627, implying a molecular formula of $C_{32}H_{28}O_{12}$, which was confirmed by the HR–ESI–MS (m/z 627.12919 [M + Na]$^+$, calcd. 627.14784) and by the ^{1}H- and ^{13}C-NMR data. The IR spectrum showed the presence of hydroxyl

(3466 cm^{-1}), ester carbonyl (1761 and 1740 cm^{-1}), and the conjugated carbonyl (1657 cm^{-1}) groups. The signal at δ 12.50 exhibited a chelated hydroxyl group with the carbonyl group. Comparison of the ^{1}H and ^{13}C NMR data of **3** with those of epiremisporine D (**2**) suggested that their structures were closely related, except that the 2′β-methoxyl group of **3** replaced the 2′α-methoxyl group of **2**. This was supported by both HMBC correlations between OMe-2′ ($δ_H$ 3.11) and C-2′ ($δ_C$ 107.6), and the ROESY correlations between OMe-2′ ($δ_H$ 3.11) and H$_β$-4′ ($δ_H$ 2.85). The relative configuration of **3** was elucidated on the basis of ROESY experiments. The ROESY cross-peaks between H-3/H-4, H-3/H-3′, H-3/H$_α$-4′, OMe-2′/H-4′, and H-3/H-16 suggested that H-3, H-4, H-3′, COOMe-2, and COOMe-2′ were α-oriented, and OMe-2′ was β-oriented. To further confirm the relative configuration of **3**, a computer-assisted 3D structure was obtained by using the molecular-modeling program CS CHEM 3D Ultra 16.0, with MM2 force-field calculations for energy minimization. The calculated distances between H-3/H-4 (2.169 Å), H-3/H-16 (2.285Å), H-3/H-3′ (2.445 Å), and OMe-2′/H$_β$-4′ (3.682Å) were all less than 4 Å (Figure 6). This was consistent with the well-defined ROESY observed for each of these H-atom pairs. Compound **3** showed similar CD Cotton effects [331.0 (Δε +4.01), 286.5 (Δε −7.51), 261.5 (Δε +19.77), 230.5 (Δε −4.98), and 207.5 (Δε +12.68) nm], compared to the literature data [16]. Thus, **3** possessed a 2*S*,3*R*,2′*S*,3′*S*-configuration. The ^{1}H- and ^{13}C-NMR resonances were fully assigned by ^{1}H–^{1}H COSY, ROESY (Figure 7a), HSQC, and HMBC (Figure 7b) experiments. On the basis of the above data, the structure of **3** was elucidated, as shown in Figure 1, and named epiremisporine E.

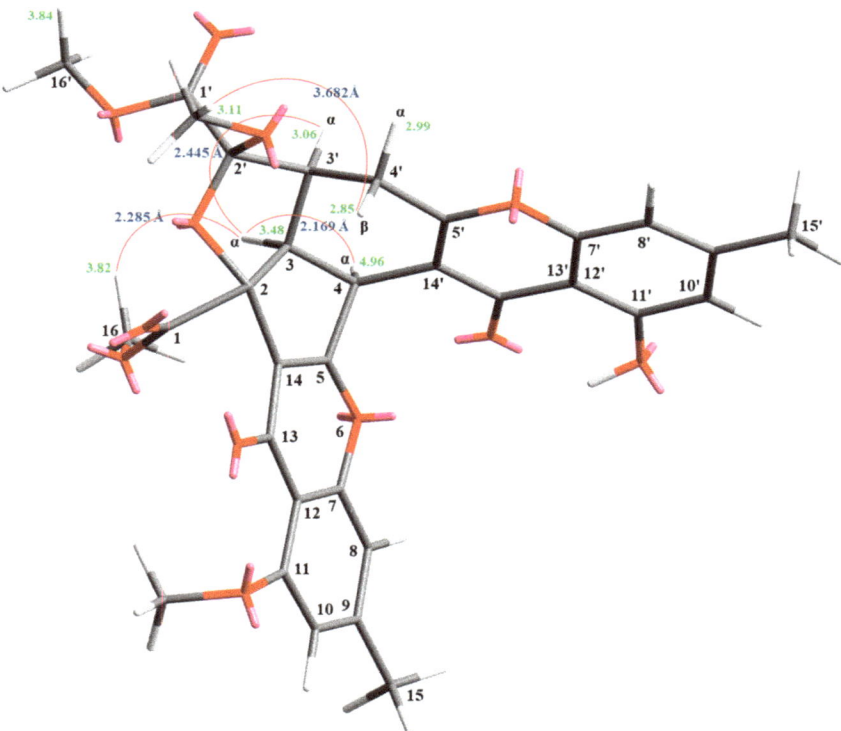

Figure 6. Selected ROESY correlations and the relative configuration of **3**.

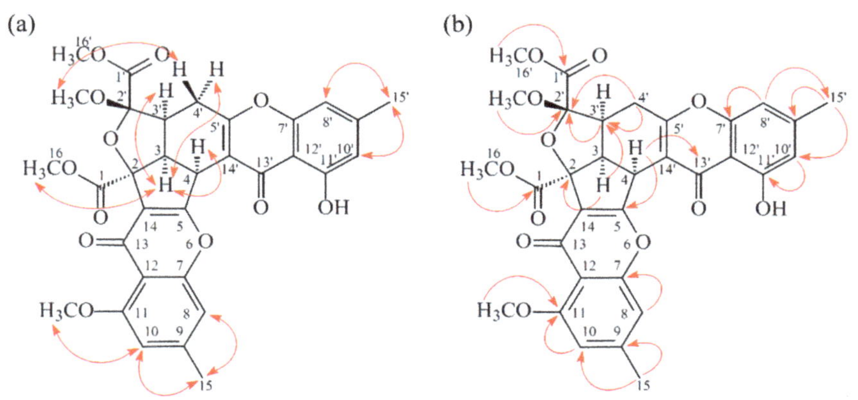

Figure 7. Key ROESY (**a**) and HMBC (**b**) correlations of **3**.

The correlations between the dihedral angles (H3'-C3'-C4'-H4'α and H3'-C3'-C4'-H4'β) and the vicinal coupling constants ($J_{3',4'\alpha}$ and $J_{3',4'\beta}$) of compounds **1–3** and related analogues [16] are summarized in Table 1. The dihedral angles were calculated by using the molecular-modeling program CS CHEM 3D Ultra 16.0, with the MM2 force-field calculations for energy minimization. The correlations between dihedral angles (H3'-C3'-C4'-H4'α and H3'-C3'-C4'-H4'β) and vicinal coupling constants ($J_{3',4'\alpha}$ and $J_{3',4'\beta}$) of compounds **1–3** were consistent with the Karplus relationship. The 2'S,3'S-configuration slightly decreased the $J_{3',4'\beta}$ value from 11.3~12.8 to 8.3~10.3 compared to the 2'R,3'S-configuration. These data could also support the structural confirmation of the new compounds **1–3**.

Table 1. The correlations between dihedral angles and vicinal coupling constants of compounds **1–3** and related analogues [16].

Compounds	Dihedral Angles (H3'-C3'-C4'-H4'α)	$J_{3',4'\alpha}$ (Hz)	Dihedral Angles (H3'-C3'-C4'-H4'β)	$J_{3',4'\beta}$ (Hz)
1 (2'R,3'S)	50.7°	5.3	169.8°	12.8
2 (2'R,3'S)	51.1°	5.4	170.2°	12.7
3 (2'S,3'S)	54.8°	4.7	173.9°	8.3
Epiremisporine B (2'R,3'S)	53.9°	5.9	173.5°	12.5
Epiremisporine B (2'S,3'S)	54.7°	6.4	173.8°	10.1
Epiremisporine B1 (2'R,3'S)	54.2°	6.6	173.8°	11.3
Epiremisporine B1 (2'S,3'S)	56.0°	6.5	175.2°	10.3
Remisporine B (2'S,3'R)	178.8°	12.2	61.0°	4.3

2.3. Structure Identification of the Known Isolated Compounds

The known isolated compounds were readily identified by a comparison of physical and spectroscopic data (UV, IR, ^{1}H-NMR, [α]$_D$, and MS) with corresponding authentic samples or literature values. They included epiremisporine B (**4**) [16] (Figures S31–S34; Tables S1 and S2), penicitrinone A (**5**) [15,28] (Figures S35 and S36), 8-hydroxy-1-methoxycarbonyl-6-methylxanthone (**6**) [10] (Figures S37 and S38), and isoconiochaetone C (**7**) [16] (Figures S39 and S40).

2.4. Biological Studies

2.4.1. Inhibitory Activities on Neutrophil Pro-Inflammatory Responses

The anti-inflammatory effects of the isolated compounds from *Penicillium citrinum* were evaluated by their ability to suppress formyl-L-methionyl-L-leucyl-L-phenylalanine (fMLP)-induced $O_2^{\bullet-}$ generation by human neutrophils. The anti-inflammatory activity data are shown in Table 2. The clinically used anti-inflammatory agent, ibuprofen, was used as the positive control. From the results of our anti-inflammatory tests, epiremisporine D (**2**), epiremisporine E (**3**), epiremisporine B (**4**), and penicitrinone A (**5**) exhibited inhibition (IC_{50} values ≤ 8.28 μM) of superoxide anion generation by human neutrophils, in response to fMLP. Thus, our study suggests *Penicillium citrinum* and its isolated compounds (especially **2**, **3**, **4**, and **5**) could be further developed as potential candidates for the treatment or prevention of various inflammatory diseases.

Table 2. Inhibitory effects of compounds **1–7** from *Penicillium citrinum* on superoxide anion generation by human neutrophils, in response to fMLP.

Compounds	IC_{50} (μM) [a]
Epiremisporine C (**1**)	>50
Epiremisporine D (**2**)	6.39 ± 0.40 [e]
Epiremisporine E (**3**)	8.28 ± 0.29 [d]
Epiremisporine B (**4**)	3.62 ± 0.61 [e]
Penicitrinone A (**5**)	2.67 ± 0.10 [e]
8-Hydroxy-1-methoxycarbonyl-6-methylxanthone (**6**)	>50
Isoconiochaetone C (**7**)	38.35 ± 0.21 [c]
Ibuprofen [b]	27.85 ± 3.56 [c]

[a] Concentration necessary for 50% inhibition (IC_{50}). [b] Ibuprofen (a fMLP receptor antagonist) was used as a positive control. Results are presented as average ± SEM ($n = 3$). Values are expressed as average ± SEM ($n = 3$). [c] $p < 0.05$; [d] $p < 0.01$; [e] $p < 0.001$ compared with the control.

2.4.2. Cytotoxic Effects and Selectivity of Compounds 1–7

In this study, the cytotoxic activities of seven compounds (**1–7**) against A549 (human lung carcinoma) and HT-29 (human colon carcinoma) cells were studied; shown in Table 3. Among the isolated compounds, compounds **3**, **4**, and **5** exhibited potent cytotoxic activities with IC_{50} values of 43.82 ± 6.33, 32.29 ± 4.83, and 49.15 ± 6.47 μM against A549 cells, respectively. In addition, compound **4** exhibited cytotoxic activities with an IC_{50} value of 50.88 ± 2.29 μM against HT-29 cells. According to the data in Table 2, compounds **3** and **5** showed selective cytotoxicity against A549 cancer cells. Among the chromone derivatives (**1–4**), epiremisporine B (**4**) (with 2′-hydroxy group) exhibited a more effective cytotoxic activity than its analogue, epiremisporines C–E (**1–3**) (without 2′-hydroxy group) against the A549 and HT-29 cells. New compound, epiremisporines E (**3**) (with 2′β-methoxyl group) exhibited a stronger anticancer activity than its analogues, epiremisporines C and D (**1** and **2**) (with 2′α-methoxyl group) against A549 cells.

Table 3. Cytotoxic effects of compounds **1–7** against A549 and HT-29 cells.

Compounds	IC$_{50}$ (μM) [a]	
	A549	HT-29
Epiremisporine C (**1**)	>100	>100
Epiremisporine D (**2**)	>100	>100
Epiremisporine E (**3**)	43.82 ± 6.33 [c]	>100
Epiremisporine B (**4**)	32.29 ± 4.83 [c]	50.88 ± 2.29 [c]
Penicitrinone A (**5**)	49.15 ± 6.47	>100
8-Hydroxy-1-methoxycarbonyl-6-methylxanthone (**6**)	>100	>100
Isoconiochaetone C (**7**)	>100	>100
5-FU [b]	12.52 ± 2.02 [d]	40.92 ± 3.93 [d]

[a] The IC$_{50}$ values were calculated from the slope of dose-response curves (SigmaPlot). Values are expressed as mean ± SEM (n = 3). [c] $p < 0.05$; [d] $p < 0.01$ compared with the control. [b] 5-Fluorouracil (5-FU) was used as a positive control.

2.4.3. New Compound 3 Inhibited Proliferation of A549 Cells

The known compounds, epiremisporine B (**4**) [16] and penicitrinone A (**5**) [28], were reported to exhibit anticancer activities in previous studies. Epiremisporine E (**3**) was selectively tested for clonogenic assay as it is a new compound and possesses cytotoxic activity against A549. The effect of compound **3** on colony formation of A549 cells was examined using the clonogenic assay (Figure 8). The A549 cell colonies were visualized as blue discs, through crystal violet staining. It was clearly observed that compound **3** (25 μM) significantly reduced the colony formation of A549 cells. Moreover, compound **3** almost completely inhibited the colony formation at 50 μM.

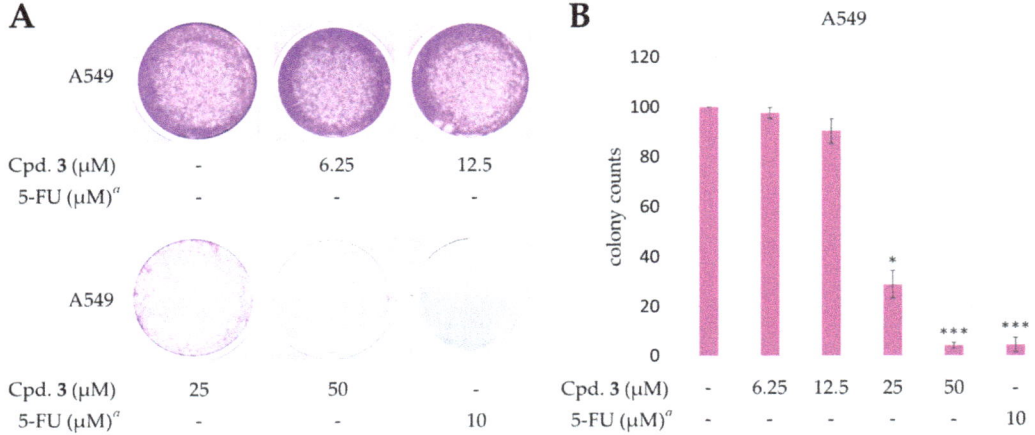

Figure 8. Effect of epiremisporine E (**3**) on the colony formation of A549 cells. (**A**) The effect of **3** against A549 cell colony formation. Clonogenicity was evaluated by the monolayer colony formation assay. Representative images show the blue colonies of A549 cells stained with crystal violet. (**B**) Histogram presentation of A549 cell colony quantification. * $p < 0.05$; *** $p < 0.001$ compared with the control. [a] 5-Fluorouracil (5-FU) was used as a positive control.

2.4.4. Effects of Epiremisporine E (3) and Epiremisporine B (4) on Protein Expressions of Pro-caspase 3 and Cleaved-caspase 3 in A549 Cells

Caspase 3 activation is a hallmark of apoptosis. Caspase 3 activation involves the cleavage of pro-caspase 3 (the inactive precursor form of caspase 3), leading to the formation of cleaved-caspase 3 (which is the active caspase 3). Upon apoptosis, the pro-caspase 3 would decrease and the cleaved-caspase 3 would increase accordingly. We further investigated whether epiremisporine E (3) and epiremisporine B (4) were able to influence these enzymatic activities of caspase 3. The results showed that compounds 3 and 4 suppressed pro-caspase 3 and increased the cleaved-caspase 3 (Figures 9 and 10). Furthermore, compounds 3 and 4 markedly induced apoptosis of A549 cells through caspase 3-dependent pathways.

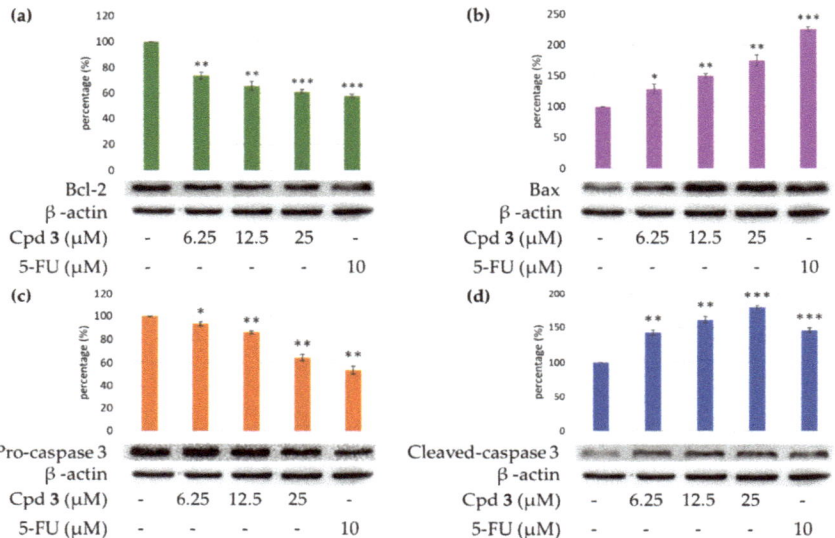

Figure 9. Western blot analysis for Bcl-2 (a), Bax (b), pro-caspase 3 (c), and cleaved-caspase 3 (d) in each group. Treatment with epiremisporine C (3) significantly reduced the expression levels of Bcl-2 and pro-caspase 3, and increased the expression levels of Bax and cleaved-caspase 3. Asterisks indicate significant differences (* $p < 0.05$, ** $p < 0.01$, and *** $p < 0.001$) compared with the control group.

2.4.5. Effects of Compounds 3 and 4 on Protein Expressions of Bax and Bcl-2 in A549 Cells

To determine whether compounds 3 and 4 could influence the expression of proteins related to A549 cells apoptosis, compounds 3 and 4 (6.25, 12.5, and 25 μM) were added to A549 cells. Figures 9 and 10 showed that the expression level of pro-apoptotic protein, bax was obviously higher with 25 μM treatment of compound 3 or 4 than with 12.5 or 6.25 μM treatment. On the contrary, the cells treated with 25 μM of compound 3 or 4 showed higher Bcl-2 (anti-apoptotic protein) expression than that treated with 12.5 or 6.25 μM. The results showed that compounds 3 and 4 suppressed the expression of Bcl-2 and increased bax expression.

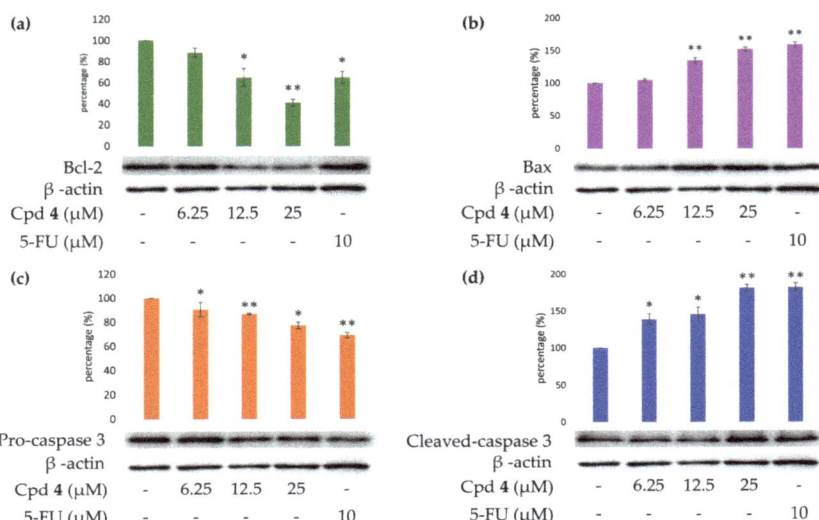

Figure 10. Western blot analysis for Bcl-2 (**a**), Bax (**b**), pro-caspase 3 (**c**), and cleaved-caspase 3 (**d**) in each group. Treatment with epiremisporine B (**4**) significantly reduced the expression levels of Bcl-2 and pro-caspase 3, and increased the expression levels of Bax and cleaved-caspase 3. As-terisks indicate significant differences (* $p < 0.05$ and ** $p < 0.01$) compared with the control group.

3. Experimental Section

3.1. General Procedures

Optical rotations were measured using a Jasco P-2000 polarimeter (Japan Spectroscopic Corporation, Tokyo, Japan) in CHCl$_3$. Circular dichroism (CD) spectra were obtained on a J-715 spectropolarimeter (Jasco, Easton, MD, USA). Ultraviolet (UV) spectra were obtained on a Hitachi U-2800 Double Beam Spectrophotometer (Hitachi High-Technologies Corporation, Tokyo, Japan). Infrared (IR) spectra (neat or KBr) were recorded on a Shimadzu IRAffinity-1S FT-IR Spectrophotometer (Shimadzu Corporation, Kyoto, Japan). Nuclear magnetic resonance (NMR) spectra, including correlation spectroscopy (COSY), rotating frame nuclear Overhauser effect spectroscopy (ROESY), heteronuclear multiple-bond correlation (HMBC), and heteronuclear single-quantum coherence (HSQC) experiments, were acquired using a BRUKER AVIII-500 or a BRUKER AVIII-600 spectrometer (Bruker, Bremen, Germany), operating at 500 or 600 MHz (^{1}H) and 125 or 150 MHz (^{13}C), respectively, with chemical shifts given in the ppm (δ), using CDCl$_3$ as an internal standard (peak at 7.263 ppm in ^{1}H NMR and 77.0 ppm in ^{13}C NMR spectrum). Electrospray ionization (ESI) and high-resolution electrospray ionization (HRESI)-mass spectra were recorded on a Bruker APEX II Mass Spectrometer (Bruker, Bremen, Germany). Silica gel [70–230 mesh (63–200 µm) and 230–400 mesh (40–63 µm), Merck] was used for column chromatography (CC). Silica gel 60 F-254 (Merck, Darmstadt, Germany) was used for thin-layer chromatography (TLC) and preparative thin-layer chromatography (PTLC).

3.2. Fungal Material

The fungal strain *Penicillium citrinum* BCRC 09F458 was isolated from waste water, which was collected from Hazailiao, Dongshi, Chiayi, Taiwan, in 2009. The fungal strain was identified as *Penicillium citrinum* (family Trichocomaceae) by the BCRC center, based on cultural and anamorphic data. The rDNA-ITS (internal transcribed spacer) region was used for further identification. After searching the GenBank database through BLAST (nucleotide sequence comparison program), it was found to have a 100% similarity to *P. citrinum*. *P. citrinum* BCRC 09F458 was stored in the Biological Resources Collection and Research Center (BCRC) of the Food Industry Research and Development Institute (FIRDI).

Cultivation and Preparation of the Fungal Strain

We kept *P. citrinum* BCRC 09F0458 on potato dextrose agar (PDA), and cultivated the strain on PDA at 25 °C for one week, and finally harvested the spores with sterile water. The spores (5×10^5) were seeded into 300 mL shake flasks containing 50 mL RGY medium (3% rice starch, 7% glycerol, 1.1% polypeptone, 3% soybean powder, 0.1% $MgSO_4$, and 0.2% $NaNO_3$), and cultivated with shaking (150 rpm) at 25 °C, for 3 days. After the mycelium enrichment step, an inoculum mixing 100 mL mycelium broth and 100 mL RGY medium was inoculated into plastic boxes (25 cm × 30 cm) containing 1.5 kg sterile rice and cultivated at 25 °C for producing rice, and the above mentioned RGY medium was added for maintaining the growth. After 21 days of cultivation, the rice was harvested, and used as a sample for further extraction.

3.3. Extraction and Isolation

The rice of the *P. citrinum* BCRC 09F0458 (1.5 kg) was extracted with 95% EtOH (3 × 10 L, 3 d each) at room temperature. The ethanol extract was concentrated under reduced pressure, and was partitioned with *n*-BuOH/H_2O (1:1, v/v) to afford *n*-BuOH soluble fraction (36.2 g), H_2O soluble fraction (13.0 g), and insoluble fraction (500 mg). The *n*-BuOH fraction (fraction A, 36.2 g) was purified by column chromatography (CC) (1.6 kg of silica gel, 70–230 mesh ((63–200 μm); *n*-hexane/EtOAc 25:1–0:1, 1500 mL) to afford 13 fractions: A1–A13. Fraction A2 (1.54 g) was subjected to medium pressure liquid chromatography (MPLC) (69 g of silica gel, 230–400 mesh (40–63 μm); *n*-hexane/acetone 1:0–0:1, 700 mL-fractions) to give 11 subfractions: A2-1–A2-11. Fraction A2-6 (126 mg) was further purified by semipreparative normal-phase high performance liquid chromatography (HPLC) (silica gel; *n*-hexane/dichloromethane/EtOAc, 6:3:1) to obtain 8-hydroxy-1-methoxycarbonyl-6-methylxanthone (**6**) (14.9 mg). Fraction A6 (1.18 g) was subjected to MPLC (53 g of silica gel, 230–400 mesh (40–63 μm); *n*-hexane/acetone 1:0–0:1, 500 mL-fractions) to give 13 subfractions: A6-1–A6-13. Fraction A6-9 (150 mg) was further purified by preparative TLC (silica gel; *n*-hexane/EtOAc, 1:9) to afford penicitrinone A (**5**) (18.3 mg). Fraction A9 (1.44 g) was subjected to MPLC (65 g of silica gel, 230–400 mesh (40–63 μm)); dichloromethane/EtOAc 1:0–2:3, 650 mL-fractions) to give 12 subfractions: A9-1–A9-12. Fraction A9-6 (128 mg) was further purified by preparative TLC (silica gel; *n*-hexane/acetone, 3:2) to afford epiremisporine C (**1**) (12.2 mg). Fraction A10 (0.98 g) was subjected to MPLC (44 g of silica gel, 230–400 mesh (40–63 μm); *n*-hexane/acetone 1:0–0:1, 450 mL-fractions) to give 10 subfractions: A10-1–A10-10. Fraction A10-4 (120 mg) was further purified by preparative TLC (silica gel; *n*-hexane/EtOAc, 7:3) to afford isoconiochaetone C (**7**) (11.2 mg). Fraction A11 (2.38 g) was subjected to MPLC (107 g of silica gel, 230–400 mesh (40–63 μm); *n*-hexane/acetone 1:0–0:1, 1000 mL-fractions) to give 14 subfractions: A11-1–A11-14. Fraction A11-2 (138 mg) was further purified by semipreparative normal-phase HPLC (silica gel; *n*-hexane/EtOAc, 1:1) to afford epiremisporine D (**2**) (14.6 mg). Fraction A11-4 (168 mg) was further purified by preparative TLC (silica gel; dichloromethane/methanol, 19:1) to afford epiremisporine B (**4**) (23.8 mg). Fraction A12 (1.28 g) was subjected to MPLC (58 g of silica gel, 230–400 mesh (40–63 μm); *n*-hexane/EtOAc 1:0–0:1, 600 mL-fractions) to give 10 subfractions: A12-1–A12-10. Fraction A12-1 (122 mg) was further purified by preparative TLC (silica gel; *n*-hexane/dichloromethane/acetone, 5:3:2) to afford epiremisporine E (**3**) (13.7 mg).

Epiremisporine C (**1**): $[\alpha]_D^{25}$ = +527.6° (*c* 0.22, $CHCl_3$); UV (MeOH) λ_{max} nm (log ε): 241 (4.35), 326 (3.50) nm; ^{1}H NMR data, see Table 4; ^{13}C NMR data, see Table 5.

Table 4. ^{1}H NMR data (500 MHz, CDCl$_3$) for **1–3**.

Position	1	2	3
		δ_H (J in Hz)	
3	3.87 (dd, 8.9, 8.6)	3.77 (dd, 8.7, 8.6)	3.48 (dd, 10.5, 8.9)
4	5.21 (d, 8.9)	5.14 (d, 8.9)	4.96 (d, 8.9)
8	6.67 (br s)	6.76 (br s)	6.81 (br s)
10	6.62 (br s)	6.58 (br s)	6.59 (br s)
15	2.33 (s)	2.36 (s)	2.38 (s)
16	3.83 (s)	3.78 (s)	3.82 (s)
3′	2.86 (ddd, 12.8, 8.6, 5.3)	2.82 (ddd, 12.7, 8.6, 5.4)	3.06 (ddd, 10.5, 8.3, 4.7)
4′α	2.58 (dd, 15.6, 5.3)	2.55 (dd, 15.5, 5.4)	2.99 (dd, 18.6, 4.7)
4′β	2.37 (dd, 15.6, 12.8)	2.36 (dd, 15.5, 12.7)	2.85 (dd, 18.6, 8.3)
8′	6.69 (br s)	6.69 (br s)	6.69 (br s)
10′	6.70 (br s)	6.69 (br s)	6.68 (br s)
15′	2.42 (s)	2.41 (s)	2.42 (s)
16′	3.87 (s)	3.84 (s)	3.84 (s)
11-OH	12.11 (br s)	-	-
11-OMe	-	3.91 (s)	3.91 (s)
2′-OMe	3.50 (s)	3.51 (s)	3.11 (s)
11′-OH	12.30 (br s)	12.36 (s)	12.50 (s)

Table 5. ^{13}C NMR data (125 MHz, CDCl$_3$) for **1–3**.

Position	1	2	3
		δ_C, Type	
1	170.8, C	171.2, C	170.5, C
2	91.2, C	91.7, C	91.6, C
3	46.9, CH	46.8, CH	44.0, CH
4	36.6, CH	36.1, CH	37.3, CH
5	168.3, C	164.7, C	166.4, C
7	157.2, C	159.1, C	159.2, C
8	108.3, CH	110.7, CH	110.9, CH
9	147.4, C	145.2, C	145.1, C
10	113.1, CH	108.4, CH	108.3, CH
11	160.9, C	160.0, C	159.9, C
12	109.0, C	112.9, C	112.6, C
13	179.0, C	173.7, C	173.9, C
14	118.8, C	121.7, C	121.2, C
15	22.2, CH$_3$	22.1, CH$_3$	22.1, CH$_3$
16	53.1, CH$_3$	52.9, CH$_3$	53.1, CH$_3$
1′	166.7, C	167.1, C	168.5, C
2′	111.1, C	111.0, C	107.6, C
3′	48.4, CH	48.4, CH	43.3, CH
4′	27.1, CH$_2$	27.1, CH$_2$	25.5, CH$_2$
5′	165.5, C	165.5, C	165.4, C
7′	156.0, C	156.1, C	155.9, C
8′	107.6, CH	107.5, CH	107.3, CH
9′	147.7, C	147.5, C	147.3, C
10′	112.7, CH	112.6, CH	112.2, CH
11′	160.5, C	160.5, C	160.4, C
12′	108.5, C	108.5, C	108.3, C
13′	179.7, C	179.8, C	180.6, C
14′	112.8, C	113.0, C	111.7, C
15′	22.4, CH$_3$	22.4, CH$_3$	22.4, CH$_3$
16′	52.8, CH$_3$	52.6, CH$_3$	52.8, CH$_3$
11-OMe	-	56.3, CH$_3$	56.4, CH$_3$
2′-OMe	52.7, CH$_3$	52.7, CH$_3$	52.2, CH$_3$

Epiremisporine D (**2**): $[\alpha]_D^{25}$ = +526.8° (*c* 0.10, CHCl$_3$); UV (MeOH) λ_{max} nm (log ε): 237 (4.25), 317 (3.52) nm; ^{1}H NMR data, see Table 4; ^{13}C NMR data, see Table 5.

Epiremisporine E (**3**): $[\alpha]_D^{25}$ = +561.3° (*c* 0.09, CHCl$_3$); UV (MeOH) λ_{max} nm (log ε): 235 (4.30), 315 (3.54) nm; ^{1}H NMR data, see Table 4; ^{13}C NMR data, see Table 5.

Epiremisporine B (**4**): Yellow amorphous powder; $[\alpha]_D^{25}$ = +523.6° (*c* 0.16, CHCl$_3$); ^{1}H NMR data, see Table S1; ^{13}C NMR data, see Table S2; HRESIMS: *m*/*z* 599.11558 [M + Na]$^+$ (calcd. for C$_{30}$H$_{24}$O$_{12}$ + Na, 599.11654).

Penicitrinone A (**5**): Orange crystalline powder; $[\alpha]_D^{25}$ = +102.6° (*c* 0.12, MeOH); ^{1}H NMR (600 MHz, CDCl$_3$) δ 1.32 (3H, d, *J* = 7.2 Hz, Me-4), 1.33 (3H, d, *J* = 7.0 Hz, Me-3′), 1.42 (3H, d, *J* = 6.4 Hz, Me-2′), 1.44 (3H, d, *J* = 6.7 Hz, Me-3), 2.11 (3H, s, Me-5), 2.21 (3H, s, Me-4′), 3.12 (1H, qd, *J* = 7.2, 0.9 Hz, H-4), 3.16 (1H, qd, *J* = 7.0, 4.1 Hz, H-3′), 4.61 (1H, qd, *J* = 6.4, 4.1 Hz, H-2′), 4.96 (1H, qd, *J* = 6.7, 0.9 Hz, H-3), 6.37 (1H, s, H-7), 8.33 (1H, br s, OH-5′); HRESIMS: *m*/*z* 381.17094 [M + H]$^+$ (calcd. for C$_{23}$H$_{24}$O$_5$ + H, 381.17020).

8-Hydroxy-1-methoxycarbonyl-6-methylxanthone (**6**): Yellow amorphous solid; ^{1}H NMR (600 MHz, CDCl$_3$) δ 2.44 (3H, s, Me-6), 4.03 (3H, s, COOMe-1), 6.64 (1H, br d, *J* = 1.4 Hz, H-5), 6.76 (1H, br d, *J* = 1.4 Hz, H-7), 7.31 (1H, dd, *J* = 7.3, 1.1 Hz, H-2), 7.53 (1H, dd, *J* = 8.5, 1.1 Hz, H-4), 7.74 (1H, dd, *J* = 8.5, 7.3 Hz, H-3), 12.15 (1H, s, OH-8); HRESIMS: *m*/*z* 285.07730 [M + H]$^+$ (calcd. for C$_{16}$H$_{12}$O$_5$ + H, 285.07630).

Isoconiochaetone C (**7**): Colorless needles (MeOH), m.p. 99–100.5 °C; $[\alpha]_D^{25}$ = +79.3° (*c* 0.18, MeOH); ^{1}H NMR (600 MHz, CDCl$_3$) δ 2.15 (1H, dddd, *J* = 14.0, 8.5, 2.5, 1.4 Hz, H$_\beta$-2), 2.32 (1H, dddd, *J* = 14.0, 9.4, 7.4, 6.8 Hz, H$_\alpha$-2), 2.40 (3H, s, Me-8), 2.77 (1H, ddd, *J* = 18.0, 9.4, 2.5 Hz, H$_\beta$-3), 3.17 (1H, dddd, *J* = 18.0, 8.5, 7.4, 1.4 Hz, H$_\alpha$-3), 3.50 (3H, s, OMe-1), 4.94 (1H, dt, *J* = 6.8, 1.4 Hz, H-1), 6.63 (1H, br s, H-9), 6.71 (1H, br s, H-7), 12.55 (1H, s, OH-10); HRESIMS: *m*/*z* 247.09688 [M + H]$^+$ (calcd. for C$_{14}$H$_{14}$O$_4$ + H, 247.09703).

3.4. Biological Assay

The anti-inflammatory effects of the isolated compounds from *Penicillium citrinum* were evaluated by suppressing fMLP-induced $O_2^{\bullet-}$ generation by human neutrophils. In addition, anti-cancer activity was evaluated by cytotoxicity assay and Western blot analysis.

3.4.1. Preparation of Human Neutrophils

Human neutrophils from the venous blood [21] of healthy, adult volunteers (20–35 years old) were isolated using a standard method of dextran sedimentation, prior to centrifugation in a Ficoll Hypaque gradient and hypotonic lysis of erythrocytes, as previously described [29]. Purified neutrophils containing >98% viable cells, as determined by the trypan blue exclusion method, were resuspended in HBSS buffer at pH 7.4 and were maintained at 4 °C, prior to use [30].

3.4.2. Measurement of $O_2^{\bullet-}$ Generation

The assay for measurement of $O_2^{\bullet-}$ generation was based on the SOD-inhibitable reduction of ferricytochrome c [31]. In brief, neutrophils (1 × 10^6 cells/mL) pretreated with the various test agents at 37 °C for 5 min were stimulated with fMLP (1 μmol/L) in the presence of ferricytochrome c (0.5 mg/mL). Extracellular $O_2^{\bullet-}$ production was assessed with a UV spectrophotometer at 550 nm (Hitachi U-3010, Tokyo, Japan). The percentage of superoxide inhibition of the test compound was calculated as the percentage of inhibition = {(control − resting) − (compound − resting)}/(control − resting) × 100. The software SigmaPlot was used for determining the IC$_{50}$ values [30].

3.4.3. Chemicals and Antibodies

Fluorouracil (5-FU) and bovine serum albumin (BSA) were purchased from Sigma-Aldrich (St. Louis, MO, USA). The antibodies against Bcl-2, Bax, and β-actin were purchased from Cell Signaling Technology (Danvers, MA, USA). Caspase-3 was obtained from GeneTex International Corporation (Hsinchu, Taiwan).

3.4.4. Cells and Culture Medium

A549 (human lung carcinoma) and HT-29 (human colon carcinoma) cells were kindly provided by Prof. T. M. Hu and Prof. Y. Su, respectively, of National Yang-Ming University, Taipei, Taiwan.

All cell lines were cultured in Dulbecco's modified Eagle's medium supplemented with 10% fetal bovine serum (FBS), 100 U/mL penicillin, 100 µg/mL streptomycin, 2 µM L-glutamine, and 1 mM sodium pyruvate. The cells were incubated in an atmosphere of 37 °C and 5% CO_2 and passaged twice a week. Cells were stored in liquid nitrogen at −155 °C. After the cells were thawed, the experiment was completed before 30 generations. The purpose was to minimize experimental errors. The compound stock solution was stored in DMSO at a concentration of 10 mM and stored at −20 °C, and finally melted immediately before use.

3.4.5. Cytotoxicity Assay

A MTT colorimetric assay was used to determine cell viability. The assay was modified from that of Mosmann [32]. MTT reagent (0.5 mg/mL) was added onto the attached cells mentioned above (100 µL per 100 µL culture) and incubated at 37 °C for 3 h. Then, DMSO was added and the amount of colored formazan metabolite formed was measured by absorbance at 570 nm, using an ELISA plate reader (µ Quant). The optical density of formazan formed in control (untreated) cells was taken as 100% viability.

3.4.6. Clonogenic Assay

The clonogenic assay followed as previously described with slight changes [33]. For the clonogenic assay, cells at a density of 3000 cells/well were seeded in 6-well plates for 24 h. Next, the cells were treated with compound 3 or vehicle (DMSO) and allowed to form colonies for 14 days. Colonies were washed with PBS, and the cells attached to the plastic surface were fixed in 99% MeOH for 30 min and stained with 0.2% crystal violet for 15 min. The stained cells were quantified using the ImageJ software (BioTechniques, NY, USA).

3.4.7. Western Blotting Analysis

Western blot analysis was performed according to the method previously reported [34]. In brief, A549 (1×10^5 cells) was seeded into 6 wells plate and grown until 85–90% confluent. Then, different concentrations (3.125, 6.25, 12.5, 25, and 50 µM) of compounds 3 and 4 were added. Cells were collected and lysed by radioimmunoprecipitation assay (RIPA) buffer. Lysates of total protein were separated by 12.5% sodium dodecyl sulfate-polyacrylamide gels and transferred to polyvinylidene difluoride (PVDF) membranes. After blocking, the membranes were incubated with anti-Bax, anti-Bcl-2 (Cell Signaling Inc., Danvers, MA, USA), anti-caspase-3, and anti-β-actin (GeneTex Inc., Irvine, CA, USA) primary antibodies at 4 °C overnight. Then, each membrane was washed with Tris-buffered saline containing 0.1% Tween 20 (TBST) and incubated with horseradish peroxidase (HRP)-conjugated secondary antibodies at room temperature, for 1 h, while shaking. Finally, each membrane was developed using an enhanced chemiluminescence (ECL) detection kit, and the images were visualized by ImageQuant LAS 4000 Mini biomolecular imager (GE Healthcare, MA, USA). The band densities were quantified using the ImageJ software (BioTechniques, NY, USA).

3.4.8. Statistical Analysis

All data are expressed as mean ± SEM. Statistical analysis was carried out using Student's t-test. A probability of 0.05 or less was considered to be statistically significant. Microsoft Excel 2019 was used for the statistical and graphical evaluation. All experiments were performed at least 3 times.

4. Conclusions

Three novel (**1–3**) and four known compounds were isolated and identified from *Penicillium citrinum*. Among the isolated compounds, compounds **2–5** could significantly inhibit fMLP-induced $O_2^{\bullet-}$ generation, with IC_{50} values ≤ 8.28 μM. These isolated compounds are worth further research, as promising new leads for developing anti-inflammatory agents. Furthermore, compounds **3** and **4** markedly induced apoptosis of A549 cells through the mitochondrial- and caspase 3-dependent pathways (Figure 11). This suggests that compounds **3** and **4** are worth further investigation and might be expectantly developed as the candidates for the treatment or prevention of non-small cell lung cancer and liver cancer.

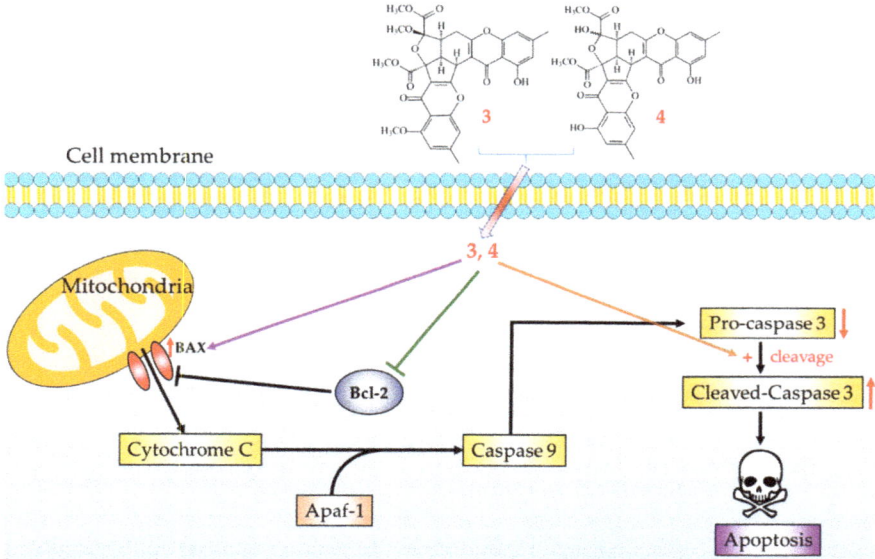

Figure 11. Schematic diagram for cancer cell apoptosis mechanism of compounds **3** and **4** in A549 cells.

Supplementary Materials: The following are available online at https://www.mdpi.com/1660-3397/19/1/25/s1, Figures S1–S10: HRESIMS, CD, 1D, and 2D NMR spectra for epiremisporine C (**1**). Figures S11–S20: HRESIMS, CD, 1D, and 2D NMR spectra for epiremisporine D (**2**). Figures S21–S30: HRESIMS, CD, 1D, and 2D NMR spectra for epiremisporine E (**3**). Figures S31–S34: HRESIMS, CD, ^1H and ^{13}C NMR spectra for (**4**). Figures S35 and S36: HRESIMS, ^1H NMR spectra for penicitrinone A (**5**). Figures S37 and S38: HRESIMS, ^1H NMR spectra for 8-hydroxy-1-methoxycarbonyl-6-methylxanthone (**6**). Figures S39 and S40: HRESIMS, ^1H NMR spectra for isoconiochaetone C (**7**) Figure S41: CD and ECD spectra of epiremisporine B. Tables S1 and S2: ^1H and ^{13}C NMR spectrum for **4** and epiremisporine B. Table S3: The ROESY correlations for compounds **1–3**.

Author Contributions: Y.-C.C. performed the isolation and structure elucidation of the constituents and prepared the manuscript. C.-H.C. and H.-R.L. conducted the bioassay and analyzed the data. M.-J.C. and M.-D.W. performed the cultivation and preparation of the fungal strain. S.-L.F. analyzed bioassay data. J.-J.C. planned, designed, and organized all of the research of this study and reviewed the manuscript. All authors read and approved the final version of the manuscript.

Funding: This research received no external funding.

Institutional Review Board Statement: Not applicable.

Informed Consent Statement: Not applicable.

Data Availability Statement: The data presented in this study are available in the main text and the supplementary materials of this article.

Acknowledgments: This research was supported by grants from the Ministry of Science and Technology (MOST), Taiwan (No. MOST 109-2320-B-010-029-MY3 and MOST 106-2320-B-010-033-MY3), awarded to J.-J. Chen. We gratefully thank Shou-Ling Huang and Iren Wang for the assistance in NMR experiments of the Instrumentation Center at NTU which is supported by the Ministry of Science and Technology, Taiwan.

Conflicts of Interest: The authors declare no conflict of interest.

References

1. Blunt, J.W.; Copp, B.R.; Keyzers, R.A.; Munro, M.H.G.; Prinsep, M.R. Marine natural products. *Nat. Prod. Rep.* **2015**, *32*, 116–211. [CrossRef] [PubMed]
2. Kiuru, P.; D'Auria, M.V.; Muller, C.D.; Tammela, P.; Vuorela, H.; Yli-Kauhaluoma, J. Exploring marine resources for bioactive compounds. *Planta Med.* **2014**, *80*, 1234–1246. [CrossRef] [PubMed]
3. Bao, J.; Wang, J.; Zhang, X.Y.; Nong, X.H.; Qi, S.H. New furanone derivatives and alkaloids from the co-culture of marine-derived fungi *Aspergillus sclerotiorum* and *Penicillium citrinum*. *Chem. Biodivers.* **2016**, *14*, 327–335.
4. Huang, G.L.; Zhou, X.M.; Bai, M.; Liu, Y.X.; Zhao, Y.L.; Luo, Y.P.; Niu, Y.Y.; Zheng, C.J.; Chen, G.Y. Dihydroisocoumarins from the mangrove-derived fungus *Penicillium citrinum*. *Mar. Drugs* **2016**, *14*, 177–185. [CrossRef]
5. Ibrar, M.; Ullah, M.W.; Manan, S.; Farooq, U.; Rafiq, M.; Hasan, F. Fungi from the extremes of life: An untapped treasure for bioactive compounds. *Appl. Microbiol. Biotechnol.* **2020**, *104*, 2777–2801. [CrossRef]
6. Khan, S.A.; Hamayun, M.; Yoon, H.; Kim, H.Y.; Suh, S.J.; Hwang, S.K.; Kim, J.M.; Lee, I.J.; Choo, Y.S.; Yoon, U.H.; et al. Plant growth promotion and *Penicillium citrinum*. *BMC Microbiol.* **2008**, *8*, 231–241. [CrossRef]
7. Kong, F.; Carter, G.T. Remisporine B, a novel dimeric chromenone derived from spontaneous Diels-Alder reaction of remisporine A. *Tetrahedron Lett.* **2003**, *44*, 3119–3122. [CrossRef]
8. Liu, Q.Y.; Zhou, T.; Zhao, Y.Y.; Chen, L.; Gong, M.W.; Xia, Q.W.; Ying, M.G.; Zheng, Q.H.; Zhang, Q.Q. Antitumor effects and related mechanisms of penicitrinine A, a novel alkaloid with a unique spiro skeleton from the marine fungus *Penicillium citrinum*. *Mar. Drugs* **2015**, *13*, 4733–4753. [CrossRef]
9. Liu, F.A.; Lin, X.; Zhou, X.; Chen, M.; Huang, X.; Yang, B.; Tao, H. Xanthones and quinolones derivatives produced by the deep-sea-derived fungus *Penicillium sp.* SCSIO Ind16F01. *Molecules* **2017**, *22*, 1999. [CrossRef]
10. Lösgen, S.; Magull, J.; Schulz, B.; Draeger, S.; Zeeck, A. Isofusidienols: Novel chromone-3-oxepines produced by the endophytic fungus *Chalara sp.*. *Eur. J. Org. Chem.* **2008**, 698–703. [CrossRef]
11. Meng, L.H.; Liu, Y.; Li, X.M.; Xu, G.M.; Ji, N.Y.; Wang, B.G. Citrifelins A and B, citrinin adducts with a tetracyclic framework from cocultures of marine-derived isolates of *Penicillium citrinum* and *Beauveria felina*. *J. Nat. Prod.* **2015**, *78*, 2301–2305. [CrossRef] [PubMed]
12. Mossini, S.A.; Kemmelmeier, C. Inhibition of citrinin production in *Penicillium citrinum* cultures by neem [*Azadirachta indica* A. Juss (meliaceae)]. *Int. J. Mol. Sci.* **2008**, *9*, 1676–1684. [CrossRef] [PubMed]
13. Sabdaningsih, A.; Liu, Y.; Mettal, U.; Heep, J.; Riyanti; Wang, L.; Cristianawati, O.; Nuryadi, H.; Sibero, M.T.; Marner, M.; et al. A new citrinin derivative from the Indonesian marine sponge-associated fungus *Penicillium citrinum*. *Mar. Drugs* **2020**, *18*, 227–239. [CrossRef]
14. Shen, H.D.; Wang, C.W.; Chou, H.; Lin, W.L.; Tam, M.F.; Huang, M.H.; Kuo, M.L.; Wang, S.R.; Han, S.H. Complementary DNA cloning and immunologic characterization of a new *Penicillium citrinum* allergen (Pen c 3). *J. Allergy Clin. Immunol.* **2000**, *105*, 827–833. [CrossRef]
15. Wakana, D.; Hosoe, T.; Itabashi, T.; Okada, K.; de Campos Takaki, G.M.; Yaguchi, T.; Fukushima, K.; Kawai, K.I. New citrinin derivatives isolated from *Penicillium citrinum*. *J. Nat. Med.* **2006**, *60*, 279–284. [CrossRef]
16. Xia, M.W.; Cui, C.B.; Li, C.W.; Wu, C.J.; Peng, J.X.; Li, D.H. Rare chromones from a fungal mutant of the marine-derived *Penicillium purpurogenum* G59. *Mar. Drugs* **2015**, *13*, 5219–5236. [CrossRef] [PubMed]
17. Zheng, C.J.; Huang, G.L.; Xu, Y.; Song, X.M.; Yao, J.; Liu, H.; Wang, R.P.; Sun, X.P. A new benzopyrans derivatives from a mangrove-derived fungus *Penicillium citrinum* from the South China Sea. *Nat. Prod. Res.* **2016**, *30*, 821–825. [CrossRef] [PubMed]
18. Zheng, C.J.; Liao, H.X.; Mei, R.Q.; Huang, G.L.; Yang, L.J.; Zhou, X.M.; Shao, T.M.; Chen, G.Y.; Wang, C.Y. Two new benzophenones and one new natural amide alkaloid isolated from a mangrove-derived fungus *Penicillium citrinum*. *Nat. Prod. Res.* **2019**, *33*, 1127–1134. [CrossRef]
19. Witko-Sarsat, V.; Rieu, P.; Descamps-Latscha, B.; Lesavre, P.; Halbwachs-Mecarelli, L. Neutrophils: Molecules, functions and pathophysiological aspects. *Lab. Invest.* **2000**, *80*, 617–653. [CrossRef]
20. Ennis, M. Neutrophils in asthma pathophysiology. *Curr. Allergy Asthma Rep.* **2003**, *3*, 159–165. [CrossRef]
21. Borregaard, N. The human neutrophil. Function and dysfunction. *Eur. J. Haematol. Suppl.* **1988**, *41*, 401–413. [CrossRef] [PubMed]

22. Roos, D.; van Bruggen, R.; Meischl, C. Oxidative killing of microbes by neutrophils. *Microbes Infect.* **2003**, *5*, 1307–1315. [CrossRef] [PubMed]
23. Vane, J.R.; Mitchell, J.A.; Appleton, I.; Tomlinson, A.; Bishop-Bailey, D.; Croxtall, J.; Willoughby, D.A. Inducible isoforms of cyclooxygenase and nitric-oxide synthase in inflammation. *Proc. Natl. Acad. Sci. USA* **1994**, *91*, 2046–2050. [CrossRef]
24. Hsiao, A.J.; Chen, L.H.; Lu, T.H. Ten leading causes of death in Taiwan: A comparison of two grouping lists. *J. Formos. Med. Assoc.* **2015**, *114*, 679–680. [CrossRef] [PubMed]
25. Yip, K.W.; Reed, J.C. Bcl-2 family proteins and cancer. *Oncogene* **2008**, *27*, 6398–6406. [CrossRef] [PubMed]
26. Mohan, S.; Abdelwahab, S.I.; Kamalidehghan, B.; Syam, S.; May, K.S.; Harmal, N.S.; Shafifiyaz, N.; Hadi, A.H.; Hashim, N.M.; Rahmani, M.; et al. Involvement of NF-κB and Bcl2/Bax signaling pathways in the apoptosis of MCF7 cells induced by a xanthone compound pyranocycloartobiloxanthone A. *Phytomedicine* **2012**, *19*, 1007–1015. [CrossRef] [PubMed]
27. Vucicevic, K.; Jakovljevic, V.; Colovic, N.; Tosic, N.; Kostic, T.; Glumac, I.; Pavlovic, S.; Karan-Djurasevic, T.; Colovic, M. Association of Bax expression and Bcl2/Bax ratio with clinical and molecular prognostic markers in chronic lymphocytic leukemia. *J. Med. Biochem.* **2016**, *35*, 150–157. [CrossRef] [PubMed]
28. Wu, C.J.; Yi, L.; Cui, C.B.; Li, C.W.; Wang, N.; Han, X. Activation of the silent secondary metabolite production by introducing neomycin-resistance in a marine-derived *Penicillium purpurogenum* G59. *Mar. Drugs* **2015**, *13*, 2465–2487. [CrossRef] [PubMed]
29. English, D.; Andersen, B.R. Single-step separation of red blood cells. Granulocytes and mononuclear leukocytes on discontinuous density gradients of Ficoll-Hypaque. *J. Immunol. Methods* **1974**, *5*, 249–252. [CrossRef]
30. Chen, L.C.; Liao, H.R.; Chen, P.Y.; Kuo, W.L.; Chang, T.H.; Sung, P.J.; Wen, Z.H.; Chen, J.J. Limonoids from the seeds of *Swietenia macrophylla* and their anti-inflammatory activities. *Molecules* **2015**, *20*, 18551. [CrossRef]
31. Babior, B.M.; Kipnes, R.S.; Curnutte, J.T. Biological defense mechanisms. The production by leukocytes of superoxide, a potential bactericidal agent. *J. Clin. Invest.* **1973**, *52*, 741–744. [CrossRef] [PubMed]
32. Mosmann, T. Rapid colorimetric assay for cellular growth and survival: Application to proliferation and cytotoxicity assays. *J. Immunol. Methods* **1983**, *65*, 55–63. [CrossRef]
33. Su, M.; Zhao, C.; Li, D.; Cao, J.; Ju, Z.; Kim, E.L.; Young-Suk, J.; Jung, J.H. Viriditoxin stabilizes microtubule polymers in SK-OV-3 cells and exhibits antimitotic and antimetastatic potential. *Mar. Drugs* **2020**, *18*, 445. [CrossRef] [PubMed]
34. Huang, C.Y.; Chang, T.C.; Wu, Y.J.; Chen, Y.; Chen, J.J. Benzophenone and benzoylphloroglucinol derivatives from *Hypericum sampsonii* with anti-inflammatory mechanism of otogirinin A. *Molecules* **2020**, *25*, 4463. [CrossRef] [PubMed]

Sample Availability: Samples of the compounds are available from the authors.

MDPI
St. Alban-Anlage 66
4052 Basel
Switzerland
Tel. +41 61 683 77 34
Fax +41 61 302 89 18
www.mdpi.com

Marine Drugs Editorial Office
E-mail: marinedrugs@mdpi.com
www.mdpi.com/journal/marinedrugs

www.ingramcontent.com/pod-product-compliance
Lightning Source LLC
LaVergne TN
LVHW070634100526
838202LV00012B/803